JAIKRISHNADAS AYURVEDA SERIES
No. 58

ŚĀRṄGADHAR-SAṂHITĀ

(A treatise on Āyurveda)

By

ŚĀRṄGADHARA

Translated in English
by
Āyurveda-Vidwān
PROF. K. R. SRIKANTHA MURTHY
L. A. M. S., H. P. A.
Principal,
Gov. College of Indian Medicine
Bangalore.
Fellow, The Royal Asiatic Society (London).

CHAUKHAMBHA ORIENTALIA
A House of Oriental and Antiquarian Books
VARANASI

Publishers :

CHAUKHAMBHA ORIENTALIA

Post Box No. 1032

Gokul Bhawan, K. 37/109

Gopal Mandir Lane, Golghar, Maidagin

VARANASI - 221001 (U.P.) India

Telephone: (0542) 2333476, 2334356

Fax No. (0542) 2334356

Telegram: Gokulotsav

E-mail: covns@sify.com

Fifth Edition : 2003

Price : [illegible]

Printers– CHARU PRINTERS, Gopal Mandir Lane, VARANASI-1

INTRODUCTION

Ancient treatises of Ayurveda have been broadly classified into two groups viz., the Brihat trayee (greater triad) and the Laghu trayee (lesser triad); Charaka Samhita, Sushruta Samhita and Ashtanga Sangraha[1] are the Brihat trayee while Madhava Nidana, Sharngadhara Samhita and Bhavaprakasha are the Laghu trayee. Brihat trayee are great in respect of their authors, antiquity and originality. Laghu trayee are the works of later authors and are, more or less, compilations without much originality. But in view of their containing the quintessence of the Brihat trayee in easy diction, the Laghu trayee are also being studied by students and practioners of Ayurveda since long in our country. Sharngadhara Samhita, the second of this category is a very popular treatise.

Date of the treatise :

Sharngadhara Samhita is assigned to the early part of 14th century A. D. based on the following points :

(a) Chakrapanidatta and Ḍalhana, the two famous commentators of Charaka and Sushruta Samhitas respectively who lived during 11th century A. D. are ignorant of either Sharngadhara or his Samhita.

(b) Hemadri, the celebrated commentator of Ashtanga Hridaya who belonged to 13th—14th century A. D. has referred to Sharngadhara Samhita in his commentary.[2]

(c) Bopadeva who flourished during the early part of the 14th century A. D. as the protege of Hemadri, is said to have written a commentary on Sharngadhara Samhita.[3]

Authorship :

As there is no personal information of the author in the text, except his name as Sharngadhara and as the later commentators of the treatise are also silent on this point, differences of opinion exists among scholars in identifying the

---

1. Some scholars count Ashtanga Hridaya in place of Ashtanga Sangraha. But considering the volume and merit of the two it is most appropriate to include Ashtanga Sangraha in the Brihat trayee, than Ashtanga Hridaya.
2. Ayurveda Rasayana Commentary on Ash. Hri. Sut. 5/73.
3. Aufrecht—Catalogus Catalogorum—Part I & Weber-Catalogue of Berlin, 1853.

real author. It seems Sharngadhara was a very popular name in medieval India, as we come across many of them, as authors of treatises : Aufrecht mentions about eight of them.[1] For the present study, it is enough if we consider the following personalities who lived during the period of 13th–14th century A.D. or near about.

1. Sharngadhara—author of this Samhita.
2. Sharngadhara—author of S. Trishati or Jwara Trishati.
3. Sharngadhara—author of S. Paddhati.
4. Sharnga Deva—author of Sangeeta Ratnakara.

A glimpse into each of these texts, will have to be made to clear the confusion about the correct identification.

Sharngadhara Samhita :

(a) Except giving out his name as the author at the commencement of the text,[2] he has not furnished any information about himself or his other works.

(b) The language and style of composition of the text, both being insipid, give room to doubt the erudition of the author in Sanskrit and Ayurveda.

(c) The text predominantly deals with Bhaishajya Kalpana (pharmacy and pharmaceutics). Brief narration of basic principles, anatomy and physiology, methods of diagnosis of diseases, and enumeration of diseases though found in the first section, does not reflect profound knowledge of the author.

Sharngadhara Trishati :

Also known as Jwara Trishati is a small treatise with three hundred verses describing the Nidana (aetiology) Lakshanas (symptomatology) and Chikitsa (Therapeutics) of different kinds of fevers. The author says that he is the son of Devaraja, belonging to Nagara Brahman community of Gujarat and he is a disciple of Swami Vaikunthashrama. He has not mentioned any other text on Ayurveda written by him. Vaidya Vallabhabhatta has written a commentary on this Trishati.[3]

---

1. Aufrecht—Catalogus Catalogorum.
2. Sharngadhara Samhita, I-1-2.
3. Trishati along with the commentary has been published in 1937 by M/s. Khemaraj Shrikrishnadas, Bombay.

Sharngadhara Paddhati :

Sharngadhara Paddhati is an anthology of Sanskrit poetry. At the commencement of the text, the author gives his personal data as follows :

> "When Raja Hammera of Chahumana dynasty was reigning at Shakambari Desha, he had as his Chief Courtier, a Brahman scholar by name Raghava Deva. He had three sons—Gopala, Damodara and Devadasa. The second son Damodara had also three sons—Sharngadhara, Lakshmidhara and Krishna. I, Sharangadhara, have composed this text collecting verses from earlier scholars[1]..... "

Historians place Raja Hammera Chouhan as the Hindu king of Ranthambhor in Rajasthan who was vanquished by Allauddin Khilji in 1299–1301 A.D. So the author of this Paddhati will have to be placed in the latter part of 14th century or even early 15th century A. D. and not earlier.

The author has collected interesting and important verses on different subjects from earlier reputed treatises. Bulk of the text is reserved for Ethics (subhashita on vidya prashamsa, pandita prashamsa, guna, dhana, dana, dharma prashamsa), riddles of language (prahelika), Anyokti (parables), description of seasons (ritu Varnana), Koutuka (magic), Shakuna (omens), Kala Jnana (foretelling), Rajaneeti (state craft), Dhanurveda (science of warfare), Gandharva Veda (music and dance), Ayurveda (medical science) for pashu (veterinary medicine), Vriksha (horticulture) and Nara (human medicine), Bhootavidya (demonology), Vishapaharana (toxicology), Rasayana Kalpa (preparation of medicines and elixirs), Arishta Jnana (signs of death), Shareera (cosmic and human body), Yoga especially Hatha Yoga and Moksha (liberation) have all been dealt with. Vrikshayurveda (horticulture and plant medicine) gets the major share under Ayurveda. The verses dealing with treatment of human beings are few and do not belong to Charaka, Sushruta or Vagbhata, the three ancient authorities on Ayurveda. The verses describing Shareera (anatomy) numbering about 65 are taken from a text called 'Yogarasayana' and bear little resemblance to Shareera found in Ayurvedic texts. The author does not mention the name of any scholar or treatise of Ayurveda whereas he names a large number of poets (including one or two of his own name). Majority of the verses being the composition of others,

---

1. The first edition of this book with 4,689 verses was published in 1988 by the Department of Public Instructions, Bombay Presidency, edited by Mr. Peter Peterson, Professor of Sanskrit and Principal, Elphinston College, Bombay.

it is difficult to estimate the contribution of the author himself. As a good compiler he has brought out a valuable encyclopaedic anthology. He does not refer to any other book written by him and his lack of insight into ancient texts of Ayurveda is conspicuous.

Sangeeta Ratnakara :

Sangeeta Ratnakara is a treatise on music. Its author Sharngadeva was the son of Shodala and grandson of Bhaskara; belonging to the Vrishagana gotra of Brahamanas of Kashmir ; having migrated to South India and settled at Devagiri in Karnataka. Shodala was the minister and army commander of Yadava King Bilhana and his son Singhana (1210–1248 A.D.).

Sharngadeva was a profound scholar in many branches of knowledge such as Sangeeta (music), Ayurveda (medicine), Vedanta (philosophy) and many more. He has indicated his authorship of many books on different subjects, of which Sangeeta Ratnakara and Adhyatma Viveka stand out pre-eminent as authoritative texts. According to his own statement in Sangeeta Ratnakara, he was a scholar, philosopher, musician and physician and "that he satisfied the needy in these fields".[1]

Sangeeta Ratnakara exhaustively deals with all aspects of musicology and is ranked as an authoritative text on the subject. Composed in verses of different metres with pleasant diction, fine vocabulary and vast information, the book bears testimony to the great erudition of the author both in language and subject.

In a chapter called 'Pindotpatti Prakarana', the author describes the doctrines of panchamahabhootas, composition of the human body, formation and development of the Embrayo, Trigunas, Pancha Vayus, Doshas–Dhatus, Malas–Sushumna, Shatchakras, Nadis and their functions.

Description of Swarayantra (voice box), mechanism of sound production and methods to gain control over it are lucidly explained. These descriptions, very closely, correlate with those found in Samhitas of Charaka and Sushruta, proving the author's deep knowledge of Ayurveda. He has not mentioned the names of his books on Ayurveda but according to his own statement, he has written books on this subject. But till today no such book has been found.

---

1. Introductory verses in Chapter I.

Different views on authorship :

The following are the views of scholars entitled for authoritative opinion.

1. Aufrecht opines that the authors of S. Samhita and S. Paddhati are one and the same person.[1]
2. Parashuram Shastry Vidyasagar, the editor of S. Samhita published by Nirnayasagar Press, Bombay, in his introduction[2] also holds the same view and further identifies him as Sharngadhara son of Damodara based upon the colophon found in the manuscript which he edited.
3. C. G. Kashikar states that the author of Samhita, Paddhati, Trishati and another work on Rasa Shastra by name Sharngadhara Sangraha (not traced so far) is the same person and that he was a Gujarati Nagar Brahman.[3]
4. Priyavrata Sharma opines that S. Samhita and S. Paddhati are the works of two different persons.[4]
5. There are some scholars who hold the view that S. Samhita is to be ascribed to the author of Sangeeta Ratnakara assuming the term Sharngadeva as a variant of Sharngdhara and this will substantiate the statement of Sharngadeva about his authorship of book on Ayurveda also.
6. Majority of Ayurvedists without going into discussion, simply subscribe to the current popular view that Sharngadhara son of Damodara is the author of S. Samhita.

Difficulties in correct identification :

Attempting at correct identification of the authors of these texts, the reviewer faces the following problems and finds it difficult to arrive at a satisfactory solution :—

1. Absence of personal narration of his life and works by the author or by later commentators of S. Samhita.

---

1. Aufrecht—Catalogus Catologorum, Part I, p. 643.
2. Sanskrit Introduction to S. Samhita, Nirnaya Sagar Press, Bombay, 1920.
3. C. G. Kashikar—Supplementary notes appended to English translation of Jolius Jolly's 'Indian Medicine'.
4. Priyavrata Sharma—Ayurveda Ka Vaigyanik Itihasa.

2. Absence of colophon mentioning the details of the author in the manuscript of S. Samhita first edited by Kaviraj Pyarimohansengupta[1] and presence of a colophon mentioning "Sharangadhara son of Damodara as the author" in the manuscripts of S. Samhita edited by Parashuram Shastry Vidyasagar.[2]
3. Likewise, the assumption, that the author of S. Paddhati and the author of S. Samhita are one and the same and identifying him as son of Damodara is also not satisfactory since the author of Paddhati is glaringly ignorant of classical texts of Ayurveda.
4. Non-availability of Bopadeva's commentary on S. Samhita which might have given some information about Sharngadhara.
5. Non-mention of names of books on Ayurveda said to be written by Sharngadeva, author of Sangeeta Ratnakara and not finding of any such book till now. Alluding the authorship of S. Samhita which is a small insipid text to Sharngadeva taking the names as variants, will be nothing short of an insult to the wide knowledge and high standard of Sharngadeva. His book on Ayurveda, if at all, will definitely stand equal in comparison to Sangeeta Ratnakara.

In the face of the divergent views and difficulties described so far, it is better to keep this question open till such time when further research on the subject brings out some more facts. For the present, it will be prudent on our part to consider the author of S. Samhita as a person distinct from all others; and whose whereabouts are not known.

Nature and contents of S. Samhita :

The Samhita is designed to serve as a practitioner's hand book as the author himself states.[3] Written in simple and easy language the book consists of 32 chapters with 2,600 verses in all; the first section with 7 chapters and 585 verses, the second with 12 chapters and 1,261 verses and the third section with 13 chapters and 682 verses.[4]

Prathama Khanda (first section) has one chapter each for Paribhasha (weights and measures), Bhaishajyakhyana (time for medicine, collection of drugs,

---

1. S. Samhita—first edition—by Pyarimohansengupta, Calcutta.
2. S. Samhita—Parashuram Shastry Vidyasagar, Nirnaya Sagar Press, Bombay, 1920.
3. S. Samhita III—13—128.
4. These numbers of verses are as found in the present book and fall short by about 40.

seasonal effects, etc.,), Nadiparikshadi Vidhi (examination of pulse and other methods of diagnosis of diseases), Deepanapachanadi (definitions of pharmacological terms), Kaladikakhyana (anatomy and physiology), Aharadi Vidhi (digestion of food, human constitution, etc.,) and Roga ganana (enumeration of diseases).

Madhyama Khanda (second section) describes the composition, method of preparation and uses of different kinds of recipes. It has one chapter each for Swarasa (fresh juice), Quatha (decoctions), Phanta (infusions), Hima (cold infusions), Kalka (wet pill), Choorna (powders), Gutika (pills), Avaleha (confections), Sneha (oils and ghee), Sandhana (fermented liquids), Dhatushuddhi (purification of minerals and metals) and Rasa Oushadhas (mercurial recipes).

Uttara Khanda—the third and last section explains the different kinds of treatment in separate chapters viz., Sneha (oleation), Sweda (sudation), Vamana (emesis), Virechana (purgation), Sneha basti (oil enema), Nirooha basti (decoction enema), Uttara basti (vaginal and vesical douches), Nasya (nasal medications), Dhoomapana (inhalation of vapour of smoke), Gandoosha (mouth gargles), Lepa (topical applications), Shonita Visruti (blood letting) and Netra prasadana (eye salves, collyriums, etc.).

According to the author's own statament :

"All the recipes are those formulated by ancient seers, used and found effective by reputed physicians.[1] Many treatises have been written by scholars imbibing the gems from the ocean of Ayurveda and this Samhita is written by collecting information—a little from such texts–for the benefit of physicians.[2]

Merits and demerits :

The following are the special merits of the treatise :

(a) It is the first Ayurvedic treatise to describe Nadi-pariksha (examination of pulse) as a method of diagnosis of diseases.

(b) It is the first book describing the mechanism of respiration by making use of new terms like Ambara-Peeyoosha, Vishnupadamrita (both to mean oxygen) and Jeevaraktashaya (to mean heart).

(c) Clear definitions of pharmacological terms are found only in this text, so also the method of preparation of all types of recipes.

1. S. Samhita I-1-2.
2. Ibid—III-13-125 to 127.

(d) Opium and some other new drugs have been incorporated into Ayurvedic materia medica through this treatise.

(e) A new technique of introducing drugs directly into the blood stream through an artificial wound (Soochikabharana Rasa Prayoga) is found for the first time in this book.

(f) Snayuka Krimi Roga (guinea worm infection) has been recognised for the first time through this text.

(g) Recipes found herein are simple, easy to prepare and effacious and hence make the treatise a good practitioner's hand-book.

(h) The treatise is the best example of the condition of Ayurveda in medieval India, as will be described further.

The following are the demerits of the treatise :

(a) Names of the five kaphas vary slightly from those found in earlier texts viz., Kledana (for Kledaka), Snehana (Tarpaka), Rasana (Bodhaka), Avalambana (Avalambaka), Shleshmaka (Sleshaka).

(b) Sweda (sweat), Danta (teeth), Kesha (hairs) and Ojas (essence of dhatus) are named as Upadhatus (secondary issues).

(c) The treatise is not a comprehensive one dealing with all aspects of Ayurveda but treats Bhaishajya Kalpana (Pharmaceutics), in detail in second section and procedures of many Therapies in the third.

These demerits are negligible both in number and importance and can be overlooked.

Commentaries :

The first Sanskrit commentary on this Samhita is said to be that of Bopadeva (13th–14th century A. D.) son of Keshava Pandita. Both of them were the proteges of Hemadri, the celebrated minister of Yadava King Mahadeva and his son Ramadeva of Devagiri in Karnataka. Unfortunately this commentary has not been published so far. Some, even doubt the existence of such a commentary on the basis of chronology. Aufrecht has made a mention of it in his catalogue and also as found in Weber's catalogue of Berlin.[1]

The second commentary known as "Sharngadhara Deepika" is by Vaidya Adamalla belonging to Srivastavya sect and son of Bhava Simha who was the court

---

1. Aufrecht – Catalogus Catalogorum, Part I of Weber's Catalogue of Manuscripts, Berlin, 1853.

physician of Raja Jaitrasimha of Hastikantipuri (in Gujarat) during 14th century A. D. It is available in full, provides additional information regarding synonyms of drugs and clarification on many moot points. It is quite elaborate and has been published.

The third commentary known as "Goodarth Deepika" is the work of Kashirama Vaidya belonging to Bharadwaja Saraswata sect. He lived at Salimabad (now in Uttar Pradesh) during the period of Sultan Shah Salim who ruled from Delhi and Agra in the 16th century A. D. This commentary is brief and resembles that of Adamalla in many respects. This has also been printed.

The fourth commentary known as "Ayurveda Deepika" is by Rudra Bhatta son of Koneri Bhatta. More details of his life and works are not known. He is assigned to 17th century A. D. This commentary is very concise and at present available only for second and third sections of the Samhita.

Translations :

Sharngadhara Samhita has been translated into almost all major Indian languages by many scholars, but not into English or other European languages so far. The present attempt is the first in this direction.

Ayurveda in medieval India :

Sharngadhara Samhita can be better appreciated with a background knowledge of Ayurveda in medieval India.

The condition of India during the medieval period (800 A. D. to 1500 A.D.) was very chaotic and even pathetic. The great Hindu empires had disintegrated into small kingdoms, their kings were weaklings who spent all their energy in fighting among themselves rather than fighting unitedly with the muslims. The aggresive muslim invaders succeeded in establishing their sultanates and began consolidating power. They being invaders cared for nothing Indian, except the wealth which they got in plenty. They looted temples, burnt down institutions of learning along with their precious libraries, executed the scholars and forcebly converted the common people to Islam. The encouragement to ancient Hindu learning which a few Hindu kings continued to give was no match to the large destruction. Scholars became few and many of them migrated to villages for fear of persecution. They could carry with them very little of their precious literature and preserve them. A few scholars here and there taught their sons or disciples the knowledge they had and such instances helped to keep the knowledge in families as hereditary tradition. Sons and disciples of many scholars were not fit to receive such knowledge. Most of the manuscripts of ancient books which were either of birch bark or palm leaves became 'dead wood' to them but 'delicious food' to ants and vermins.

The condition of the society was thoroughly unconducive for any advancement in literary or scientific fields. All that the scholars of the day could do was to preserve what little literature remained with them, compile everything which came to their knowledge in whatever manner and pass them on to posterity. Hence we find no authoritative or original literature but only small compilations most of which are insipid and peurile.

The society consisting of people of different regions, religions, castes and creeds, was heterodox both in culture and way of life. Hindu religion had become very much eroded of its theological, spiritual and ethical values. Confusion and misunderstanding of religious concepts and practices loomed large in the minds of the Hindus and the common man was at the mercy of any influence-benign or malignant. Devoid of definite direction people indulged in pursuit of happiness by whatever means, fair or foul. All they desired was easy and quick result. Hectic search for new methods of obtaining pleasure and power made for the upsurge of 'Tantrism' and its different cults among Hindus, Buddhists, Jains and many others.

Some of the important principles of Tantrism are—(a) there are two powerful principles in Nature—the male and the female, all the things in the universe can either be male or female, (b) bringing about the union of male and female principles, vis a vis, substances, new substances can be created by transformation, (c) by some special techniques and divine grace man can also gain extra-ordinary powers, such as capacity of creation and destruction, capacity to travel in the sky and reach other worlds, transform his mortal body into an immortal one and attain liberation from cycle of births and deaths.

Based on these assumptions, there grew a new type of worship of Gods. Hindus identified Lord Shiva as the chief "male" principle and his consort Parvati as the "female" principle. Shiva was worshipped in his fierceful forms (Bhairava, Kala, Kalamukha, Lakuleesha, Natha, etc.,) and Parvati as Shakti (Chandi, Chamundi, Durga, Sati, etc.,). Later on Ganapati and many other minor deities also were included into the Tantric pantheon. The method of worship adopted by the Tantriks was totally different from the traditional one. Indulgence in the

Pancha "Ma" Karas–mamsa (meat), madya (alcoholic beverages), maithuna (sexual intercourse), mudra (yogic postures) and mantra (meditation with chanting of specific syllables) was ordained to be followed. Surrendering to a teacher and earning his grace was essential for success. Blood was to be offered to gods. These and many such unholy, immoral and abhoric practices made these worships frightful and the society could not tolerate it for long. Tantriks withdrew themselves to forests and other places away from society and pursued their practices secretly.

Tantrism did not confine itself to the field of religion only, but even entered into the field of some sciences like Loha Vidya (metallurgy), Rasayana Vidya (alchemy), Yoga etc. Among them, Rasayana Tantra was the foremost and drew a large number of learned men into its fold. Mercury (Rasa) was named as the semen of Shiva and identified as the male principle. Sulpher was called as the seed of Parvati and identified as the female principle. By worshipping these two substances, combining them and subjecting them into eighteen different processes along with admixture of herbs, minerals, salts, poisons, etc., a Rasayana–Elixir, could be prepared which would not only transform base metals into gold but also the mortal human body into an immortal one. These techniques known as Rasa Vidya held many scholars and rich men by its glamour and lure of gold for nearly six to seven centuries. In spite of perseverant and hard endeavour for a long time by a large number of alchemists supported by kings and nobles, this did not yield, the much aspired elixir. With dismal failure these alchemical practices began to dwindle slowly but remained alive till the 18th century A. D.

All the alchemical knowledge did not altogether become a waste. Many of the chemical compounds produced during these processes were found to possess medicinal properties and could be used with great advantage in the treatment of diseases. Alchemists soon learnt Ayurveda and began to use these chemical compounds as medicines. Mercurial and metallic recipes were incorporated into Ayurvedic materia medica. Rasayana Vidya became a part of Ayurveda from about the 12th century A. D. under the name 'Rasa Shastra'. Its vast literature still retains the features of Tantrism. Ayurvedic books written after 12th century A. D. have in them a large number of mercurial recipes along with herbal recipes.

Another notable feature in the field of medicine is the inclusion of aphrodisiacs or sex tonics into therapeutics. Muslim rulers indulged themselves in sex and wished to retain their sexual prowess despite their age. To this end they made it mandatory on the part of the physicians of their courts to invent new aphrodisiac drugs. Thus we find medieval medical treatises containing many new drugs used for this purpose, though the science of aphrodisiacs was a part of Ayurveda many centuries earlier.

From about the 14th century A. D. and onwards an uneasy calm came to prevail in the country. Muslim rulers especially Mugals having stabilised their power fairly well, found time to personal pleasures and aggrandizement. They built mosques and forts of massive proportions, laid highways, maintained pleasure gardens and enacted many laws for the welfare of the people. They invited scholars of literature and other branches of knowledge from Arabia, Persia, Iran and other muslim countries and maintained in their courts. A few Indian scholars were also recognised and given this honour. A large number of books on religion philosophy, medicine and some other secular sciences were written by them. Translations of ancient Sanskrit texts into Persian or Arabic was undertaken in a big way, making for exchange of ideas. Modern scholars entitled for authoritative opinion consider that the quantum and richness of Indian wisdom borrowed by muslim scholars was greater than what they gave to their Indian counterpart. Little though it might be, Indian literature incorporated new things into its domain. This applies to the field of Ayurveda also, and all the books of this period reflect this trend in having some ideas and drugs borrowed by Unani system of medicine.

Sharngadhara Samhita stands as a best example of Ayurvedic literature of medieval India having all the features so far described.

Acknowledgments :

In preparing this book, I have received help in copying the manuscripts from my student Dr. Manonmani, in preparing the appendices from Dr. M. Eswara Reddy, Lecturer, Taranath Government Ayurvedic College, Bellary, Dr. T. R. Anandalwar, Lecturer, Government College of Indian Medicine, Bangalore. I am obliged to them for this valuable help. I thank to Smt. V. Vani Shastry, Bellary and Sri M. R. Seshadri for their neat typing.

I am equally thankful to my wife Smt. Lalithamma, many of my friends, colleagues and students who are the sources of encouragement and inspiration to me.

I am beholden to M/s. Chaukhambha Orientalia, Varanasi, the reputed publishers of Sanskrit literature, especially Ayurveda, for including this book in their series.

Bangalore, **K. R. Srikanta Murthy**
1984

CONTENTS

Uttara Khaṇḍa (Third Section)

शार्ङ्गधरसंहिता

ŚĀRṄGADHARA-SAṂHITĀ

(TEXT WITH ENGLISH TRANSLATION)

Prathama Khaṇḍa (First Section)

प्रथमोऽध्यायः

CHAPTER 1

Paribhāṣā (Definitions, Weights and Measures etc.)

मंगलाचरणम्

श्रियं स दद्याद्भवतां पुरारिर्यदङ्गतेजः प्रसरे भवानी ।
विराजते निर्मलचन्द्रिकायां महौषधीव ज्वलिता हिमाद्रौ ॥ १ ॥

May Lord Purāri, (Shiva), in whose brilliance shines Bhavānī, just as wonderful herbs shine in the moonlight spread on the slopes of the Himālayas, grant us prosperity (1).

प्रसिद्धयोगा मुनिभिः प्रयुक्ताश्चिकित्सकैर्ये बहुशोऽनुभूताः ।
विधीयते शार्ङ्गधरेण तेषां सुसंग्रहः सज्जनरञ्जनाय ॥ २ ॥

Such of the famous recipes which the sages formulated and found effective by the physicians from repeated usage, are herein collected by Śārṅgadhara (author) for the benefit of all good men (2).

हेत्वादिरूपाकृतिसात्म्यजातिभेदैः समीक्ष्यातुरसर्वरोगान् ।
चिकित्सितं कर्षणबृंहणाख्यं कुर्वीत वैद्यो विधिवत्सुयोगैः ॥ ३ ॥

Having diagnosed the disease first, by correct understanding of its cause, prodromal symptoms, characteristic features and variety from a detailed examination of the patient, the physician should adopt either a karṣaṇa chikitsā (therapy of thinning the body) or Bṛṃhaṇa chikitsā (therapy of fattening the body) with the use of effective recipes (3).

दिव्यौषधीनां बहवः प्रभेदा वृन्दारकाणामिव विस्फुरन्ति ।
ज्ञात्वेति संदेहमपास्य धीरैः संभावनीया विविधप्रभावाः ॥ ४ ॥

Innumerable are the varieties of potent herbs which shine like gods; physicians should acquire infalliable knowledge of their various properties (4).

स्वाभाविकागन्तुककायिकान्तरा रोगा भवेयुः किल कर्मदोषजाः ।
तच्छेदनार्थं दुरितापहारिणः श्रेयोमयान्योगवरान्नियोजयेत् ॥ ५ ॥

Diseases arise from many causes such as swābhāvika (natural), āgantuka (external agents), kāyikāntara (internal agents), karmadoṣa (past sins) and others. To get rid of them and obtain happiness, the physician should make use of efficacious recipes. (5).

प्रयोगानागमात्सिद्धान्प्रत्यक्षादनुमानतः । सर्वलोकहितार्थाय वक्ष्याम्यनतिविस्तरान् ॥ ६ ॥

I am going to describe briefly in these pages, such recipes which are extolled by the scriptures and found effective by the personal experience and logical reasoning for the benefit of the people of the world at large (6).

प्रथमं परिभाषा स्याद्भैषज्याख्यानकं तथा । नाडीपरिक्षादिविधिस्ततो दीपनपाचनम् ॥ ७ ॥
ततः कलादिकाख्यानमाहारादिगतिस्तथा । रोगाणां गणना चेति पूर्वखण्डोऽयमीरितः ॥ ८ ॥

In the first khaṇḍa (section) the first chapter deals with paribhāṣā (definition) followed by six chapters dealing with bhaiṣajya vyākhyāna (principles of pharmacy), nāḍī parīkshādi vidhi (examination of pulse, etc.), dīpanapāchanādi (pharmacological definitions), kalādi ākhyāna (description of structures of the body), āhārādi gati (digestion and fate of food) and roga gaṇanā (enumeration of diseases) respectively (7–8).

स्वरसः क्वाथफाण्टौ च हिमः कल्कश्च चूर्णकम् । तथैव गुटिकालेहौ स्नेहः सन्धानमेव च ॥ ९ ॥
धातुशुद्धी रसाश्चैव खण्डोऽयं मध्यमः स्मृतः ।

The madhyama khaṇḍa (second section) has twelve chapters dealing with the preparation of swarasa (fresh juice, aqueous extract), qwātha (decoction), phāṇṭa (hot infusion), hima (cold infusion), kalka (paste), chūrṇa (powder), guṭikā (pill), leha (confection), sneha (lipid preparation), sandhāna (fermented preparation), dhātu shuddhi (purification of minerals and metals) and rasas (metallic recipes) (9–10).

स्नेहपानं स्वेदविधिर्वमनं च विरेचनम् ॥ १० ॥
ततस्तु स्नेहबस्तिः स्यात्ततश्चापि निरूहणम् । ततश्चाप्युत्तरो बस्तिस्ततो नस्यविधिर्मत ॥ ११ ॥
धूमपानविधिश्चैव गण्डूषादिविधिस्तथा । लेपादीनां विधिः ख्यातस्तथा शोणितविस्रुतिः ॥ १२ ॥
नेत्रकर्मप्रकारश्च खण्डः स्यादुत्तरस्त्वयम् ।
द्वात्रिंशत्संमिताध्यायैर्युक्तेयं संहिता स्मृता ॥ १३ ॥
षड्विंशतिशतान्यत्र श्लोकानां गणितानि च ।

The uttara khaṇḍa (third section) has thirteen chapters dealing with therapies like snehapāna (oleation), sweda vidhi (sudation), vamana (emesis), virechana (purgation), snehabasti (oil enema), nirūhaṇa (decoction enema), uttara basti (urethral and vaginal douches), nasya vidhi (nasal medication), dhūmapāna (inhalation, fumigation), gaṇḍūṣa vidhi (gargles and mouth washes), lepa vidhi (external applications), shoṇita visruti (blood letting), netra karma

(ophthalmic therapy). Thus this treatise has 32 (thirty two) chapters containing 2600 verses in total (10–14).

अथ मागधपरिभाषा—

न मानेन विना युक्तिर्द्रव्याणां जायते क्वचित् ॥ १४ ॥
अतः प्रयोगकार्यार्थं मानमत्रोच्यते मया ।

System of weights and measures will be described first without which dealing with drugs and recipes will be impractical (14–15).

मागधीयं मानम्—

त्रसरेणुर्बुधैः प्रोक्तस्त्रिंशता परमाणुभिः ॥ १५ ॥
त्रसरेणुस्तु पर्यायनाम्ना वंशी निगद्यते ।
जालान्तरगते भानौ यत्सूक्ष्मं दृश्यते रजः ॥ १६ ॥
तस्य त्रिंशत्तमो भागः परमाणुः स कथ्यते । जालान्तरगतैः सूर्यकरैर्वंशी विलोक्यते ॥१७॥

One by thirtieth part of a paramāṇu is called a trasareṇu. It is also known as vaṃshī. The minutest particle of dust visible in a beam of sunlight, if divided into thirty parts and one part taken out of it equals the paramāṇu (15–17).

षड्वंशीभिर्मरीचिः स्यात्ताभिः षड्भिस्तु राजिका । तिसृभी राजिकाभिश्च सर्षपः प्रोच्यते बुधैः ॥ १८ ॥
यवोऽष्टसर्षपैः प्रोक्तो गुञ्जा स्यात्तच्चतुष्टयम् । षड्भिस्तु रक्तिकाभिः स्यान्माषको हेमधान्यकौ ॥ १९ ॥
माषैश्चतुर्भिः शाणः स्याद्धरणः स निगद्यते । टङ्कः स एव कथितस्तद्द्वयं कोल उच्यते ॥ २० ॥
क्षुद्रको वटकश्चैव द्रङ्क्षणः स निगद्यते ।
कोलद्वयं च कर्षः स्यात्स प्रोक्तः पाणिमानिका ॥ २१ ॥
अक्षं पिचुः पाणितलं किंचित्पाणिश्च तिन्दुकम् । बिडालपदकं चैव तथा षोडशिका मता ॥ २२ ॥
करमध्यो हंसपदं सुवर्णं कवलग्रहः । उदुम्बरं च पर्यायैः कर्ष एव निगद्यते ॥ २३ ॥
स्यात्कर्षाभ्यामर्धपलं शुक्तिरष्टमिका तथा । शुक्तिभ्यां च पलं ज्ञेयं मुष्टिराम्रं चतुर्थिका ॥ २४ ॥
प्रकुञ्चः षोडशी बिल्वं पलमेवात्र कीर्त्यते ।
पलाभ्यां प्रसृतिर्ज्ञेया प्रसृतश्च निगद्यते ॥ २५ ॥
प्रसृतिभ्यामञ्जलिः स्यात्कुडवोऽर्धशरावकः । अष्टमानं च स ज्ञेयः कुडवाभ्यां च मानिका ॥२६॥
शरावोऽष्टपलं तद्वज्ज्ञेयमत्र विचक्षणैः ।
शरावाभ्यां भवेत्प्रस्थश्चतुः प्रस्थैस्तथाढकम् ॥ २७ ॥
भाजनं कंसपात्रं च चतुःषष्टिपलं च तत् ।
चतुर्भिराढकैर्द्रोणः कलशो नल्वणोऽर्मणः ॥ २८ ॥
उन्मानश्च घटो राशिर्द्रोणपर्यायसंज्ञकाः । द्रोणाभ्यां शूर्पकुम्भौ च चतुःषष्टिशरावकाः ॥ २९ ॥
शूर्पाभ्यां च भवेद्द्रोणी वाही गोणी च सा स्मृता ।
द्रोणीचतुष्टयं खारी कथिता सूक्ष्मबुद्धिभिः ॥ ३० ॥
चतुःसहस्रपलिका षण्णवत्यधिका च सा ।
पलानां द्विसहस्रं च भार एकः प्रकीर्तितः ॥ ३१ ॥

तुला पलशतं ज्ञेया सर्वत्रैवैष निश्चयः ।
माषटङ्काक्षबिल्वानि कुडवः प्रस्थमाढकम् ॥ ३२ ॥
राशिर्गोणी खारिकेति यथोत्तरचतुर्गुणाः ।

Six vaṃshīs (trasareṇus) make one marīchi, six marīchis make one rājikā; three rājikās make one sarṣapa, eight sarṣapas make a yava; four yavas make one guñjā (also known as raktikā); six raktikās make one māṣā (also known as hema, dhānyaka); four māṣās make one shāṇa (also known as dharaṇa, ṭaṅka), two shāṇas make one kola (also known as kshudraka, vaṭaka, draṅkshaṇa); two kolas make one karṣa (also known as pāṇimānikā, aksha, pichu, pāṇitala, kinchit-pāṇi, tinduka, biḍālapadaka, ṣoḍashikā, karamadhya, haṃsapada, suvarṇa, kavala-graha and udumbara); two karṣas make one ardhapala (also known as shukti, aṣṭamikā); two shuktis make a pala (also known as muṣṭi, āmra, chaturthaka, prakuñcha, ṣoḍashī, bilwa); two palas make one prasṛti (prasṛta); two prasṛtis make one añjali (also known as kuḍava, ardhasharāva, aṣṭamāna); two kuḍavas make one mānikā (also known as sharāva, aṣṭapala); two sharāvas make one prastha; four prasthas make one āḍhaka (also known as bhājana, kaṃsapātra) which is equivalent to sixty-four palas. Four āḍhakas make one droṇa (also known as kalasha, nalvaṇa, māna, unmāna, ghaṭa, rāshī); two droṇas make one shūrpa (also known as kumbha, and equivalent to sixtyfour sharāvas); two shūrpas make one droṇī (also known as vāhī, goṇī); four droṇīs make one khārī (equivalent to 4960 palas); two thousand palas make one bhāra; one hundred palas is popular everywhere as a tulā. Māṣā, ṭaṅka, aksha, bilwa, kuḍava, prastha, āḍhaka, rāshī, goṇī and khārī are quadruples in successive order (18–33).

गुञ्जादिमानमारभ्य यावत्स्यात्कुडवस्थितिः ॥ ३३ ॥
द्रवार्द्रशुष्कद्रव्याणां तावन्मानं समं मतम् ।
प्रस्थादिमानमारभ्य द्विगुणं तद्द्रवार्द्रयोः ॥ ३४ ॥
मानं तथा तुलायाश्च द्विगुणं न क्वचित्स्मृतम् ।

In compounding a recipe the quantity of both the green drugs and dry drugs should be the same if their prescribed quantity ranges from guñjā to kuḍava and from tulā and above; whereas if from prastha to tulā green drugs and liquids should be taken double the prescribed quantity but not so upwards of tulā (33–35).

मृद्वृक्षवेणुलोहादेर्भाण्डं यच्चतुरङ्गुलम् ॥ ३५ ॥
विस्तीर्णं च तथोच्चं च तन्मानं कुडवं वदेत् ।

The quantity that fills a vessel of 4 aṅgulis in each of its length, breadth and height, prepared out of mud, wood, bamboo or metal is one "kuḍava" (35–36).

यदौषधं तु प्रथमं यस्य योगस्य कथ्यते ॥ ३६ ॥
तन्नाम्नैव स योगो हि कथ्यतेऽत्र विनिश्चयः ।

A recipe receives its name usually from the first drug in its compositon (36-337).

अथ कालिङ्गपरिभाषा ।

स्थितिर्नास्त्येव मात्रायाः कालमग्निं वयो बलम् ॥ ३७ ॥
प्रकृतिं दोषदेशौ च दृष्ट्वा मात्रां प्रकल्पयेत् ।
यतो मन्दाग्नयो ह्रस्वा हीनसत्त्वा नराः कलौ ॥ ३८ ॥
अतस्तु मात्रा तद्योग्या प्रोच्यते सुज्ञसम्मता ।
यवो द्वादशभिर्गौरसर्षपैः प्रोच्यते बुधैः ॥ ३९ ॥
यवद्वयेन गुञ्जा स्यात्त्रिगुञ्जो वल्ल उच्यते । माषो गुञ्जाभिरष्टाभिः सप्तभिर्वा भवेत्कचित् ॥ ४० ॥
स्याच्चतुर्माषकैः शाणः स निष्कष्टङ्क एव च । गद्याणो माषकैः षड्भिः कर्षः स्याद्दशमाषिकः ॥४१॥
चतुष्कर्षैः पलं प्रोक्तं दशशाणमितं बुधैः । चतुष्पलैश्च कुडवं प्रस्थाद्याः पूर्ववन्मताः ॥ ४२ ॥
कालिङ्गं मागधं चेति द्विविधं मानमुच्यते ॥ ४३ ॥
कालिङ्गान्मागधं श्रेष्ठं मानं मानविदो विदुः ।

Determination of weights and measures of drugs is not rigid. The physicians should decide it taking into consideration the kāla (season), agni (digestive-capacity), vaya (age), bala (strength), prakṛti (constitution), doṣas (humors) and desha (habitat). As the people of Kaliyuga (the present era) are poor in their digestive capacity, physical stature and mental power, the follc v-ing dosage will be more suitable; twelve gaurasarṣapas make one yava, two yavas make one guñjā, three guñjās make one valla, eight guñjās (in some places seven) make one māṣā; four māṣās make one shāṇa (also known as niṣka, ṭaṅka); six māṣās make one gadyāṇa, ten māṣās make one karṣa, four karṣas make one pala (equivalent to ten shāṇas); four palas make one kuḍava; from prastha onwards there is no difference from the earlier. Kaliṅga and Māgadha are the two systems of weights and measures in vogue, of which the Magadhan system is considered best (37–44).

नवान्येव हि योज्यानि द्रव्याण्यखिलकर्मसु । विना विडङ्गकृष्णाभ्यां गुडधान्याज्यमाक्षिकैः ॥४४॥
गुडूची कुटजो वासा कूष्माण्डं च शतावरी । अश्वगन्धा सहचरी शतपुष्पा प्रसारिणी ॥ ४५ ॥
प्रयोक्तव्या सदैवार्द्रा द्विगुणा नैव योजयेत् ।

On all occasions fresh drugs only should be used except viḍaṅga, kṛṣṇā, guḍa, dhānya, ājya and mākshika. Guḍūchī, kuṭaja, vāsā, kūṣmāṇḍa, shatāvarī, ashwagandhā, sahacharī, shatapuṣpā and prasāriṇī—these should always be used in green state but need not be taken in double the prescribed quantity (44–46).

शुष्कं नवीनं यद्द्रव्यं योज्यं सकलकर्मसु ॥ ४६ ॥
आर्द्रं च द्विगुणं युञ्ज्यादेष सर्वत्र निश्चयः ।

On all occasions the drugs which are dry and fresh should be selected and in case of green drugs they should be taken in double the prescribed quantity (46–47).

कालेऽनुक्त प्रभातं स्यादङ्गेऽनुक्ते जटा भवेत् ॥ ४७ ॥
भागेऽनुक्ते तु साम्यं स्यात्पात्रेऽनुक्ते च मृण्मयम् । द्रवेऽनुक्ते जलं ग्राह्यं तैलेऽनुक्ते तिलोद्भवम् ॥४८॥

If in a recipe, the time of consuming it is not mentioned, mornings are to be presumed as ideal; if the part of the plant to be used is not mentioned, roots are to be selected, if proportion is not mentioned equal quantity is to be presumed, if the kind of the vessel for preparing is not mentioned earthen one is best; if the liquid to be used is not specified water is to be used; if oil is not specified tilataila (sesame oil) is to be selected (47–48).

एकमप्यौषधं योगे यस्मिन्यत्पुनरुच्यते । मानतो द्विगुणं कार्यं तद्द्रव्यं तत्त्वदर्शिभिः ॥ ४९ ॥

If in a recipe a drug is mentioned twice, experts prescribe its inclusion in double the quantity (49).

चूर्णस्नेहासवा लेहाः प्रायशश्चन्दनान्विताः । कषायलेपयोः प्रायो युज्यते रक्तचन्दनम् ॥ ५० ॥

If chandana is included in a recipe of chūrṇa (powder), sneha (oil or ghee) or āsava (fermented liquor), śweta chandana (the white variety) only is to be used; whereas in the preparation of kaṣāya (decoction) and lepa (topical application) rakta chandana (red variety) is usually used (50).

गुणहीनं भवेद्वर्षादूर्ध्वं तद्रूपमौषधम् । मासद्वयात्तथा चूर्णं हीनवीर्यत्वमाप्नुयात् ॥ ५१ ॥
हीनत्वं गुटिकालेहौ लभेते वत्सरात्परम् । हीनाः स्युर्घृततैलाद्याश्चतुर्मासाधिकात्तथा ॥ ५२ ॥
ओषध्यो लघुपाकाः स्युर्निर्वीर्या वत्सरात्परम् । पुराणाः स्युर्गुणैर्युक्ता आसवा धातवो रसाः ॥ ५३ ॥

Generally, medicinal recipes lose their potency after one year of their preparation; chūrṇas (powders) after two months, guṭikās (pills) and lehyas (confections) after one year; ghṛtas and taila (ghee, oils) after four months; recipes which are digested easily and quickly become poor in action after one year; while āsavas (fermented liquors) and dhātus (metal and mineral recipes) become more potent as they become old (51–53).

व्याधेरयुक्तं यद्द्रव्यं गणोक्तमपि तत्त्यजेत् । अनुक्तमपि युक्तं योजयेत्तत्र तद्बुधः ॥ ५४ ॥

If in a prescription, drugs included are inappropriate for the diseases, the wise physician should omit them, and can include drugs suitable for the disease even though not mentioned in the prescription (54).

आग्नेया विन्ध्यशैलाद्याः सौम्यो हिमगिरिर्मतः । अतस्तदौषधानि स्युरनुरूपाणि हेतुभिः ॥ ५५ ॥
अन्येष्वपि प्ररोहन्ति वनेषूपवनेषु च ।

Herbs grown in the Vindhya mountains are āgneya (heat producing) while those growing in the Himalayas are saumya (coolant), hence they should be so choosen as are suited to the person. Plants growing in other forests will have the qualities of the place (55–56).

गृह्णीयात्तानि सुमनाः शुचिः प्रातः सुवासरे ॥ ५६ ॥
आदित्यसंमुखो मौनी नमस्कृत्य शिवं हृदि । साधारणधराद्द्रव्यं गृह्णीयादुत्तराश्रितम् ॥ ५७ ॥

The physician who is pure in mind and clean in body should collect the herbs during sunshine praying to Lord Shiva in silence; herbs growing in northerly direction are to be collected (56–57).

वल्मीककुत्सितानूपश्मशानोषरमार्गजाः । जन्तुवह्निहिमव्याप्ता नौषध्यः कार्यसिद्धिदाः ॥ ५८ ॥

Herbs growing on anthills, dirty places, marshy land, burial ground, salty soil, roads and those which have been infested with worms, affected by fire and snow will not yield the desired effect (58).

शरद्यखिलकार्यार्थं ग्राह्यं सरसमौषधम् । विरेकवमनार्थं च वसन्तान्ते समाहरेत् ॥ ५९ ॥

Sharat ṛtu (October, November) is the best time for collection of herbs for all types of preparations, but for herbs which are for vamana (emesis) and virechana (purgation) the best time is the end of Vasanta ṛtu (February-March) (59).

अतिस्थूलजटा याः स्युस्तासां ग्राह्यास्त्वचो बुधैः । गृह्णीयात्सूक्ष्ममूलानि सकलान्यपि बुद्धिमान् ॥६०॥
न्यग्रोधादेस्त्वचो ग्राह्याः सारः स्याद्बीजकादितः । तालीसादेश्च पुष्पाणि फलं स्यात्त्रिफलादितः ॥६१॥
धातक्यादेश्च पुष्पाणि स्नुह्यादेः क्षीरमाहरेत् ।

The root bark is to be collected in case of big roots whereas in case of tender ones the entire root system is collected; in case of big trees like nyagrodha etc., their outer bark is to be collected; in case of trees like bījaka etc., their pith; in case of tālīsa etc., their leaves; in case of triphalā etc., their fruits; in case of dhātakī etc., their flowers and in case of snuhi etc. their sap (60–62).

इति श्रीदामोदरसूनुना शार्ङ्गधरेण विरचितायां शार्ङ्गधरसंहितायां पूर्वखण्डे
परिभाषा नाम प्रथमोऽध्यायः ॥ १ ॥

Thus ends the first chapter of first section.

द्वितीयोऽध्यायः

CHAPTER 2

Bhaiṣajya Vyākhyāna (Principles of Pharmacy)

अथ भैषज्याख्यानकाध्यायः—

भैषज्यमभ्यवहरेत्प्रभाते प्रायशो बुधः । कषायांश्च विशेषेण तत्र भेदस्तु दर्शितः ॥ १ ॥
ज्ञेयः पञ्चविधः कालो भैषज्यग्रहणे नृणाम् । किञ्चित्सूर्योदये जाते तथा दिवसभोजने ॥ २ ॥
सायन्तने भोजने च मुहुश्चापि तथा निशि ।

Medicines are generally administered in the morning specially so the kaṣāyas (decoctions). Sunrise, the time of midday meal, night meal, frequent intervals, and bed-time : these are the five suitable times for the administration of medicines (1–3).

प्रायः पित्तकफोद्रेके विरेकवमनार्थयोः ॥ ३ ॥
लेखनार्थं च भैषज्यं प्रभाते तत्समाहरेत् । एवं स्यात्प्रथमः कालो भैषज्यग्रहणे नृणाम् ॥ ४ ॥

In diseases of kapha and pitta and for the purpose of vamana (emesis), vireka (purgation) and lekhana (scarification) medicines should be administered in the mornings. This is the first period for the administration of medicines (3–4).

भैषज्यं विगुणेऽपाने भोजनाग्रे प्रशस्यते । अरुचौ चित्रभोज्यैश्च मिश्रं रुचिरमाहरेत् ॥ ५ ॥
समानवाते विगुणे मन्देऽग्नावग्निदीपनम् । दद्याद्भोजनमध्ये च भैषज्यं कुशलो भिषक् ॥ ६ ॥
व्यानकोपे च भैषज्यं भोजनान्ते समाहरेत् । हिक्काक्षेपककम्पेषु पूर्वमन्ते च भोजनात् ॥ ७ ॥

एवं द्वितीयकालश्च प्रोक्तो भैषज्यकर्मणि ।

In diseases of apānavāta, medicines are given just before midday meal, in cases of aruchi (anorexia) they should be given mixed with morsels of food, in disorders of samānavāta, for agni dīpana (kindling of digestion) medicines are best given in the middle of the meal, in disorders of vyānavāta, end of the meal is best; in diseases like hikkā (hiccough), ākshepaka (convulsions) and kampa (tremors) both times (before and after meals). This is the second period for the administration of medicines (5–8).

उदाने कुपिते वाते स्वरभङ्गादिकारिणि ॥ ८ ॥
ग्रासे ग्रासान्तरे देयं भैषज्यं सान्ध्यभोजने । प्राणे प्रदुष्टे सान्ध्यस्य भुक्तस्यान्ते च दीयते ॥ ९ ॥
औषधं प्रायशो धीरैः कालोऽयं स्यात्तृतीयकः ।

In disorders of udānavāta and diseases like swarabhaṅga (hoarseness) etc, medicines are given between each morsel of night meal; in disorders of prāṇavāta it should be after the meal. This is the third period (8–10).

मुहुर्मुहुश्च तृट्छर्दिहिक्काश्वासगरेषु च ॥ १० ॥
साम्नं च भेषजं दद्यादिति कालश्चतुर्थकः ।

In diseases like tṛṭ (thirst), chardi (vomiting), hikkā (hiccough), śwāsa (dyspnoea) and gara (homicidal poisoning) medicines are to be given at frequent intervals or along with food. This is the fourth period (10–11).

ऊर्ध्वजत्रुविकारेषु लेखने बृंहणे तथा ॥ ११ ॥
पाचनं शमनं देयमनन्नं भेषजं निशि । इति पञ्चमकालः स्यात् प्रोक्तो भैषज्यकर्मणि ॥ १२ ॥

In diseases of the head and for lekhana (curetting action), bṛṃhaṇa (strengthening and fattening action), pāchana (digestive action) and shamana (palliative action) medicines should be given on empty stomach at night. This is the fifth period (11–12).

द्रव्ये रसो गुणो वीर्यं विपाकः शक्तिरेव च । संबन्धेन क्रमादेताः पञ्चावस्थाः प्रकीर्तिताः ॥ १३ ॥

Rasa (taste), guṇa (properties and qualities), virya (potency), vipāka (post-digestive action) and shakti (special effect) are the five inter-related working factors in a drug (13).

रसः— मधुरोऽम्लः पटुश्चैव कटुतिक्तकषायकाः । इत्येते षड्रसाः ख्याता नानाद्रव्यसमाश्रिताः ॥ १४ ॥
धराम्बुक्ष्मानलजलज्वलनाकाशमारुतैः । वाय्वग्निक्ष्मानिलैर्भूतद्वयैः रसभवः क्रमात् ॥ १५ ॥

Madhura (sweet), amla (sour), paṭu (salt), kaṭu (pungent), tikta (bitter) and kaṣāya (astringent) are the six rasas (tastes) present in various materials. These tastes are formed from the combination of two mahābhūtas in the following way; dharā (pṛthvi) and ambu (ap) create madhura rasa (sweet taste); kshmā (pṛthvi) and anala (teja) create amla (sour); jala (ap) and jwalana (tejas) create lavaṇa (salt); ākāsha and maruta create kaṭu (pungent); vāyu and agni (tejas) tikta (bitter) while kshmā (pṛthvī) and anila (vāyu) create kaṣāya (astringent) (14–15).

गुणाः—गुरुः स्निग्धश्च तीक्ष्णश्च रूक्षो लघुरिति क्रमात् । धराम्बुवह्निपवनव्योम्नां प्रायो गुणाः स्मृताः॥१६॥
पश्वेवान्तर्भवन्त्यन्ये गुणेषु गुणसञ्चयाः ।

Guru (heavyness), snigdha (unctousness), tīkshṇa (penetrating effect), rūksha (dryness) and laghu (lightness) are the properties of dharā (pṛthvī), ambu (ap), vahni (tejas), pavana (vāyu) and vyoma (ākāsha) respectively. All other properties are included under these five only (16–17).

वीर्यम्–वीर्यमुष्णं तथा शीतं प्रायशो द्रव्यसंश्रयम् ॥ १७ ॥
तत्सर्वमग्नीषोमीयं दृश्यते भुवनत्रये । अत्रैवान्तर्भविष्यन्ति वीर्याण्यन्यानि यान्यपि ॥ १८ ॥

All the substances of the three worlds are either āgneya (hot) or saumya (coolant) predominantly. So the vīryas (potency) are only two viz., ūṣṇa (hot) and shīta (cold), any other vīrya, if at all, is included in any one of these two (17–18).

विपाकः-त्रिधा विपाको द्रव्यस्य स्वाद्वम्लकटुकात्मकः । मिष्टः पटुश्च मधुरमम्लोऽम्लं पच्यते रसः ॥१९॥
कषायकटुतिक्तानां पाकः स्यात्प्रायशः कटुः । मधुराज्जायते श्लेष्मा पित्तमम्लाच्च जायते ॥२०॥
कटुकाज्जायते वायुः कर्माणीति विपाकतः ।

Vipāka (post-digestive effect) of all substaces are only three viz., swādu (sweet), amla (sour) and kaṭu (pungent). The vipāka of madhura (sweet) and lavaṇa (salt) substances will be madhura (sweet); that of amla substance will be amla (sour); while those of kaṣāya (astringent), kaṭu (pungent) and tikta (bitter) will be kaṭu (pungent). Madhura vipāka produces ślesma (kapha), amla vipāka produces pitta and kaṭu vipāka produces vāta (19–21).

प्रभावः-प्रभावस्तु तथा धात्री लकुचस्य रसादिभिः ॥ २१ ॥
समापि कुरुते दोषं नियतस्य विनाशनम् ।

Prabhāva is a special effect as seen from the example of dhātrī and lakucha; though both are similar in their rasa, guṇa, vīrya and vipāka, dhātrī alleviates all the tridoṣas whereas lakucha will not (21–22).

कश्चित्तु केवलं द्रव्यं कर्म कुर्यात्प्रभावतः ॥ २२ ॥
ज्वरं हन्ति शिरोबद्धा सहदेवीजटा यथा । कश्चिद्रसो गुणो वीर्यं विपाकः शक्तिरेव च ॥ २३ ॥
कर्म स्वं स्वं प्रकुर्वन्ति द्रव्यमाश्रित्य ये स्थिताः ।

Some drugs act by their own (total effect of all its properties) for example the root of sahadevī cures jwara (fever) if tied on the head. Some others act by virtue of their rasa (taste), some by their guṇas (properties), some by their vīrya (potency), some others by their vipāka and yet others by their shakti (prabhāva)--special effect present in them (22–24).

चयकोपशमा यस्मिन्दोषाणां संभवन्ति हि ॥ २४ ॥
ऋतुषट्कं तदाख्यातं रवे राशिषु संक्रमात् ।

Movement of the Sun from one stellar constellation to the other makes for the six ṛtus (seasons) during which the tridoṣas undergo chaya (mild increase), prakopa (profound increase) and shamana (decrease to normal) (24–25).

ग्रीष्मो मेषवृषौ प्रोक्तौ प्रावृड्मिथुनकर्कयोः ॥ २५ ॥
सिंहकन्ये स्मृता वर्षास्तुलावृश्चिकयोः शरत् । धनुर्ग्राहौ च हेमन्तो वसन्तः कुम्भमीनयोः ॥ २६ ॥

When the Sun is in Meṣa (Aries) and Vṛṣabha (Taurus) constellations it is Grīṣma ṛtu (summer, April–May); in Mithuna (Gemini) and Karka (cancer) it is Prāvṛṭ (June—July); in Siṃha (Leo) and Kanyā (Virgo) it is Varṣā (rainy season, August—September); in Tulā (Libra) and Vṛśchika (Scorpio) it is Sharat (Autumn, October—November); in Dhanu (Sagitarrus) and Grahi (Copricorn) it is Hemanta (Winter, December—January); in Kumbha (Aquarius) and Mīna (piscus) it is Vasanta (Spring, February--March) (25-26).

ग्रीष्मे संचीयते वायुः प्रावृट्काले प्रकुप्यति । वर्षासु चीयते पित्तं शरत्काले प्रकुप्यति ॥ २७ ॥
हेमन्ते चीयते श्लेष्मा वसन्ते च प्रकुप्यति । प्रायेण प्रशमं याति स्वयमेव समीरणः ॥ २८ ॥
शरत्काले वसन्ते च पित्तं प्रावृडृतौ कफः ।
कार्तिकस्य दिनान्यष्टावष्टावाग्रयणस्य च ॥ २९ ॥
यमदंष्ट्रा समाख्याता स्वल्पभुक्तो हि जीवति ।

Vāyu undergoes chaya (mild increase) during Grīṣhma and prakopa (profound increase) during Prāvṛṭ; pitta undergoes chaya during Varṣā and prakopa during Sharat; kapha undergoes chaya during Hemanta and prakopa during Vasanta ṛtu. Vāyu attains prashama (decrease to normal) of its own accord in Sharat; pitta in Vasanta; and kapha in Prāvṛṭ. The (last) eight days of Kārtika māsa (third week of November) and the (first) eight days of Agrahāyaṇa (fourth week of November) are known as Yamadaṃṣṭra kāla. During this period one can be healthy if he takes only small quantities of food (27-30).

चयकोपशमा दोषा विहाराहारसेवनैः ॥ ३० ॥
समानैर्यान्त्यकालेऽपि विपरीतैर्विपर्ययम् । लघुरूक्षमिताहारादतिशीताच्छ्रमात्तथा ॥ ३१ ॥
प्रदोषे कामशोकाभ्यां भीचिन्तारात्रिजागरैः । अभिघातादपां गाहाज्जीर्णेऽन्ने धातुसंक्षयात् ॥३२॥
वायुः प्रकोपं यात्येभिः प्रत्यनीकैश्च शाम्यति ।

The doṣas attain chaya (mild increase), kopa (profound increase) and prashamana (decrease back to normal) even in other sessons due to indulgence in vihāra (activities) and āhāra (foods) which are either similar or dissimilar respectively to their nature and qualities. Vāyu attains prakopa by ingestion of foods which are laghu (light), rūksha (dry), mita (very less), ati śita (very cold); by shrama (physical exertion), kāma (lust), shoka (grief), bhi (fright), chintā (worry); in the evenings, by rātri jāgaraṇa (keeping awake at nights), abhighāta (injury); bathing in cold water; after the digestion of food, and dhātu kshaya (depletion or loss of body tissues). It attains prashama by the opposites of the above (30-33).

विदाहिकटुकाम्लोष्णभोज्यैरत्युष्णसेवनात् ॥ ३३ ॥
मध्याह्ने क्षुत्तृषो रोजाज्जीर्यत्यन्नेऽर्धरात्रके । पित्तं प्रकोपं यात्येभिः प्रत्यनीकैश्च शाम्यति ॥ ३४ ॥

Pitta undergoes prakopa by ingestion of foods which are vidāhī (producing burning inside the stomach), kaṭu (pungent), amlā (sour), ūṣṇa (hot), exposure to heat of fire, sun etc ; during midday, the suppression of hunger and thirst; during the period of digestion and midnight. It attains shamana by the opposites of the above (33-34).

मधुरस्निग्धशीतादिभोज्यैर्दिवसनिद्रया । मन्देऽग्नौ च प्रभाते च भुक्तमात्रे तथाऽश्रमात् ॥ ३५ ॥
श्लेष्मा प्रकोपं यात्येभिः प्रत्यनीकैश्च शाम्यति ॥ ३६ ॥

Kapha attains prakopa by foods which are madhura (sweet), snigdha (oily, fatty), shīta (cold); by day sleep, physical inactivity, poor digestive power, in the mornings and immediately after the meal. It undergoes prashama by the opposites of the above (35-36).

इति दामोदरसूनुना शार्ङ्गधरेण विरचितायां श्रीशार्ङ्गधरसंहितायां
पूर्वखण्डे भैषज्याख्यानकं नाम द्वितीयोऽध्यायः ॥ २ ॥

Thus ends the second chapter.

तृतीयोध्यायः

CHAPTER 3

Nāḍī Parīkshādi Vidhi (Examination of Pulse etc.)

अथ नाडीपरीक्षादिविधिरध्यायः

करस्याङ्गुष्ठमूले या धमनी जीवसाक्षिणी । तच्चेष्टया सुखं दुःखं ज्ञेयं कायस्य पण्डितैः ॥ १ ॥

The pulse at the wrist signifies the presence of life. The physician should recognise health and ill health of a person from its activities (1).

नाडी धत्ते मरुत्कोपे जलौकासर्पयोर्गतिम् । कुलिङ्गकाकमण्डूकगतिं पित्तस्य कोपतः ॥ २ ॥
हंसपारावतगतिं धत्ते श्लेष्मप्रकोपतः ।
लावतित्तिरवर्तीनां गमनं संनिपाततः ॥ ३ ॥
कदाचिन्मन्दगमना कदाचिद्वेगवाहिनी ।
द्विदोषकोपतो ज्ञेया

During vātaprakopa (increase of vāta) the movement of the pulse resembles the movement of jalaukā (leech) or sarpa (snake); during the prakopa of pitta it will be like the movement of kuliṅga (sparrow), kāka (crow) and maṇḍūka (frog); during kapha prakopa it resembles the movement of hamsa (swan) or pārāvata (pigeon); in sannipāta (increase of all the three doṣas together) it will be like the movement of lāva (bustard quail), tittira (grey partridge) and vārtāka (button quail) bird. In case of increase of any two doṣas it will be some times very slow and some times very quick (2–4).

हन्ति च स्थानविच्युता ॥ ४ ॥
स्थित्वा स्थित्वा चलति या सा स्मृता प्राणनाशिनी । अतिक्षीणा च शीता च जीवितं हन्त्यसंशयम् ॥५॥
ज्वरकोपेण धमनी सोष्णा वेगवती भवेत् । कामक्रोधाद्वेगवहा क्षीणा चिन्ताभयप्लुता ॥ ६ ॥
मन्दाग्नेः क्षीणधातोश्च नाडी मन्दतरा भवेत् । असृक्पूर्णा भवेत्कोष्णा गुर्वी सामा गरीयसी ॥ ७ ॥
लघ्वी वहति दीप्ताग्नेस्तथा वेगवती मता । सुखितस्य स्थिरा ज्ञेया तथा बलवती स्मृता ॥ ८ ॥
चपला क्षुधितस्यापि तृप्तस्य वहति स्थिरा ।

Pulse which has moved away from its normal place, which stops and starts again, which is very thin (feeble) and cold signifies death. Nāḍī attains increased rate and warmth in cases of jwara (fever), during emotions of kāma (lust) and krodha (anger); its rate decreases during chintā (worry) and bhaya (fright). In conditions of mandāgni (poor digestive capacity) and kshīṇa dhātu (loss or impoverishment of body tissues) it is very slow and feeble; whereas it will be warm when full with blood, in the state of sāma (accumulation of toxins) it will be hard and tense. It will be light and quick when the digestive capacity is powerful; during hunger it is unsteady and attains steadyness after food. During health it is steady and forceful (5–8).

दूताः स्वजातयोऽव्यङ्गाः पटवो निर्मलाम्बराः । सुखिनोऽश्ववृषारूढाः शुभ्रपुष्पफलैर्युताः ॥ ९ ॥
सुजातयः सुचेष्टाश्च सजीवदिशि संश्रिताः । भिषजं समये प्राप्ता रोगिणः सुखहेतवे ॥ १० ॥
वैद्याह्वानाय दूतस्य गच्छतो रोगिणः कृते ॥ ११ ॥
न शुभं सौम्यशकुनं प्रदीप्तं च सुखावहम् । चिकित्सां रोगिणः कर्तुं गच्छतो भिषजः शुभम् ॥ १२ ॥
यात्रेयं सौम्यशकुनं प्रोक्तं दीप्तं न शोभनम् ।

Dūta (messenger who comes to call the physician) is considered auspicious if he is of the same caste as the patient, who himself is not sick, who is active, is wearing clean dress, happily riding on horse or bull, adorned with flowers and fruits, coming from an auspicious direction and who has arrived in proper time. Such a messenger portends restoration of health of the patient. If the messenger sees auspicious omens on his way it is bad to the patient whereas seeing inauspicious omens is good. If the physician sees auspicious omen on his way to the patient's house it is good for the patient whereas seeing inauspicious omen is bad (9–12).

निजप्रकृतिवर्णाभ्यां युक्तः सत्त्वेन संयुतः ॥ १३ ॥
चिकित्स्यो भिषजा रोगी वैद्यभक्तो जितेन्द्रियः ।

A patient is considered ideal for therapy if he possesses the features of a good prakṛti (constitution), varṇa (colour) and satwa (mental make up), who is obedient to the physician and has control over his senses (13).

स्वप्नेषु नग्नान्मुण्डांश्च रक्तकृष्णाम्बरावृतान् ॥ १४ ॥
व्यङ्गांश्च विकृतान्कृष्णान्सपाशान्सायुधानपि । बध्नतो निघ्नतश्चापि दक्षिणां दिशमाश्रितान् ॥ १५ ॥

महिषोष्ट्रखरारूढांस्त्रीपुंसो यस्तु पश्यति । स स्वस्थो लभते व्याधिं रोगी यात्येव पञ्चताम् ॥ १६ ॥
अधो यो निपतत्युच्चाज्जलेऽग्नौ वा विलीयते । श्वापदैर्हन्यते योऽपि मत्स्याद्यैर्गिलितो भवेत् ॥ १७ ॥
यस्य नेत्रे विलीयेते दीपो निर्वाणतां व्रजेत् । तैलं सुरां पिबेद्वापि लोहं वा लभते तिलान् ॥ १८ ॥
पक्वान्नं लभतेऽश्नाति विशेत्कूपं रसातलम् । स स्वस्थो लभते रोगं रोगी यात्येव पञ्चताम् ॥ १९ ॥
दुःस्वप्नानेवमादींश्च दृष्ट्वा ब्रूयान्न कस्यचित् । स्नानं कुर्यादुषस्येव दद्याद्धेमतिलानपः ॥ २० ॥
पठेत्स्तोत्राणि देवानां रात्रौ देवालये वसेत् । कृत्वैवं त्रिदिनं मर्त्यो दुःस्वप्नात्परिमुच्यते ॥ २१ ॥

Sight of men or women, naked or shaven head, wearing red or black garments, of distorted limbs, of unusual shape, very black in colour, holding rope or weapons; engaged in roping or killing others, occupying southern direction, riding on buffalo, camel or donkey are inauspicious dreams. If a healthy person sees them he becomes diseased and if a sick person sees them he surely dies. Like wise is the case with seeing himself falling down from a height, drowning in water, being consumed by fire, killed by dogs, swallowed by fish; flame burning inside his eyes without its brilliance, drinking oil or intoxicating drinks, acquiring iron vessels, sessamum or cooked food and eating them, and entering deep pit. Having seen such bad dreams one should not reveal them to others, but take bath before dawn, chant prayers to gods, give gifts of gold and sessamum and stay in a temple at night. This done for three days the person gets over the ill effects of inauspicious dreams (14–21).

स्वप्नेषु यः सुरान्भूपाञ्जीवतः सुहृदो द्विजान् । गोसमिद्धाग्नितीर्थानि पश्येत्सुखमवाप्नुयात् ॥ २२ ॥
तीर्त्वा कलुषनीराणि जित्वा शत्रुगणानपि । आरुह्य सौधगोशैलकरिवाहान्सुखी भवेत् ॥ २३ ॥
शुभ्रपुष्पाणि वासांसि मांसमत्स्यफलानि च । प्राप्यातुरः सुखी भूयात्स्वस्थो धनमवाप्नुयात् ॥ २४ ॥
अगम्यागमनं लेपो विष्ठया रुदितं मृतिः । आममांसाशनं स्वप्ने धनारोग्याप्तये विदुः ॥ २५ ॥
जलौका भ्रमरी सर्पो मक्षिका वापि यं दशेत् । रोगी स भूयादुल्लाघः स्वस्थो धनमवाप्नुयात् ॥ २६ ॥

Sight of Gods, kings and friends who are alive, brahmins, cow, burning fire, places of pilgrimage in dreams brings about health and happiness. Coming out of polluted water, gaininig victory over foes, climbing palaces, mountains, riding on bullock, elephant or other conveyances bestows health. Sight of flowers, clean cloths, mutton, fish and fruits if seen by a sick person portend relief from disease, if seen by a healthy person, portend wealth. Doing a forbidden act, besmeared with filth, weeping, dying and eating raw flesh—if these are dreamt, they portend wealth and health. Seeing of leeches, bees, serpents or honey-bees biting him, if dreamt by a sick person portends relief from disease and if seen by a healthy one portends acquisition of wealth (22–26).

इति श्रीदामोदरसूनुना शार्ङ्गधरेण विरचितायां शार्ङ्गधरसंहितायां
नाडीपरीक्षादिविधिरध्यायः ॥ ३ ॥

Thus ends the third chapter.

चतुर्थोऽध्यायः

CHAPTER 4

Dīpanapāchanādi Kathanam (Pharmacological definitions)

अथ दीपनपाचनाध्यायः

पचेन्नामं वह्निकृच्च दीपनं तद्यथा मिशिः । पचत्यामं न वह्निं च कुर्याद्यत्तद्धि पाचनम् ॥ १ ॥
नागकेशरवद्विद्याच्चित्रो दीपनपाचनः ।

Drugs which do not cook the undigested food (not helping digestion) but only kindle the gastric fire are known as dīpana (appetisers); for example mishi. Drugs which cook the undigested food but do not kindle the appetite are known as pāchana (digestives); for example nāgakeśara. Drugs which possess both these actions are dīpana-pāchana; for example chitraka (1–2).

न शोधयति न द्वेष्टि समान् दोषांस्तथोद्धतान् ॥ २ ॥
समीकरोति विषमाञ्शमनं तद्यथाऽमृता ।

Drugs which bring down the increased doṣa to normal without expelling them out and not interfering with the doṣas which are normal are called shamana (palliatives); for example amṛtā (2–3).

कृत्वा पाकं मलानां यद्भित्त्वा बन्धमधो नयेत् ॥ ३ ॥
तच्चानुलोमनं ज्ञेयं यथा प्रोक्ता हरीतकी ।

Drugs which expel out flatus and faeces after proper digestion and thus removing the obstruction are known as anulomana (aperients); for example harītakī (3–4).

पक्तव्यं यदपक्त्वैव श्लिष्टं कोष्ठे मलादिकम् ॥ ४ ॥
नयत्यधः स्रंसनं तद्यथा स्यात्कृतमालकः ।

Drugs which expel the faeces and other wastes with or without proper digestion are sraṃsana (laxatives) ; for example kṛtamālaka (4–5).

मलादिकमबद्धं च बद्धं वा पिण्डितं मलैः ॥ ५ ॥
भित्त्वाधः पातयति तद्भेदनं कटुकी यथा ।

Drugs which break up the faecal mass and expel it out forcibly are known as bhedana (purgatives); for example kaṭukī (5–6).

विपक्वं यदपक्वं वा मलादि द्रवतां नयेत् ॥ ६ ॥
रेचयत्यपि तज्ज्ञेयं रेचनं त्रिवृता यथा ।

Drugs which make the faeces watery and expel out forcibly either formed or not formed into a mass are rechana (cathartics); for example trivṛtā. (6–7)

अपक्वपित्तश्लेष्माणौ बलादूर्ध्वं नयेत्तु यत् ॥ ७ ॥
वमनं तद्धि विज्ञेयं मदनस्य फलं यथा ।

Drugs which bring out the raw pitta and kapha from the stomach through the mouth by force are vamana (emetics); for example madanaphala (7–8).

स्थानाद्बहिर्नयेदूर्ध्वमधो वा मलसंचयम् ॥ ८ ॥
देहसंशोधनं तत्स्याद्देवदालीफलं यथा ।

Drugs which dislodge the body wastes from their places and expel them forcibly either in upward or downward direction are deha saṃshodhana (purifiers of the body); for example devadālī phala (8–9).

श्लिष्टान्कफादिकान्दोषानुन्मूलयति यद्बलात् ॥ ९ ॥
छेदनं तद्यथा क्षारा मरिचानि शिलाजतु ।

Drugs which scratch out the adherant kapha and other wastes from their places are chedana (scarificants); for example kshāras (alkalies), maricha and shilājatu (9–10).

धातून्मलान्वा देहस्य विशोष्योल्लेखयेच्च यत् ॥ १० ॥
लेखनं तद्यथा क्षौद्रं नीरमुष्णं वचा यवाः ।

Drugs which expel the dhātus (tissues) and malas (wastes) of the body after drying up their moisture are known as lekhana (mild dehydrants); for example, honey, hot water, vacha and yava (10–11).

दीपनं पाचनं यत्स्यादुष्णत्वाद्द्रवशोषकम् ॥ ११ ॥
ग्राहि तच्च यथा शुण्ठी जीरकं गजपिप्पली ।

Drugs which possess dīpanapāchana properties and also dry up the moisture of the tissues and wastes of the body are grāhī (water absorbants); for example shuṇṭhī, jīraka and gajapippalī (11–12).

रौक्ष्याच्छैत्यात्कषायत्वाल्लघुपाकाच्च यद्भवेत् ॥ १२ ॥
वातकृत्स्तम्भनं तत्स्याद्यथा वत्सकटुण्टुकौ ।

Drugs which increase vāta by their rūksha (dry), shīta (cold), kaṣāya (astringent) and laghupāka (undergoing quick digestion) properties are sthambhana (constipating); for example vatsaka and ṭuṇṭuka (12–13).

रसायनं च तज्ज्ञेयं यज्जराव्याधिनाशनम् ॥ १३ ॥
यथाऽमृता रुदन्ती च गुग्गुलुश्च हरीतकी ।

Drugs which ward off old age and diseases are rasāyanas (tonics, rejuvenators, elixirs); for example amṛtā, rudantī, guggulu, harītakī (13–14).

यस्माद्द्रव्याद्भवेत्स्त्रीषु हर्षो वाजीकरं च तत् ॥ १४ ॥
यथा नागबलाद्याः स्युर्बीजं च कपिकच्छुजम् ।

Drugs which increase sexual desire are vājīkara (aphrodisiacs); for example, nāgabalā and kapikacchu bīja (14–15).

यस्माच्छुक्रस्य वृद्धिः स्याच्छुक्रलं च दुच्यते ॥ १५ ॥
यथाऽश्वगन्धा मुसली शर्करा च शतावरी । दुग्धं माषाश्च भल्लातफलमज्जामलानि च ॥ १६ ॥
प्रवर्तकानि कथ्यन्ते जनकानि च रेतसः । प्रवर्तनी स्त्री शुक्रस्य रेचनं बृहतीफलम् ॥ १७ ॥
जातीफलं स्तम्भकं च शोषणी च हरीतकी ।

Drugs which increase the quantity of śukra (semen) are śukrala (semenogogues); for example, aśwagandhā, musalī, sharkarā and shatāvarī kṣīra, māṣa. Bhallātaka-phalamajjā and āmalakī not only increase semen but also help in ejaculating it out. Woman is the stimulator of the semen, fruits of bṛhatī expel it, jātīphala withholds it longer, while harītakī dries it up (15–18).

देहस्य सूक्ष्मछिद्रेषु विशेद्यत्सूक्ष्ममुच्यते ॥ १८ ॥
तद्यथा सैन्धवं क्षौद्रं निम्बतैलं रुबूद्भवम् ।

Drugs which enter into even the minutest pores of the body are called sūkṣma (subtle); for example, saindhava, kṣaudra, nimba taila and rubu taila (18–19).

पूर्वं व्याप्याखिलं कायं ततः पाकं च गच्छति ॥ १९ ॥
व्यवायि तद्यथा भङ्गा फेनं चाहिसमुद्भवम् ।

Drugs which act very quickly in the body first by spreading all over and undergoing change later are vyavāyī; for example, bhaṅga, ahiphena (19–20).

सन्धिबन्धांस्तु शिथिलान्यत्करोति विकाशि तत् ॥ २० ॥
विश्लेष्यौजश्च धातुभ्यो यथा क्रमुककोद्रवाः ।

Drugs which weaken the joints by dislodging the ojas from the tissues are vikāśī; for example, kramuka, kodrava (20–21).

बुद्धिं लुम्पति यद्द्रव्यं मदकारी तदुच्यते ॥ २१ ॥
तमोगुणप्रधानं च यथा मद्यं सुरादिकम् । व्यवायि च विकाशि स्यात्सूक्ष्मं छेदिमदावहम् ॥ २२ ॥
आग्नेयं जीवितहरं योगवाहि स्मृतं विषम् ।

Drugs possessing tamoguṇa predominantly and cause derangement of the mind are called madakārī (intoxicants); for example Surā and other alcoholic beverages.

Drugs which possess vyavāyī, vikāśī, sūkṣma, chedana, and madakārī properties are āgneya and yogavāhī in nature and bring about death; for example, viṣa (poison) (21–22).

निजवीर्येण यद्द्रव्यं स्रोतोभ्यो दोषसंचयम् ॥ २३ ॥
निरस्यति प्रमाथि स्यात्तद्यथा मरिचं वचा । पैच्छिल्याद्गौरवाद्द्रव्यं रुद्ध्वा रसवहाःशिराः ॥ २४ ॥
धत्ते यद्गौरवं तत्स्यादभिष्यन्दि यथा दधि ॥ २५ ॥

Drugs which remove the accumulated doṣas from the cell pores by their own specific action are pramāthi; for example, maricha, vacha.

Drugs which by their picchila (unctous), guru (heavy) properties block the passages of rasavaha srotas (tissue pores) thereby causing heavyness of the body or organ are abhiṣyandi (obstructants); for example, dadhi (curds) (23–25).

इति श्रीदामोदरसूनुना शार्ङ्गधरेण विरचितायां शार्ङ्गधरसंहितायां सूत्रस्थाने
दीपनपाचनाऽध्यायश्चतुर्थः ।

Thus ends the fourth chapter.

पञ्चमोऽध्यायः

CHAPTER 5

Kalādikākhyāna—Shārīram (Anatomy and Physiology)

अथ कलादिकाख्यानाध्यायः

(धात्वाशयान्तरस्थस्तु यः क्लेदस्त्वधितिष्ठति । देहोष्मणा विपक्वो यः सा कलेत्यभिधीयते ॥ १ ॥)
कलाः सप्ताशयाः सप्त धातवः सप्त तन्मलाः । सप्तोपधातवः सप्त त्वचः सप्त प्रकीर्तिताः ॥ १ ॥
त्रयो दोषा नवशतं स्नायूनां संधयस्तथा । दशाऽधिकं च द्विशतमस्थ्नां च त्रिशतं तथा ॥ २ ॥
सप्तोत्तरं मर्मशतं सिराः सप्तशतं तथा । चतुर्विंशतिराख्याता धमन्यो रसवाहिकाः ॥ ३ ॥
मांसपेश्यः समाख्याता नृणां पञ्चशतं बुधैः । स्त्रीणां च विंशत्यधिकाः कण्डराश्चैव षोडश ॥ ४ ॥
नृदेहे दश रन्ध्राणि नारीदेहे त्रयोदश । एतत्समासतः प्रोक्तं विस्तरेणाधुनोच्यते ॥ ५ ॥

The components of the human body, in short, are : kalās, āshayas, dhātus, dhātumalas, upadhātus, and twak each seven; three doṣas, nine hundred snāyus, two hundred and ten sandhis, three hundred asthis, hundred and seven marmas, seven hundred śirās, twentyfour rasavaha dhamanīs, five hundred māṃsapeshīs in males and twenty more in females, sixteen kaṇḍarās, nine dwāras in males and thirteen in females; these will be elaborated further on (1–5).

मांसासृङ्मेदसां तिस्रो यकृत्प्लीह्नोश्चतुर्थिका । पञ्चमी च तथाऽन्त्राणां षष्ठी चाग्निधरा मता ॥ ६ ॥
रेतोधरा सप्तमी स्यादिति सप्त कलाः स्मृताः ।

The moisture present in the dhātus (tissues) undergoes transformation by the heat of the body and forms into structure known as kalās (lining membranes, sheaths, coverings and secreting membranes). The first three kalās are present in māṃsa (muscles), asṛk (blood) and medas (fat); the fourth is in yakṛt (liver) and plīhā (spleen), fifth is in the two antras (intestines), sixth is the agnidhara (deodenum) and the seventh retodhara (seminal tract). These are the seven kalās of the body (6–7).

श्लेष्माशयः स्यादुरसि तस्मादामाशयस्त्वधः ॥ ७ ॥
ऊर्ध्वमग्न्याशयो नाभेर्वामभागे व्यवस्थितः । तस्योपरि तिलं ज्ञेयं तदधः पवनाशयः ॥ ८ ॥
मलाशयस्त्वधस्तस्माद्वस्तिर्मूत्राशयस्त्वधः । जीवरक्ताशयमुरो ज्ञेयाः सप्ताशयास्त्वमी ॥ ९ ॥
पुरुषेभ्योऽधिकाश्चान्ये नारीणामाशयास्त्रयः । धरा गर्भाशयः प्रोक्तः स्तनौ स्तन्याशयौ मतौ ॥ १० ॥

Śleṣmāshaya (seat of kapha) is in the uras (chest), below it is in āmāshaya (stomach); above and to the left of the nābhi (umbilicus) is the agnyāshaya (liver) and below it is the tila (gall-bladder); below these is the pavanāshaya (seat of vāta), still below is malāshaya (seat of faeces), next below is the mūtrāshaya or basti (urinary bladder); jīva raktāshaya (heart) is in the uras (chest). These are the seven āshayas (organs) in men while women have three more, dharā or garbhāshaya (uterus) and two stanas or stanyāshayas (breasts) (8–10).

रसासृङ्मांसमेदोऽस्थिमज्जाशुक्राणि धातवः । जायन्तेऽन्योन्यतः सर्वे पाचिताः पित्ततेजसा ॥११ ॥
(रसाद्रक्तं ततो मांसं मांसान्मेदः प्रजायते । मेदसोऽस्थि ततो मज्जा मज्जायाः शुक्रसंभवः ॥ १२ ॥)

Rasa (chyle), asṛk (blood), māṃsa (muscle), medas (fat), asthi (bone), majjā (bone marrow) and shukra (semen) are the seven dhātus (basic tissues); each succeeding one gets formed from the preceding one, transformed by the heat or energy of pitta in the following manner; rakta gets formed from rasa, māṃsa from rakta, medas from māṃsa, asthi from medas, majjā from asthi, and shukra from majjā (11–12).

जिह्वानेत्रकपोलानां जलं पित्तं च रञ्जकम् । कर्णविड्रसनादन्तकक्षामेढ्रादिजं मलम् ॥ १३ ॥
नखनेत्रमलं वक्त्रे स्निग्धत्वं पिण्डिकास्तथा । जायन्ते सप्तधातूनां मलान्येतान्यनुक्रमात् ॥ १४ ॥
कफः पित्तं मलं खेषु प्रस्वेदो नखरोम च । नेत्रविट् त्वक्षु च स्नेहो धातूनां क्रमशो मलः ॥ १५ ॥

The moisture of the tongue, eyes, mouth, the rañjaka pitta, the excretions of the ears, eyes, tongue, teeth, axilla, genitals, nails; pimples, greasiness of the skin of the face etc. are the waste products of the dhātus (tissues) respectively. Kapha, pitta, khamalas (excretions from open orifices, tissue pores), sweda (sweat), nakha (nails), roma (hair), the lubricating material of the eyes, faeces and skin; these seven are the wastes of the seven dhātus respectively (13–15).

स्तन्यं रजश्च नारीणां काले भवति गच्छति । शुद्धमांसभवः स्नेहः सा वसा परिकीर्तिता ॥ १६ ॥
स्वेदोदन्तास्तथा केशास्तथैवोजश्च सप्तमम् । इति धातुभवा ज्ञेया एते सप्तोपधातवः ॥ १७ ॥

Stanya (breast milk) and rajas (menstrual fluid) appear and disappear according to age; vasā is the fatty material present in the māṃsadhātu (muscle); sweda (sweat), danta (teeth), kesha (hairs) and ojas—these seven are known as the upadhātus (secondary tissues) because they are produced by the dhātus (16–17).

ओजः सर्वशरीरस्थं शीतं स्निग्धं स्थिरं मतम् । सोमात्मकं शरीरस्य बलपुष्टिकरं मतम् ॥ १८ ॥

Ojas (essence of the tissues) possessing properties like sīta (cold), snigdha (greasyness) and sthira (stable) is present all over the body and confers it with bala (physical strength, power of resistance) and puṣṭi (nourishment), and is somātmaka (resembles moisture) (18).

ज्ञेयावभासिनी पूर्वं सिध्मस्थानं च सा मता । द्वितीया लोहिता ज्ञेया तिलकालकजन्मभूः ॥ १९ ॥
श्वेता तृतीया संख्याता स्थानं चर्मदलस्य च । ताम्रा चतुर्थी विज्ञेया किलासश्वित्रभूमिका ॥ २० ॥
पञ्चमी वेदनी ख्याता सर्वकुष्ठोद्भवस्ततः । विख्याता रोहिणी षष्ठी ग्रन्थिगण्डापचीस्थितिः ॥ २१ ॥
स्थूला त्वक्सप्तमी ख्याता विद्रध्यादेः स्थितिश्च सा । इति सप्तत्वचः प्रोक्ताः स्थूला व्रीहिद्विमात्रया ॥२२॥

Avabhāsinī is the name of the first layer of the skin and is the site of occurrence of sidhma (a kind of skin disease); the second layer is lohita, the site of occurrence of tilakas (moles); śweta is the third layer, the site of charmadala (a kind of skin disease); tāmra is the fourth layer, the site of kilāsa and shwitra (leucoderma); vedinī is the fifth, the site of all types of kuṣṭha (leprosy); rohiṇī is the sixth, the site of granthi, gaṇḍa and apachī (tumors and goitre); sthūla the seventh layer is the site of vidradhi (abscesses). The thickness of all these seven layers together equals to that of two vrīhis (paddy grains) (19-22).

वायुः पित्तं कफो दोषा धातवश्च मला मताः । तत्रापि पञ्चधा ख्याताः प्रत्येकं देहधारणात् ॥ २३ ॥
(शरीरदूषणाद्दोषा धातवो देहधारणात् । वातपित्तकफा ज्ञेया मलिनीकरणान्मलाः ॥ २४ ॥)

Vāyu, pitta and kapha are called doṣas (blemishes, vitiators), dhātus (supports, tissues) and malas (wastes) in different contexts : doṣas because they vitiate the body, dhātus because they support the body and malas because they contaminate it. Each is again of five divisions (23–24).

पित्तं पङ्गु कफः पङ्गुः पङ्गवो मलधातवः । वायुना यत्र नीयन्ते तत्र गच्छन्ति मेघवत् ॥ २५ ॥
पवनस्तेषु बलवान्विभागकरणान्मतः । रजोगुणमयः सूक्ष्मः शीतो रूक्षो लघुश्चलः ॥ २६ ॥
मलाशये चरेत्कोष्ठे वह्निस्थाने तथा हृदि । कण्ठे सर्वाङ्गदेशेषु वायुः पञ्चप्रकारतः ॥ २७ ॥
अपानः स्यात्समानश्च प्राणोदानौ तथैव च । व्यानश्चेति समीरस्य नामान्युक्तान्यनुक्रमात् ॥ २८ ॥

Pitta is lame (incapable of independent movement), kapha is lame, so also are the seven dhātus, all these are driven by vāyu from place to place like the clouds in the sky by the wind.

Of the three doṣas, vāyu is powerful in view of its activating others and putting them to work, is possessing rajo guṇa (activity), is sūkshma (subtle), shīta (cold), rūksha (dry), laghu (light in weight), chala (unsteady). It moves (functions) in the malāshaya (colon), agnisthāna (deodenum) and the koṣṭha (alimentary tract), hṛdaya (heart), kaṇṭha (throat) and sarvāṅga (the entire body). Apāna, samāna, prāṇa, udāna and vyāna are the names of the five divisions of samīraṇa (vāyu) respectively (25–28).

पित्तमुष्णं द्रवं पीतं नीलं सत्त्वगुणोत्तरम् । कटुतिक्तरसं ज्ञेयं विदग्धं चाम्लतां व्रजेत् ॥ २९ ॥
अग्न्याशये भवेत्पित्तमग्निरूपं तिलोन्मितम् । त्वचि कान्तिकरं ज्ञेयं लेपाभ्यङ्गादिपाचकम् ॥ ३० ॥
हृश्यं यकृति यत्पित्तं तद्रसं शोणितं नयेत् । यत्पित्तं नेत्रयुगुले रूपदर्शनकारि तत् ॥ ३१ ॥
यत्पित्तं हृदये तिष्ठेन्मेधाप्रज्ञाकरं च तत् । पाचकं भ्राजकं चैव रञ्जकालोचके तथा ॥ ३२ ॥
साधकं चेति पञ्चैव पित्तनामान्यनुक्रमात् ।

Pitta is uṣṇa (heat producing), drava (fluid), pīta (yellow), nīla (blue), kaṭu (pungent) and tikta (bitter) in taste but assumes amlatā (sourness) during vidagdha (transformation in the alimentary tract) and possesses satwa guṇa predominately. The pitta present in the agnyāshaya (also known as tila) is agnirūpa (fire like in action); the pitta present in the twak (skin) bestows lustre and absorbs the materials applied in the form of lepa (paste, ointments) and abhyaṅga (oil massage). The pitta present in the yakṛt (liver) is responsible for converting rasa (chyle) into rakta (blood); that present in the eyes makes vision possible, that present in the hṛdaya (heart, brain) is responsible for medhā (intelligence) and prajñā (consciousness); pāchaka, bhrājaka, rañjaka, ālochaka and sādhaka are the names of these pittas respectively (29–32).

कफः स्निग्धो गुरुः श्वेतः पिच्छिलः शीतलस्तथा ॥ ३३ ॥
तमोगुणाधिकः स्वादुर्विदग्धो लवणो भवेत् । कफश्चामाशये मूर्ध्नि कण्ठे हृदि च संधिषु ॥ ३४ ॥
तिष्ठन्करोति देहेषु स्थैर्यं सर्वाङ्गपाटवम् । क्लेदनः स्नेहनश्चैव रसनश्चावलम्बनः ॥ ३५ ॥
श्लेष्मकश्चेति नामानि कफस्योक्ताऽनुक्रमात् ।

Kapha is snigdha (unctuous), guru (heavy), śweta (white), picchila (slimy), shīta (cold), swādu (sweet) but lavaṇa (salty) during vidagdha (transformation) and possesses tamoguṇa predominantly. Kapha is located in the āmāshaya (stomach), mūrdhā (head), kaṇṭha (throat), hṛdaya (heart), sandhis (joints). It confers stability and strength to the body. Kledana, snehana, rasana, avalambana and śleṣmaka are the names of the five divisions of kapha respectively (33–35).

स्नायवो बन्धनं प्रोक्ता देहे मांसास्थिमेदसाम् ॥ ३६ ॥
सन्धयश्चाङ्गसन्धानाद्देहे प्रोक्ताः कफान्विताः । आधारश्च तथासाराः कायेऽस्थीनि बुधा विदुः ॥ ३७ ॥

Snāyus (tendons) are so called because they bind the māmsa (muscles), asthis (bones) and medas (fat). Sandhis (joints) are the junctions of bones and are the seat of kapha, they help to keep the body parts together. Asthis (bones) are the supports of the body, so say the wise (36-37).

मर्माणि जीवाधाराणि प्रायेण मुनयो जगुः ।
संधिबन्धनकारिण्यो दोषधातुवहाः सिराः ॥ ३८ ॥
धमन्यो रसवाहिन्यो धमन्ति पवनं तनौ । मांसपेश्यो बलाय स्युरवष्टम्भाय देहिनाम् ॥ ३९ ॥
प्रसारणाकुञ्चनयोरङ्गानां कण्डरा मताः ।

Marmas (vital spots) are places in which life resides, so say the sages. Śirās (veins) bind the parts together and transport the doṣas and dhātus. Dhamanīs (arteries) carry rasadhātu all over the body and fill it with air. Māṃsapeshīs (muscles) confer strength and working capacity to the body. Kaṇḍarās (big tendons) help in expansion and contraction of the various parts (38–39).

नासानयनकर्णानां द्वे द्वे रन्ध्रे प्रकीर्तिते ॥ ४० ॥
मेहनापानवक्त्राणामेकैकं रन्ध्रमुच्यते । दशमं मस्तके प्रोक्तं रन्ध्राणीति नृणां विदुः ॥ ४१ ॥
स्त्रीणां त्रीण्यधिकानि स्युः स्तनयोर्गर्भवर्त्मनः । सूक्ष्मच्छिद्राणि चान्यानि मतानि त्वचि जन्मिनाम् ॥४२॥

The body has ten large orifices viz., one in each of the eyes, nose and ears; one in the urethra, one of the rectum, one of the mouth and the tenth is in the head. Women have three more; one each in the two breasts and the third in the uterus. There are innumerable minute pores in the skin (40–42).

तद्वामे फुप्फुसप्लीहौ दक्षिणाङ्गे यकृन्मतम् । उदानवायोराधारः फुप्फुसः प्रोच्यते बुधैः ॥ ४३ ॥
रक्तवाहिशिरामूलं प्लीहा ख्याता महर्षिभिः । यकृद्रञ्जकपित्तस्य स्थानं रक्तस्य संश्रयः ॥ ४४ ॥
जलवाहिशिरामूलं तृष्णाच्छादनकं तिलम् । वृक्कौ पुष्टिकरौ प्रोक्तौ जठरस्थस्य मेदसः ॥ ४५ ॥
वीर्यवाहिशिराधारौ वृषणौ पौरुषावहौ । गर्भाधानकरं लिङ्गमयनं वीर्यमूत्रयोः ॥ ४६ ॥

On the left are placed the puppusa (lung) and the plīhā (spleen), while on the right is the yakṛt (liver). The learned say that puppusa is the seat of udāna vāyu, plīhā is the source of raktavāhī śirās (veins), yakṛt is the seat of rañjaka pitta and also the store house of rakta (blood). Tila (pancreas) is the seat of jalavāhī śirās (channels of water) and so satiates thirst. The two vṛkkas (kidneys) nourish the medas (fat) of the abdomen. The two vṛṣaṇas (testes) are the source of vīryavāhī śirās (seminal channels) and responsible for manliness. Liṅga (penis) is the organ of reproduction and also the passage for both semen and urine (43–46).

हृदयं चेतनास्थानमोजसश्चाश्रयो मतम् ।
शिरा धमन्यो नाभिस्थाः सर्वा व्याप्य स्थितास्तनुम् । पुष्णन्ति चानिशं वायोः संयोगात्सर्वधातुभिः ४७
नाभिस्थः प्राणपवनः स्पृष्ट्वा हृत्कमलान्तरम् ॥ ४८ ॥
कण्ठाद्बहिर्विनिर्याति पातुं विष्णुपदामृतम् । पीत्वा चाम्बरपीयूषं पुनरायातिवेगतः ॥ ४९ ॥
प्रीणयन्देहमखिलं जीवयञ्जठरानलम् । शरीरप्राणयोरेव संयोगादायुरुच्यते ॥ ५० ॥
कालेन तद्वियोगाच्च पञ्चत्वं कथ्यते बुधैः ।
न जन्तुः कश्चिदमरः पृथिव्यां जायते क्वचित् । अतोमृत्युरवार्यः स्यात् किंतु रोगान्निवारयेत् ॥ ५१ ॥

Hṛdaya (heart) is the seat of chetana (life, soul) and also of ojas (essence of the dhātus). Śirās and dhamanīs (veins and arteries) arise from the nābhi (umbilicus) spread throughout the body and supply air to the dhātus (tissues) constantly. The prāṇa vāyu located near the nābhi (umbilicus) moves upward to the hṛdaya (heart) and comes out of the throat to drink the Viṣṇupadāmṛta (nectar of the atmosphere viz., oxygen) and having partaken it moves quickly inside to enliven the entire body and kindle the gastric fire (digestive power). Because of this combination of vāyu (air) and sharīra (body), āyu (life) is existing. When they get separated in course of time, pañchatwa (death) supervenes. No animal is immortal in this world; death is unavoidable whereas diseases can be avoided (47–51).

याप्यत्वं याति साध्यस्तु याप्यो गच्छत्यसाध्यताम् । जीवितं हन्त्यसाध्यस्तु नरस्याऽप्रतिकारिणः ।५२।
धर्मार्थकाममोक्षणां शरीरं साधनं यतः । अतो रुग्भ्यस्तनुं रक्षेन्नरः कर्मविपाकवित् ॥ ५३ ॥
धातवस्तन्मला दोषा नाशयन्त्यसमास्तनुम् । समाः सुखाय विज्ञेया बलायोपचयाय च ॥ ५४ ॥

If not treated in proper time sādhya (easily curable) diseases become yāpya (chronic), yāpya one becomes asādhya (incurable) and asādhya (incurable) ones destroy life. The body is the instrument for the attainment of Dharma, Artha, Kāma and Mokṣa; so it has to be protected from diseases and the evil effects of the actions of past lives. Dhātus (tissues), their malas (wastes) and doṣas destroy the body when they become abnormal but protect it with health, strength and growth when they are normal (52–54).

अथ सृष्टिक्रमः

जगद्योनेरनिच्छस्य चिदानन्दैकरूपिणः । पुंसोऽस्ति प्रकृतिर्नित्या प्रतिच्छायेव भास्वतः ॥ ५५ ॥
अचेतनादि चैतन्ययोगेन परमात्मनः । अकरोद्विश्वमखिलमनित्यं नाटकाकृति ॥ ५६ ॥
प्रकृतिर्विश्वजननी पूर्वं बुद्धिमजीजनत् ॥ ५७ ॥
इच्छामयीं महद्रूपामहङ्कारस्ततोऽभवत् । त्रिविधः सोऽपि संजातो रजःसत्त्वतमोगुणैः ॥ ५८ ॥
तस्मात्सत्त्वरजोयुक्तादिन्द्रियाणि दशाभवन् । मनश्च जातं तान्याहुः श्रोत्रत्वङ्नयनं तथा ॥ ५९ ॥
जिह्वाघ्राणवचोहस्तपादोपस्थगुदानि च । पञ्च बुद्धीन्द्रियाण्याहुः प्राक्तनानीतराणि च ॥ ६० ॥
कर्मेन्द्रियाणि पञ्चैव कथ्यन्ते सूक्ष्मबुद्धिभिः ।

The one, uninterested Puruṣa (primordial male principle) is the cause of this Universe, possesses Chit (intellect) and Ānanda (joy), is constantly accompanied by the Prakṛti (primordial female principle) like the shadow which accompanies the substance. Though Prakṛti is inactive, with the association of the active Paramātmā (Puruṣa) it has created this entire illusory and transitory Universe like a drama.

Prakṛti, the Universal Mother, desirous of creation, first gave birth to buddhi (intellect), which possessed a slightly larger form, hence called as mahat (big). Buddhi in its turn gave birth to the Ahaṅkāra (ego) which is of three kinds, possessing the three guṇas (qualities), the satwa, the rajas, and the tamas. The ten indriyas (five sense organs and five motor organs) are created later by the Ahaṅkāra possessed with the predominance of satwa and rajo guṇas; so also the manas (mind). Shrotra (ears), twak (skin), nayana (eye), jihwā (tongue), ghrāṇa (nose); vāk (organs of speech), hasta (hands), pāda (feet), upāstha (generative organ) and guda (rectum) are the ten indriyas. The first five are jñānendriyas (sensory organs) and the second five the karmendriyas (organs of work, motor organs) (55–60).

रजःसत्त्वगुणोत्कृष्टादहङ्कारादथाभवत् ॥ ६१ ॥
तन्मात्रपञ्चकं तस्य नामान्युक्तानि सूरिभिः । शब्दतन्मात्रकं स्पर्शतन्मात्रं रूपमात्रकम् ॥ ६२ ॥
रसतन्मात्रकं गन्धतन्मात्रं चेति तद्विदुः । तन्मात्रपञ्चकात्तस्मात्संजातं भूतपञ्चकम् ॥ ६३ ॥
व्योमानिलानलजलक्षोणीरूपं च तन्मतम् । शब्दः स्पर्शश्च रुपं च रसगन्धावनुक्रमात् ॥ ६४ ॥
तन्मात्राणां विशेषाः स्युः स्थूलभावमुपागताः । बुद्धीन्द्रियाणां पञ्चैव शब्दाद्या विषया मताः ॥ ६५ ॥
कर्मेन्द्रियाणां विषया भाषादानविहारिताः । आनन्दोत्सर्गकौ चैव कथितास्तत्त्वदर्शिभिः ॥ ६६ ॥

From the Ahaṅkāra, with the predominance of satwa and tamo guṇas and influence of rajo guṇa, were born the five tanmātrās (subtle elements); the shabda tanmātrā (unit of sound), the sparsha tanmātrā (unit of touch), the rūpa tanmātrā (unit of sight), the rasa tanmātrā (unit of taste) and the gandha tanmātrā (unit of smell). From these tanmātrās were born the five bhūtas (gross elements), the vyoma (space, sky), anila (air), anala (fire), jala (water) and kshoṇī (earth) which are the gross forms of the tanmātrās. Shabda (sound), sparsha (touch), rūpa (sight), rasa (taste) and gandha (smell) are the special properties of these bhūtas respectively; these are the arthas (objects) of the five sense organs in respective order. Bhāṣaṇa (speech), ādāna (holding, receiving), vihāra (locomotion), ānanda (enjoyment) and utsarga (elimination) are the functions of the karmendriyas (motor organs) respectively (61–66).

प्रधानं प्रकृतिः शक्तिर्नित्या चाविकृतिस्तथा । एतानि तस्या नामानि शिवमाश्रित्य या स्थिता ॥ ६७ ॥
महानहङ्कृतिः पञ्चतन्मात्राणि पृथक्पृथक् । प्रकृतिर्विकृतिश्चैव सप्तैतानि बुधा जगुः ॥ ६८ ॥
दशेन्द्रियाणि चित्तं च महाभूतानि पञ्च च । विकाराः षोडश ज्ञेयाः सर्वं व्याप्य जगत्स्थिताः ॥ ६९ ॥

Pradhāna, prakṛti, shakti, nitya, avikṛti are the other names of Prakṛti (female principle) which in turn stand supported by Shiva (male principle). Mahat (buddhi), Ahaṅkāra and the five tanmātrās—these seven are called, by the learned, as prakṛti-vikṛti. The ten indriyas, chitta (mind) and the five mahābhūtas—these sixteen are called as vikāras. These 24 tatwas make up for all the things of this universe (67–69).

एवं चतुर्विंशतिभिस्तत्त्वैः सिद्धे वपुर्गृहे । जीवात्मा नियतो नित्यो वसति स्वान्तदूतवान् ॥ ७० ॥
स देही कथ्यते पापपुण्यदुःखसुखादिभिः । व्याप्तो बद्धश्च मनसा कृत्रिमैः कर्मबन्धनैः ॥ ७१ ॥
कामक्रोधौ लोभमोहावहङ्कारश्च पञ्चमः । दशेन्द्रियाणि बुद्धिश्च तस्य बन्धाय देहिनः ॥ ७२ ॥
आप्नोति बन्धमज्ञानादात्मज्ञानाच्च मुच्यते । तद्दुःखयोगकृद्व्याधिरारोग्यं तत्सुखावहम् ॥ ७३ ॥

In this body composed of the above twentyfour principles resides the jīvātmā (soul, spirit) for a specific period as an emissary. He, now called dehī, becomes involved by pāpa (sin), puṇya (benevolence), sukha (happiness) and dukha (misery) and so gets entangled with the transitory bonds of human activity. Kāma (desire), krodha (anger), lobha (greed), moha (delusion), ahaṅkāra (egoism) along with ten indriyas and buddhi act as bandha (bonds) for him (jīvātmā), making him ignorant of his own self; he gets moksha (liberation, bliss) when he understands himself (as different from the body) (70–72).

Vyādhi (disease) is the cause for dukha (sorrow) while ārogya (health) brings about sukha (happiness) (73).

इति श्रीदामोदरसूनुना शार्ङ्गधरेण विरचितायां शार्ङ्गधरसंहितायां
कलादिकाख्यानाध्यायः ॥ ५ ॥

Thus ends the fifth chapter.

———

षष्ठोऽध्यायः

CHAPTER 6

Āhārādigati Kathanam (Digestion and Metabolism)

अथाहारादिगतिरध्यायः

यात्यामाशयमाहारः पूर्वं प्राणानिलेरितः । माधुर्यं फेनभावं च षड्सोऽपि लभेत सः ॥ १ ॥
अथ पाचकपित्तेन विग्धश्चाम्लतां व्रजेत् । ततः समानमरुता ग्रहणीमभिनीयते ॥ २ ॥
(षष्ठी पित्तधरा नाम या कला परिकीर्तिता । पक्वामाशयमध्यस्था ग्रहणीत्यभिधीयते ॥ ३ ॥)
ग्रहण्यां पच्यते कोष्ठवह्निना जायते कटुः । रसो भवति संपकादपक्वादामसंभवः ॥ ४ ॥
वह्नेर्बलेन माधुर्यं स्निग्धतां याति तद्रसः । पुष्णाति धातूनखिलान्सम्यक्पक्वोऽमृतोपमः ॥ ५ ॥
मन्दवह्निविदग्धश्च कटुश्चाम्लो भवेद्रसः । विषभावं व्रजेद्वापि कुर्याद्वा रोगसंकरम् ॥ ६ ॥

The food taken into the mouth is forced down by prāṇavāyu and reaches the āmāshaya (stomach). There it attains a frothy state and becomes predominantly madhura (sweet) though possessing all the six tastes in the beginning. Next it gets mixed with pāchaka pitta (digestive juices), gets transformed into amlabhāva (sourness) reaching the grahaṇī (deodenum) forced by samāna vāyu. In the grahaṇī the food gets further digested by the koṣṭhāgni (digestive fire), assumes kaṭubhāva (pungent state). After proper digestion rasa (essence) gets formed but with improper cooking (digestion), āma (undigested residue) gets formed. Rasa (essence, chyle, plasma) acquiring sweetness and unctuousness by the action of koṣṭhāgni (digestive fire) nourishes all the other dhātus (tissues) acting like nectar. If by poor digestive activity and bad transformation the rasa assumes either a kaṭu (pungent) or amla (sour) property, it acts like poison and gives rise to many diseases (1–6).

आहारस्य रसः सारः सारहीनो मलद्रवः । शिराभिस्तज्जलं नीतं बस्तौ मूत्रत्वमाप्नुयात् ॥ ७ ॥
तत्किट्टं च मलं ज्ञेयं तिष्ठेत्पक्वाशये च तत् । वलित्रितयमार्गेण यात्यपानेन नोदितम् ॥ ८ ॥
प्रवाहिणी सर्जनी च ग्राहिकेति वलित्रयम् ।

Rasa (essence, plasma) is the nutrient portion of the food, while its non-nutrient portion is called kiṭṭa (waste), the liquid waste is brought to the basti (urinary bladder) by the śirās and it assumes the name mūtra (urine); the solid waste (faeces) accumulates in the pakwāshaya (large intestine) and moves out of the body through the three folds of the rectum—the pravāhiṇī, sarjanī and grāhikā—by the action of apāna vāyu (7–8).

रसस्तु हृदयं याति समानमरुतेरितः ॥ ९ ॥
रञ्जितः पाचितस्तत्र पित्तेनायाति रक्तताम् । रक्तं सर्वशरीरस्थं जीवस्याधारमुत्तमम् ॥ १० ॥
स्निग्धं गुरु चलं स्वादु विदग्धं पित्तवद्भवेत् । पाचिता पित्ततापेन रसाद्या धातवः क्रमात् ॥ ११ ॥
शुक्रत्वं यान्ति मासेन तथा स्त्रीणां रजो भवेत् ।

Rasa reaches the hṛdaya (heart) with the help of samāna vāyu, gets transformed and coloured by pitta and becomes rakta (blood). Rakta, found all over the body, is the chief sustainer of life, possessing snigdha (unctuous), guru (heavy), chala (movement) and swādu (sweet) properties. But if it becomes vidagdha (improperly processed) it assumes the qualities of pitta. Rasa and other dhātus get transformed into shukra (semen) in about a month's time by the action of pitta; so also rajas (ovum) in women (9–11).

कामान्मिथुनसंयोगे शुद्धशोणितशुक्रजः ॥ १२ ॥
गर्भः संजायते नार्याः स जातो बाल उच्यते । आधिक्ये रजसः कन्या पुत्रः शुक्राधिके भवेत् ॥ १३ ॥
नपुंसकं समत्वेन यथेच्छा पारमेश्वरी ।

During sexual intercourse the shukra (male seed) and shoṇita (female seed) unite to form the embryo inside the (uterus of) woman to be born as a baby. During this union, predominance of shoṇita (female seed) produces a female child, that of shukra (male seed) causes a male child, while a eunuch will be born when both are equal as decided by Providence (12–13).

बालस्य प्रथमे मासि देया भेषजरक्तिका ॥ १४ ॥
अवलेहीकृतैकैव क्षीरक्षौद्रसिताघृतैः । वर्धयेत्तावदेकैकां यावद्भवति वत्सरः ॥ १५ ॥
माषैर्वृद्धिस्तदूर्ध्वं स्याद्यावत्षोडशवत्सरः । ततः स्थिरा भवेत्तावद्यावद्वर्षाणि सप्ततिः ॥ १६ ॥
ततो बालकवन्मात्रा ह्रासनीया शनैः शनैः । मात्रेयं कल्कचूर्णानां कषायाणां चतुर्गुणा ॥ १७ ॥

During the first month of life of the baby the dose of medicine to be administered should be one raktikā (guñjā seed) given with either milk, honey, sugar or ghee. With each succeeding month the dose should be increased by one rakti, till the first year when the dose will be one māṣā. Further increase will be one māṣā for each successive year till the age of sixteen years. From sixteen to seventy, the dose should be the same but after seventy it has to be gradually reduced as was the case with children. This dosage is for kalka (bolus) and chūrṇa (powders) while for kaṣāyas (decoctions) it is four times of this (14–17).

अञ्जनं च तथा लेपः स्नानमभ्यङ्गकर्म च । वमनं प्रतिमर्शश्च जन्मप्रभृति शस्यते ॥ १८ ॥
कवलः पञ्चमाद्वर्षादष्टमान्नस्यकर्म च । विरेकः षोडशाद्वर्षाद्विंशतेश्चैव मैथुनम् ॥ १९ ॥

Añjana (eye salve), lepa (external applications), snāna (bath), abhyaṅgas (oil bath), vamana (emesis) and pratimarsha nasya (nasal drops) can be prescribed even from the first day after birth. Kavala (mouth gargles) is indicated after five years of age, nasya (nasal medication) after eight, virechana (purgatives) after sixteen and sexual intercourse after twenty (18–19).

बाल्यं वृद्धिश्छविर्मेधा त्वग्दृष्टिः शुक्रविक्रमौ । बुद्धिः कर्मेन्द्रियं चेतो जीवितं दशतो ह्रसेत् ॥ २० ॥

Bālya (childhood), vṛddhi (growth), chhavi (colour and complexion), medhā (intelligence), twak (skin health), dṛṣṭi (vision), shukra (semen), vikrama (valour), buddhi (intelligence), karmendriyas (physical capacity), chetana (spirituality) and jīvita (life)—these get lost or (diminished) in successive decades (ten year period) of life (20).

अल्पकेशः कृशो रूक्षो वाचालश्चलमानसः । आकाशचारी स्वप्नेषु वातप्रकृतिको नरः ॥ २१ ॥
अकालपलितैर्व्याप्तो धीमान्स्वेदी च रोषणः । स्वप्नेषु ज्योतिषां द्रष्टा पित्तप्रकृतिको नरः ॥ २२ ॥
गम्भीरबुद्धिः स्थूलाङ्गः स्निग्धकेशो महाबलः । स्वप्ने जलाशयालोकी श्लेष्मप्रकृतिको नरः ॥ २३ ॥
ज्ञातव्या मिश्रचिह्नैश्च द्वित्रिदोषोल्बणा नराः ।

Persons who have scanty hairs, dry and thin body, who are very talkative, of unsteady mind, dream as moving in air are of vāta-prakṛti (nervous constitution). Persons who have premature grey hairs, who are very intelligent, very angry, sweat profusely, and see fire in dreams are pitta-prakṛti (bilious constitution). Persons who are steady in mind, hefty physique, smooth haired, very strong, see reservoirs of water in dreams are kapha-prakṛti (phlegmatic constitution). Persons possessing the features of two doṣas are called dwidoṣaja prakṛti (double constitution) while with the features of all the three doṣas are tridoṣaja (triple constitution) (21–23).

तमः कफाभ्यां निद्रा स्यान्मूर्च्छा पित्ततमोभवा ॥ २४ ॥
रजः पित्तानिलैर्भ्रान्तिस्तन्द्रा श्लेष्मतमोनिलैः । ग्लानिरोजःक्षयाद्दुःखादजीर्णाच्च श्रमाद्भवेत् ॥ २५ ॥

Nidrā (sleep) is the effect of tamas and kapha; mūrcchā (faint) is due to pitta and tamas, bhrānti (giddiness) is from rajas and pitta, tandrā (drowsiness) results from kapha, tamas and vāta; glāni (tiredness) is due to ojaskṣaya, dukha (grief), ajīrṇa (indigestion) and shrama (exertion) (24–25).

यः सामर्थ्येऽप्यनुत्साहस्तदालस्यमुदीर्यते ।
चैतन्यशिथिलत्वाद्यः पीत्वैकं श्वासमुद्वमेत् ॥ २६ ॥

विदीर्णवदनः श्वासं जृम्भा सा कथ्यते बुधैः । उदानप्राणयोरूर्ध्वंयोगान्मैलिकफस्रवात् ॥ २७ ॥
शब्दः संजायते नस्तः क्षुतं तत्कथ्यते बुधैः । उदानकोपादाहारस्वस्थितत्वाच्च यद्भवेत् ॥ २८ ॥
पवनस्योर्ध्वगमनं तमुद्गारं प्रचक्षते ।

Ālasya (lassitude) is disinterestedness in work though capable of doing it, jṛmbha (yawning) is expelling of air through the mouth widely opened due to weakness or tiredness of the mind; kshut (sneezing) is the sound produced in the nose by the upward movement of prāṇa and udāna vāyus and kapha in the head; udgāra (belching) is the movement of air upward from the stomach due either to increase of udāna vāyu or filling of the stomach with food (26–28).

इति श्रीदामोदरसूनुना शार्ङ्गधरेण विरचितायां शार्ङ्गधरसंहितायां
शारीरे आहारादिगतिरध्यायः ॥ ६ ॥

Thus ends the sixth chapter.

सप्तमोऽध्यायः

CHAPTER 7

Rogagaṇanā (Enumeration of Diseases)

अथ रोगगणनाध्यायः

रोगाणां गणना पूर्वं मुनिभिर्या प्रकीर्तिता । मयात्र प्रोच्यते सैव तद्भेदा बहवो मताः ॥ १ ॥

I am going to describe herein the counting of diseases as has been enumerated by the ancient sages. The diseases are of many kinds[1] (1).

पञ्चविंशतिरुद्दिष्टा ज्वरास्तद्भेद उच्यते । पृथग्दोषैस्तथा द्वन्द्वभेदेन त्रिविधः स्मृतः ॥ २ ॥
एकश्च सन्निपातेन तद्भेदा बहवो मताः । प्रायशः सन्निपातेन पञ्च स्युर्विषमज्वराः ॥ ३ ॥
सन्ततः सततश्चैव अन्येद्युष्कस्तृतीयकः । चातुर्थकश्च पञ्चैते कीर्तिता विषमज्वराः ॥ ४ ॥
तथागन्तुज्वरोऽप्येकस्त्रयोदशविधो मतः । अभिचारग्रहावेशशापैरागन्तुकस्त्रिधा ॥ ५ ॥
श्रमाच्छेदात्क्षतादाहाच्चतुर्धा घातजो ज्वरः । कामाद्भीतेः शुचो रोषाद्विषादौषधगन्धत ॥ ६ ॥
अभिषङ्गज्वराः षट् स्युरेवं ज्वरविनिश्चयः ।

Jwaras (fevers) are twenty five in number, such as, one from each of the tridoṣas, one each by the combination of two doṣas—dwandwaja, one from the combination of all the three doṣas together sannipātaja with its many subdivisions; viṣama jwaras ase usually five—santata, satata, anyedyuṣka, tṛtīyaka and chaturthaka; similarly is the āgantu jwara with thirteen kinds caused by abhichāra (witchcraft), grahavesha (evil spirits), shāpa (curse), shrama (exertion),

---

1. For modern equivalents of disease-names refer Appendix II.

cheda (injury by sharp weapons), kshata (injury by blunt weapons), dāha (burns), kāma (lust), bhaya (fear), ashucha (uncleanliness), chintā (worry), roṣa (anger), viṣa (poison), and oṣadhigandhaja (contact with pollen, strong smell etc.) (2–6).

पृथक्त्रिदोषैः सर्वैश्च शोकादामाद्भयादपि ॥ ७ ॥
अतीसारः सप्तधा स्याद्ग्रहणी पञ्चधा मता । पृथग्दोषैः सन्निपातात्तथा चामेन पञ्चमी ॥ ८ ॥
प्रवाहिका चतुर्धा स्यात्पृथग्दोषैस्तथास्रतः ।

Atisāras (diarrhoeas) are seven–vātaja, pittaja, kaphaja, sannipātaja, shokaja, āmaja and bhayaja. Grahaṇī (sprue) are five—vātaja, pittaja, kaphaja, sannipātaja and āmaja. Pravāhikā (dysentery) are four—vātaja, pittaja kaphaja, and asṛja (raktaja) (7–8).

अजीर्णं त्रिविधं प्रोक्तं विष्टब्धं वायुना मतम् ॥ ९ ॥
पित्ताद्विदग्धं विज्ञेयं कफेनामं तदुच्यते । विषाजीर्णं रसादेकं दोषैः स्यादलसस्त्रिधा ॥ १० ॥
विसूची त्रिविधा प्रोक्ता दोषैः सा स्यात्पृथक्पृथक् । दण्डकालसकश्चैक एकैव स्याद्विलम्बिका ॥ ११ ॥

Ajīrṇas (indigestion) are three—viṣṭabdha from vāta, vidagdha from pitta and āmaja from kapha, one from rasa known as viṣajīrṇa. Alasa is one from all the three doṣas; visūchī is three—vātaja, pittaja and kaphaja; daṇḍakālasaka and vilambikā are one each (9–11).

अर्शांसि षड्विधान्याहुर्वातपित्तकफास्रतः । सन्निपाताच्च संसर्गात्तेषां भेदो द्विधा मतः ॥ १२ ॥
सहजोत्तरजन्मभ्यां तथा शुष्कार्द्रभेदतः । त्रिधैव चर्मकीलानि वातात्पित्तात्कफादपि ॥ १३ ॥

Arshas (haemorrhoids) are six—vātaja, pittaja, kaphaja, raktaja, sannipātaja and saṃsargaja; further they are of two kinds—sahaja (congenital) and janmottara kālaja (acquired); shuṣka (dry) and ārdra (bleeding); charmakīlas (warts) are three—one from each doṣa (12–13).

एवं विंशतिभेदेन कृमयः स्युर्द्विधा च ते । बाह्यास्तथाभ्यन्तराः स्युस्तेषु यूका बहिश्चराः ॥ १४ ॥
लिक्षाश्चान्येऽन्तरश्चराः कफात्ते हृदयोदकाः । अन्त्रादा उदरावेष्टाश्च्युरवश्च महागुहाः ॥ १५ ॥
सुगन्धा दर्भकुसुमास्तथा रक्ताश्च मातरः । सौरसा लोमविध्वंसा रोमद्वीपा उदुम्बराः ॥ १६ ॥
केशादाश्च तथैवान्ये शकृज्जाता मकेरुकाः । लेलिहाश्च सलूनाश्च सौसुरादाः ककेरुकाः ॥ १७ ॥
तथान्यः कफरक्ताभ्यां संजातः स्नायुकः स्मृतः । व्रणस्य कृमयश्चान्ये विषमा बाह्ययोनयः ॥ १८ ॥

Kṛmis (worms) are twenty in number, of the locations–external and internal; yūkā and likshā are the two external. Internal are—hṛdayodaka,[1] antrādā, udaraveṣṭā, churava, mahāguhā, sugandhā, darbhakusuma from kapha; mātara saurasa, lomavidhwaṃsā, romadwīpā, udumbarā and keshādā from rakta; make-

1. Other Ayurvedic texts name it as Hṛdayādā.

rukā, lelihā, salūnā, sausurādā and kakerukā from puriṣa (faeces). Many other from kapha and rakta viz., snāyuka. Many other types are found which are seen in ulcers and wounds (14–18).

पाण्डुरोगाश्च पञ्च स्युर्वातपित्तकफैस्त्रिधा । त्रिदोषैर्मृत्तिकाभिश्च तथैका कामला स्मृता ॥ १९ ॥
स्यात्कुम्भकामला चैका तथैकं च हलीमकम् ।

Pāṇḍuroga (anaemia) are five—vātaja, pittaja, kaphaja, sannipātaja, mṛttikaja; kāmalā (jaundice), kumbhakāmalā and halīmaka (jaundice, chlorosis) are each one (19).

रक्तपित्तं त्रिधा प्रोक्तमूर्ध्वगं कफसंभवम् ॥ २० ॥
अधोगं मारुतं ज्ञेयं तद्द्वयेन द्विमार्गगम् ।

Raktapitta (purpura) is three—ūrdhwaga from kapha, adhoga from vāta and dwimārga from both (20).

कासाः पञ्च समुद्दिष्टास्ते त्रयस्तु त्रिभिर्मलैः ॥ २१ ॥
उरःक्षताच्चतुर्थः स्यात्क्षयाद्धातोश्च पञ्चमः । क्षयाः पञ्चैव विज्ञेयास्त्रिभिर्दोषैस्त्रयश्च ते ॥ २२ ॥
चतुर्थः सन्निपातेन पञ्चमः स्यादुरः क्षतात् । शोषाः स्युः षट्प्रकारेण स्त्रीप्रसङ्गाच्छुचो व्रणात् ॥ २३ ॥
अध्वश्रमाच्च व्यायामाद्वार्धक्यादपि जायते । श्वासाश्च पञ्च विज्ञेयाः क्षुद्रः स्यात्तमकस्तथा ॥ २४ ॥
ऊर्ध्वश्वासो महाश्वासश्छिन्नश्वासश्च पञ्चमः । कथिताः पञ्च हिक्कास्तु तास्तु क्षुद्राऽन्नजा तथा ॥ २५ ॥
गम्भीरा यमला चैव महती पञ्चमी स्मृता ।

Kāsa (cough) is five—vātaja, pittaja, kaphaja, urakshataja, and dhātukshayaja; kshaya (consumption) is also five—vātaja, pittaja, kaphaja, sannipātaja and the fifth from urakshata; shoṣa (pthisis) is six—from sexual excess, too much of worry, chronic and bad ulcers, too much of walking, tiresome exercises and from old age. Śwāsa (dyspnoea) is also five—kshudra, tamaka, ūrdhwa, mahā and chinnā. Hikkā (hiccough) is five-kshudrā, annajā, gambhīrā, yamalā, and mahatī (21–25).

चत्वारोऽग्नेर्विकाराः स्युर्विषमो वातसंभवः ॥ २६ ॥
तीक्ष्णः पित्तात्कफान्मन्दो भस्मको वातपित्तयोः । पञ्चैवारोचका ज्ञेया वातपित्तकफैस्त्रिधा ॥ २७ ॥
सन्निपातान्मनस्तापात् छर्दयः सप्तधा मताः । त्रिभिर्दोषैः पृथक्त्रिस्त्रः कृमिभिः सन्निपाततः ॥ २८ ॥
घृणया च तथा स्त्रीणां गर्भाधानाच्च जायते ।

Agni vikāra (dyspepsia) is four—viṣamāgni from vāta, tīkshṇāgni from pitta and mandāgni from kapha; bhasmaka (unsatiable appetite) from vāta and pitta together. Arochaka (anorexia) is five—vātaja, pittaja, kaphaja, sannipātaja and mānasika. Chardi (vomiting) is seven—one from each doṣa, one from their combination, one from kṛmi, one from aversion, and one of pregnant women (26–28).

स्वरभेदाः षडेव स्युर्वातपित्तकफैस्त्रयः ॥ २९ ॥
मेदसा सन्निपातेन क्षयात्षष्ठः प्रकीर्तितः ।

Swarabheda (hoarseness) is six—vātaja, pittaja, kaphaja, sannipātaja, medaja, and kshayaja (29).

तृष्णा च षड्विधा प्रोक्ता वातात्पित्तात्कफादपि ॥ ३० ॥
त्रिदोषैरुपसर्गेण क्षयाद्धातोश्च षष्ठिका ।

Tṛṣṇā (thirst) is six—vātaja, pittaja, kaphaja, sannipātaja, upasargaja and dhātukshayaja (30).

मूर्च्छा चतुर्विधा ज्ञेया वातपित्तकफैः पृथक् ॥ ३१ ॥
चतुर्थी सन्निपातेन तथैकश्च भ्रमः स्मृतः । निद्रा तन्द्रा च संन्यासो ग्लानिश्चैकैकशः स्मृताः ॥ ३२ ॥

Mūrcchā (fainting) is four—vātaja, pittaja, kaphaja sannipātaja; bhrama (dizziness) is one kind only. So also is the case with nidrā (sleep), tandrā (drowsiness) and saṅnyāsa (unconsciousness) (31–32).

मदाः सप्त समाख्याता वातपित्तकफैस्त्रयः । त्रिदोषैरसृजा मद्याद्विषादपि च सप्तमः ॥ ३३ ॥
मदात्ययश्चतुर्धा स्याद्वातात्पित्तात्कफादपि । त्रिदोषैरपि विज्ञेय एकः परमदस्तथा ॥ ३४ ॥
पानाजीर्णं तथा चैकं तथैकः पानविभ्रमः । पानात्ययस्तथा चैको दाहाः सप्त मतास्तथा ॥ ३५ ॥
रक्तपित्तात्तथा रक्तात्तृष्णायाः पित्ततस्तथा । धातुक्षयान्मर्मघाताद्रक्तपूर्णोदरादपि ॥ ३६ ॥

Mada (intoxication) is seven—vātaja, pittaja, kaphaja, tridoṣaja, asṛja, madyaja and viṣaja. Madātyaya (alcoholism) is four—vātaja, pittaja, kaphaja, and sannipātaja; pramāda is one, so also are pānājīrṇa, pānavibhrama, and pānātyaya. Dāha (feeling of burning all over the body) is seven—one each from raktapitta, rakta, tṛṣṇā, pitta, dhātukshaya, marmaghāta and the last one from accumulation of blood in the abdomen (33--36).

उन्मादाः षट् समाख्यातास्त्रिभिर्दोषैस्त्रयश्च ते । सन्निपाताद्विषाज्ज्ञेयः षष्ठो दुःखेन चेतसः ॥ ३७ ॥
भूतोन्मादा विंशतिः स्युस्ते देवाद्दानवादपि । गन्धर्वात्किंनराद्यक्षात्पितृभ्यो गुरुशापतः ॥ ३८ ॥
प्रेताच्च गुह्यकाद्वृद्धात्सिद्धाद्भूतात्पिशाचतः । जलाधिदेवतायाश्च नागाद्वै ब्रह्मराक्षसात् ॥ ३९ ॥
राक्षसादपि कूष्माण्डाकृत्यावेतालयोरपि ।

Unmāda (insanity) is six—one from each doṣa, one from their combination, one from viṣa and the sixth from unhappiness of the mind. Bhūtonmāda (insanity due to possession by evil spirits) is twenty-one each from deva, dānava, gandharva, kinnara, yaksha, pitṛ; gurushāpa (curse of the teacher), preta, guhyaka, wrath of vṛddhas, siddhas, bhūtas, pishāchas, jala devatās, nāgas, brahmarākshasa, rākshasa, kūṣmāṇḍa, kṛtyonmāda (insanity due to sorcery and witch-craft) and vetāla (37–39).

अपस्मारश्चतुर्धा स्यात्समीरात्पित्ततस्तथा ॥ ४० ॥
श्लेष्मणोऽपि तृतीयः स्याच्चतुर्थः सन्निपाततः ।

Apasmāra (epilepsy) is four—vātaja, pittaja, kaphaja and fourth from sannipāta (40).

चत्वारश्चामवाताः स्युर्वातपित्तकफैस्त्रिधा ॥ ४१ ॥
चतुर्थः सन्निपातेन—

Āmavāta (rheumatism) is four—vātaja, pittaja, kaphaja and sannipātaja (41).

शूलान्यष्टौ बुधा जगुः ।
पृथग्दोषैस्त्रिधा द्वन्द्वभेदेनै त्रिविधान्यपि ॥ ४२ ॥
आमेन सप्तमं प्रोक्तं सन्निपातेन चाष्टमम् । परिणामभवं शूलमष्टधा परिकीर्तितम् ॥ ४३ ॥
मलैयैः शूलसंख्या स्यात्तैरेव परिणामजम् । अन्नद्रवभवं शूलं जरत्पित्तभवं तथा ॥ ४४ ॥
एकैकं गणितं सुज्ञैः—

Shūla (colic) is eight—one from each doṣa, one from the combination of any two of them, the seventh from āma, and the eighth from sannipāta. Pariṇāma shūla is also eight similar to that of shūla. Annadrava shūla and the shūla coming during or after digestion of food are also one each (42–44).

उदावर्तास्त्रयोदश ।
एकः क्षुन्निग्रहात्प्रोक्तस्तृष्णारोधाद्द्वितीयकः ॥ ४५ ॥
निद्राघातात्तृतीयः स्याच्चतुर्थः श्वासनिग्रहात् । छर्दिरोधात्पञ्चमः स्यात्षष्ठः क्षवथुनिग्रहात् ॥ ४६ ॥
जृम्भारोधात्सप्तमः स्यादुद्गारग्रहतोऽष्टमः । नवमः स्यादश्रुरोधाद्दशमः शुक्रधारणात् ॥ ४७ ॥
मूत्ररोधान्मलस्यापि रोधाद्वातविनिग्रहात् । उदावर्तास्त्रयश्चैते घोरोपद्रवकारकाः ॥ ४८ ॥

Udāvarta (upward oppression) is thirteen–one each from the suppression of kshut (hunger), tṛṣṇā (thirst), nidrā (sleep), śwāsa (respiration), chardi (vomiting), kshavathu (sneezing), jṛmbha (yawning), udgāra (belching), ashru (tears), shukra (semen), mūtra (urine), mala (faeces) and vāta (flatus)—these cause many complications (45–48).

आनाहो द्विविधो ज्ञेय एकः पक्वाशयोद्भवः । आमाशयोद्भवश्चान्यः प्रत्यानाहः स कथ्यते ॥ ४९ ॥

Ānāha (distention of the abdomen, tympanitis) is two–one of pakwāshaya (colon) and other of āmāshaya (stomach) which is known as pratyānāha (49).

उरोग्रहस्तथा चैको हृद्रोगाः पञ्च कीर्तिताः ।
वातादिभिस्त्रयः प्रोक्ताश्चतुर्थः सन्निपाततः ॥ ५० ॥
पञ्चमः क्रिमिसंजातः—

Urograha (pain in the chest) is one. Hṛdroga (heart diseases) is five—one from each doṣa, one from sannipāta, and the fifth from kṛmi (worms, bacteria) (50).

तथाष्टावुदराणि च ।
वातात्पित्तात्कफात्त्रीणि त्रिदोषेभ्यो जलादपि ॥ ५१ ॥
प्लीह्नः क्षताद्बद्धगुदादष्टमं परिकीर्तितम् ।

Udara (distention of the abdomen) is eight–vātaja, pittaja, kaphaja, sannipātaja, jalaja, plīhaja, kshataja, and baddhagudaja, the eighth (51–52).

गुल्मास्त्वष्टौ समाख्याता वातपित्तकफैस्त्रयः ॥ ५२ ॥
द्वन्द्वभेदास्त्रयः प्रोक्ताः सप्तमः सन्निपाततः । रक्तादष्टमकः ख्यातो मूत्राघातास्त्रयोदश ॥ ५३ ॥

Gulma (abdominal tumour) is eight–vātaja, pittaja, kaphaja, three from the combination of any two doṣas, seventh the sannipātaja, and the eighth from rakta (blood) (52–53).

वातकुण्डलिका पूर्वं वाताष्ठीला ततः परम् । वातबस्तिस्तृतीयाः स्यान्मूत्रातीतश्चतुर्थकः ॥ ५४ ॥
पञ्चमं मूत्रजठरं षष्ठो मूत्रक्षयः स्मृतः । मूत्रोत्सर्गः सप्तमः स्यान्मूत्रग्रन्थिस्तथाष्टमः ॥ ५५ ॥
मूत्रशुक्रं तु नवमं विड्घातो दशमः स्मृतः । मूत्रासादश्चोष्णवातो बस्तिकुण्डलिका तथा ॥ ५६ ॥
त्रयोऽप्येते मूत्रघाताः पृथग्घोराः प्रकीर्तिताः ।

Mūtrāghāta (suppression of urine) is thirteen—vātakuṇḍalikā, vātāṣṭhīlā, vātabasti, mūtrātīta, mūtrajaṭhara, mūtrakshaya, mūtrotsarga, mūtragranthi, mūtrashukra, viḍvighāta, mūtrāsāda, ūṣṇavāta, bastikuṇḍalikā, each one very difficult for therapy (54–56).

मूत्रकृच्छ्राणि चाष्टौ स्युर्वातपित्तकफैस्त्रिधा ॥ ५७ ॥
सन्निपाताच्चतुर्थं स्याच्छुक्रकृच्छ्रं च पञ्चमम् । विट्कृच्छ्रं षष्ठमाख्यातं घातकृच्छ्रं च सप्तमम् ॥ ५८ ॥
अष्टमं चश्मरीकृच्छ्रं—

Mūtra kṛcchra (dysuria) is eight—vātaja, pittaja, kaphaja, sannipātaja, shukraja, viḍja, ghātaja, and the eighth from ashmarī (57–58).

चतुर्धा चाश्मरी मता ।
वातात्पित्तात्कफाच्छुक्रात् तथा मेहाश्च विंशतिः ॥ ५९ ॥

Ashmarī (urinary stone) is four–vātaja, pittaja, kaphaja, and shukraja (59).

इक्षुमेहः सुरामेहः पिष्टमेहश्च सान्द्रकः । शुक्रमेहोदकाख्यौ च लालामेहश्च शीतकः ॥ ६० ॥
सिकताख्यः शनैर्मेहो दशैते कफसंभवाः । मञ्जिष्ठाख्यो हरिद्राख्यो नीलमेहश्च रक्तकः ॥ ६१ ॥
कृष्णमेहः क्षारमेहः षडेते पित्तसंभवाः । हस्तिमेहो वसामेहो मज्जामेहो मधुप्रभः ॥ ६२ ॥
चत्वारो वातजा मेहा इति मेहाश्च विंशतिः । सोमरोगस्तथा चैकः प्रमेहपिडका दश ॥ ६३ ॥
शराविका कच्छपिका पुत्रिणी विनतालजी । मसूरिका सर्षपिका जालिनी च विदारिका ॥ ६४ ॥

विद्रधिश्च दशैताः स्युः पिडका मेहसंभवाः ।

Meha (polyuria, diabetes) is twenty-ikṣumeha, surāmeha, piṣṭameha, sāndrameha, shukrameha, udakameha, lālāmeha, shītameha, sikatāmeha, shanairmeha; these ten are by kapha. Mañjiṣṭhameha, haridrāmeha, nīlameha, raktameha, kṛṣṇameha, kshārameha; these six are by pitta. Hastimeha, vasāmeha, majjāmeha, madhumeha; these four are by vāta. Somaroga is one. Prameha-piḍakās (carbuncles) are ten—sharāvikā, kacchapikā, putriṇī, vinatā, alajī, masūrikā, sarṣapikā, jālinī, vidārikā, and vidradhi; these arise from meha (diabetes) (60–64).

मेदोदोषस्तथा चैकः शोथरोगा नव स्मृताः ॥ ६५ ॥

Medo doṣa (obesity) is one. Shotha (oedema, anasarca) is nine—one from each doṣa, three from the combination of any two doṣas, one from the combination of all the three doṣas together, one from abhighāta (injury) and one from viṣa (poison) (65).

दोषैः पृथग्द्वयैः सर्वैरभिघाताद्विषादपि वृद्धयः सप्त गदिता वातात्पित्तात्कफेन च ॥ ६६ ॥
रक्तेन मेदसा मूत्रादन्त्रवृद्धिश्च सप्तमी । अण्डवृद्धिस्तथा चैका तथैका गण्डमालिका ॥ ६७ ॥
गण्डालजी तु चैका स्यात्

Vṛddhi (scrotal enlargement) is seven—vātaja, pittaja, kaphaja, raktaja, medaja, mūtraja and the seventh is the āntraja. Aṇḍavṛddhi (enlargement of the testes) is one, so also is gandamālikā (scrofula) and gaṇḍālajī (goitre) (66-67).

ग्रन्थयो नवधा मताः । त्रिभिर्दोषैस्त्रयो रक्ताच्छिराभिर्मेदसो व्रणात् ॥६८॥
अस्थ्ना मांसेन नवमः षड्विधं स्यात्तथाबुर्दम् । वातात्पित्तात्कफाद्रक्तान्मांसादपि च मेदसः ॥ ६९ ॥
श्लीपदं च त्रिधा प्रोक्तं वातात्पित्तात्कफादपि । विद्रधिः षड्विधः ख्यातो वातपित्तकफैस्त्रयः ॥ ७० ॥

Granthi (tumours) is nine—one from each doṣa, fourth is raktaja, next each one from śirāja, medaja, vraṇaja, asthija and māṃsaja; arbudas (cancers) is six—vātaja, pittaja, kaphaja, raktaja, māṃsaja and medaja.

Shlīpada (filariasis) is three—vātaja, pittaja and kaphaja. Vidradhi (abscess) is six—vātaja, pittaja, kaphaja, raktaja, kshataja, and last from the sannipāta (68-70).

रक्तात्क्षतात्त्रिदोषैश्च व्रणाः पञ्चदशोदिताः । तेषां चतुर्धा भेदाः स्युरागन्तुर्देहजस्तथा ॥ ७१ ॥
शुद्धो दुष्टश्च विज्ञेयस्तत्संख्या कथ्यते पृथक् । वातव्रणः पित्तजश्च कफजो रक्तजो व्रणः ॥ ७२ ॥
वातपित्तभवश्चान्यो वातश्लेष्मभवस्तथा । तथा पित्तकफाभ्यां च सन्निपातेन चाष्टमः ॥ ७३ ॥
नवमो वातरक्तेन दशमो रक्तपित्ततः । श्लेष्मरक्तभवश्चान्यो वातपित्तासृगुद्भवः ॥ ७४ ॥
वातश्लेष्मासृगुत्पन्नः पित्तश्लेष्मास्रसंभवः । सन्निपातासृगुद्भूत इति पञ्चदश व्रणाः ॥ ७५ ॥

Vraṇa (ulcer) is fifteen—under four major groups viz., āgantu, dehaja, shuddha and duṣṭa; they are enumerated as follows, vātaja, pittaja, kaphaja, raktaja, vātapittaja, vātashleṣmaja, pittakaphaja, sannipātaja, ninth from vātarakta, tenth from raktapitta, next from shleṣmarakta, vātapitta and rakta, vātakapharakta, pittakapharakta and sannipātarakta (71-75).

सद्योव्रणस्त्वष्टधा स्यादविक्लृप्तविलम्बिनौ । छिन्नभिन्नप्रचलिता घृष्टविद्धनिपातितः ॥ ७६ ॥

Sadyovraṇa (traumatic ulcers) is eight—aviklṛpta, vilambina, chinna, bhinna, prachalita, ghṛṣṭa, viddha, and nipātita (76).

कोष्ठभेदो द्विधा प्रोक्तश्छिन्नान्त्रो निःसृतान्त्रकः ।

Koṣṭhabheda (perforation of the abdomen) is two—chhinnāntra and nisṛtāntra (77).

अस्थिभङ्गोऽष्टधा प्रोक्तो भग्नपृष्ठविदारितौ ॥ ७७ ॥
विवर्तितश्च विश्लिष्टस्तिर्यक्क्षिप्तस्त्वधोगतः । ऊर्ध्वगः सन्धिभग्नश्च वह्निदग्धश्चतुर्विधः ॥ ७८ ॥
प्लुष्टोऽतिदग्धो दुर्दग्धः सम्यग्दग्धः प्रकीर्तितः ।

Asthibhaṅga (fractures) is eight—bhagna, pṛṣṭha, vidārita, vivartita, vishliṣṭa, tiryak-kshipta, ūrdhwagata and sandhibhagna.

Vahnidagdha (burns and scalds) is four—pluṣṭa, atidagdha, durdagdha and samyagdagdha (77-79).

नाड्यः पञ्च समाख्याता वातपित्तकफैस्त्रिधा ॥ ७९ ॥
त्रिदोषैरपि शल्येन तथाष्टौ स्युर्भगन्दराः । शतपोनस्तु पवनादुष्ट्रग्रीवश्च पित्ततः ॥ ८० ॥

Nāḍīvraṇa (fissured ulcers like that of guenea worm) is five—vātaja, pittaja, kaphaja, tridoṣaja, and shalyaja (79–80).

परिस्रावी कफाज्ज्ञेय ऋजुर्वातकफोद्भवः । परिक्षेपी मरुत्पित्तादर्शोजः कफपित्ततः ॥ ८१ ॥
आगन्तुजातश्चोन्मार्गी शङ्खावर्तस्त्रिदोषजः ।

Bhagandara (fistula-in-ano) is eight—shataponaka from vāta, uṣṭragrīva from pitta, parisrāvī from kapha, ṛju from vātakapha, parākshepī from vātapitta, arshoja from kaphapitta, unmārgī from āgantu and shaṅkhāvarta from all the three doṣas (80-81).

मेढ्रे पञ्चोपदंशाः स्युर्वातपित्तकफैस्त्रिधा ॥ ८२ ॥
सन्निपातेन रक्ताच्च

Upadaṃsha (venereal disease specially syphilis) is five—vātaja, pittaja, kaphaja, sannipātaja and raktaja (82).

मेढ्रे शूकामयास्तथा ।
चतुर्विंशतिराख्याता लिङ्गार्शो ग्रथितं तथा ॥ ८३ ॥
निवृत्तमवमन्थश्च मृदितं शतपोनकः । अष्ठीलिका सर्षपिका त्वक्पाकश्चावपाटिका ॥ ८४ ॥

मांसपाकः स्पर्शहानिर्निरुद्धमणिरुत्तमा । मांसार्बुदं पुष्करिका संमूढपिडकालजी ॥ ८५ ॥
रक्तार्बुदं विद्रधिश्च कुम्भिका तिलकालकः । निरुद्धप्रकाशः प्रोक्तस्तथैव परिवर्तिका ॥ ८६ ॥

Shūka rogas (diseases of the penis due to poisonous applications) is twenty four—liṅgārshas, grathita, nivṛtta, avamantha, mṛdita, shataponaka, aṣṭhīlikā, sarṣapikā, twakpāka, avapāṭikā, māṃsapāka, sparshahāni, niruddhamaṇi, uttamā, māṃsārbuda, puṣkarikā, saṃmūḍapiḍaka, alajī, raktārbuda, vidradhi, kumbhikā, tilakālaka, niruddhaprakāsha and parivartikā (83-86).

कुष्ठान्यष्टादशोक्तानि वातात्कापालिकं भवेत् । पित्तेनोदुम्बरं प्रोक्तं कफान्मण्डलचर्चिके ॥ ८७ ॥
मरुत्पित्तादृष्यजिह्वं श्लेष्मवाताद्विपादिका । तथा सिध्मैककुष्ठं च किटिभं चालसं तथा ॥ ८८ ॥
कफपित्तात्पुनर्दद्रूः पामा विस्फोटकं तथा । महाकुष्ठं चर्मदलं पुण्डरीकं शतारुकम् ॥ ८९ ॥
त्रिदोषैः काकणं ज्ञेयं तथान्यच्छ्वित्रसंज्ञितम् । तथातेन पित्तेन श्लेष्मणा च त्रिधा भवेत् ॥ ९० ॥

Kuṣṭha roga (leprosy and allied skin conditions) is eighteen—kāpālika from vāta, audumbara from pitta, maṇḍala and vicharchikā from kapha, ṛṣyajihwa from vātapitta, vipādikā from kaphavāta, so also sidhma, eka kuṣṭha, kiṭibha and alasa; dadru, pāmā, visphoṭaka from kaphapitta; mahākuṣṭha, charmadala, puṇḍarīka, shatāru and kākaṇa from all the three together. Shwitra (leucoderma) is three—vātaja, pittaja, kaphaja (87-90).

क्षुद्ररोगाः षष्टिसंख्यास्तेष्वादौ शर्करार्बुदम् । इन्द्रवृद्धा पनसिका विवृतान्धालजी तथा ॥ ९१ ॥
वराहदंष्ट्रो वल्मीकं कच्छपी तिलकालकः । गर्दभी रजसा चैव यवप्रख्या विदारिका ॥ ९२ ॥
कदरो मषकश्चैव नीलिका जालगर्दभः । इरिवेल्ली जतुमणिर्गुदभ्रंशोऽग्निरोहिणी ॥ ९३ ॥
संनिरुद्धगुदः कोठः कुनखोऽनुशयी तथा । पद्मिनीकण्टकश्चिप्यमलसो मुखदूषिका ॥ ९४ ॥
कक्षा वृषणकच्छूश्च गन्धः पाषाणगर्दभः । राजिका च तथा व्यङ्गश्चतुर्धा परिकिर्तिताः ॥ ९५ ॥
वातात्पित्तात्कफाद्रक्तादित्युक्तं व्यङ्गलक्षणम् । विस्फोटाः क्षुद्ररोगेषु तेऽष्टधा परिकिर्तिताः ॥ ९६ ॥
पृथग्दोषैस्त्रयो द्वन्द्वैस्त्रिविधः सप्तमोऽसृजः । अष्टमः सन्निपातेन क्षुद्ररुक्षु मसूरिका ॥ ९७ ॥
चतुर्दशप्रकारेण त्रिभिर्दोषैस्त्रिधा च सा । द्वन्द्वजा त्रिविधा प्रोक्ता सन्निपातेन सप्तमी ॥ ९८ ॥
अष्टमी त्वग्गता ज्ञेया नवमी रक्तजा मता । दशमी मांसजा ख्याता चतस्रोऽन्याश्च दुस्तरा ॥ ९९ ॥
मेदोऽस्थिमज्जाशुक्रस्थाः क्षुद्ररोगा इतीरिताः ।

Kshudra rogas (minor diseases) are sixty–sharkarārbuda, indravṛddhā, panasikā, vivṛtā, andhālajī, varāhadaṃṣtra, valmīka, kacchapī, tilakālaka, gardabhī, rajasā, yavaprakhyā, vidārikā, kadara, maṣaka, nīlikā, jālagardabha, irivellī, jatumaṇi, gudabhraṃsha, agnirohiṇī, sanniruddhaguda, koṭha, kunakha, anushayi, padminikaṇṭaka, chipya, alasa, mukhadūṣikā, kakshā, vṛṣaṇakacchu, gandha, pāṣāṇagardabha, rājikā and vyaṅga; vyaṅga is of four kinds : vātaja, pittaja, kaphaja and raktaja; visphoṭa is of eight kinds–one from each doṣa, one each from the combination of two doṣas, seventh is raktaja and the eighth from the sannipāta; Masūrikā (pox) is fourteen kinds–one from each doṣa, three from dwandwa doṣa, seventh from sannipāta, eighth is twakgata, ninth raktaja, tenth māṃsaja, the remaining four intractible for treatment–the medaja, asthija, majjāja and the shukraja (91–99).

विसर्परोगो नवधा वातपित्तकफैस्त्रिधा ॥ १०० ॥
त्रिधा स द्वन्द्वभेदेन सन्निपातेन सप्तमः । अष्टमो वह्निदाहेन नवमश्चाभिघातजः ॥ १०१ ॥

Visarpa (erysipelas) is nine–vātaja, pittaja, kaphaja, three from dwandwa doṣas, sannipātaja, eighth from dāha and the tenth from abhighāta (100–101).

तथैकः श्लेष्मपित्ताभ्यामुदर्दः परिकीर्तितः । वातपित्तेन चैकस्तु शीतपित्तामयः स्मृतः ॥ १०२ ॥

Udarda (erythema, wheels on the skin, allergy) and shītapitta (neurotic oedema) are one each, udarda from kaphapitta and shītapitta from vātapitta (102):

अम्लपित्तं त्रिधा प्रोक्तं वातेन श्लेष्मणा तथा । तृतीयं श्लेष्मवाताभ्यां वातरक्तं तथाष्टधा ॥ १०३ ॥

Amlapitta (hyperchlorhydria) is three–vātaja, shleṣmaja and the third from shleṣmavāta (103).

वाताधिक्येन पित्ताच्च कफाद्दोषत्रयेण च । रक्ताधिक्येन दोषाणां द्वन्द्वेण त्रिविधः स्मृतः ॥ १०४ ॥

Vātarakta (gout) is eight–vātaja, pittaja, kaphaja. raktaja and three from dwandwa doṣas (104).

अशीतिर्वातजा रोगाः कथ्यन्ते मुनिभाषिताः । आक्षेपको हनुस्तम्भ ऊरुस्तम्भः शिरोग्रहः ॥ १०५ ॥
बाह्यायामोऽन्तरायामः पार्श्वशूलं कटिग्रहः । दण्डापतानकः खल्ली जिह्वास्तम्भस्तथार्दितम् ॥ १०६॥
पक्षाघातः क्रोष्टुशीर्षो मन्यास्तम्भश्च पङ्गुता । कलायखञ्जता तूनी प्रतितूनी च खञ्जता ॥ १०७ ॥
पाददहर्षो गृध्रसी च विश्वाची चापबाहुकः । अपतानो व्रणायामो वातकण्टोऽपतन्त्रकः ॥ १०८ ॥
अङ्गभेदोऽङ्गशोषश्च मिन्मिनत्वं च कल्लता । प्रत्यष्ठीलाऽष्ठीलिका च वामनत्वं च कुब्जता ॥ १०९ ॥
(अङ्गभङ्गोऽङ्गशूलं च संकोचस्तम्भरूक्षता ।) अङ्गपीडाङ्गविभ्रंशो विड्ग्रहो बद्धविट्कता ॥ ११० ॥
मूकत्वमतिजृम्भा स्यादत्युद्गारोऽन्त्रकूजनम् । वातप्रवृत्तिः स्फुरणं शिराणां पूरणं तथा ॥ १११ ॥
कम्पः कार्श्यं श्यावता च प्रलापः क्षिप्रमूत्रता । निद्रानाशः स्वेदनाशो दुर्बलत्वं बलक्षयः ॥ ११२ ॥
अतिप्रवृत्तिः शुक्रस्य कार्श्यं नाशश्च रेतसः । अनवस्थितचित्तत्वं काठिन्यं विरसास्यता ॥ ११३ ॥
(कषायवक्त्रताध्मानं प्रत्याध्मानं च शीतता । रोमहर्षश्च भीरुत्वं तोदः कण्डूरसाज्ञता ॥ ११४ ॥)
शब्दाज्ञता प्रसुप्तिश्च गन्धाज्ञत्वं दृशः क्षयः ।

Vātarogas (nervous disorders) are eighty–ākshepaka, hanustambha, ūrustambha, shirograha, bāhyāyama, antarāyāma, pārshwa shūla, kaṭigraha, daṇḍāpatānaka, khallī, jihwāstambha, ardita, pakshāghāta, kroṣṭushīrṣa, manyāstambha, paṅgutā, kalāyakhañja, tūnī, pratitūnī, khañjatā, pādaharṣa, gṛdhrasī, vishwāchī, apabāhuka, vraṇāyāma, vātakaṇṭaka, apatantraka, aṅgabheda, aṅgashoṣa, minminatwa, gadgada, pratyaṣṭhīlā, aṣṭhilā, vāmanatwa, kubjatā, aṅgapīḍa, aṅgashūla, saṅkocha, stambha, rūkshatā, aṅgabhanga, aṅgavibhraṃsha, viḍgraha, baddhaviṭkatā, mūkatwa, atijṛmbha, atyudgāra, antrakūjana, vātapravṛtti, sphuraṇa and pūraṇa of śirās, kārshya, shyāvatā, pralāpa, kshipramūtratā, nidrānāsha, swedanāsha, durbalatwa, balakshaya, atipravṛtti of shukra, kārshya, retonāsha, anavasthitachittatwa, kāṭhinya, virasāsyatā, kaṣāyavakratā, ādhmāna, pratyādhmāna, shītatā, romaharṣa, bhīrutwa, toda, kaṇḍū, rasājñatā, shabdājñatā, prasupti, gandhājñāna and dṛṣṭi kshaya (105–114).

अथ पित्तभवा रोगाश्चत्वारिंशदिहोदिताः ॥ ११५ ॥
धूमोद्गारो विदाहः स्यादुष्णाङ्गत्वं मतिभ्रमः । कान्तिहानिः कण्ठशोषो मुखशोषोऽल्पशुक्रता ॥
तिक्तास्यताम्लवक्त्रत्वं स्वेदस्रावोऽङ्गपाकता । क्लमो हरितवर्णत्वमतृप्तिः पीतगात्रता ॥ ११७ ॥
रक्तद्रावोऽङ्गदरणं लोहगन्धास्यता तथा । दौर्गन्ध्यं पीतमूत्रत्वमरतिः पीतविट्कता ॥ ११८ ॥
पीतावलोकनं पीतनेत्रता पीतदन्तता । शीतेच्छा पीतनखता तेजोद्वेषोऽल्पनिद्रता ॥ ११९ ॥
कोपश्च गात्रसादश्च भिन्नविट्कत्वमन्धता । उष्णोच्छ्वासत्वमुष्णत्वं मूत्रस्य च मलस्य च ॥ १२० ॥
तमसो दर्शनं पीतमण्डलानां च दर्शनम् । निःसहत्वं च पित्तस्य चत्वारिंशद्रुजाः स्मृताः ॥ १२१ ॥

Pittarogas are forty–dhūmodgāra, vidāha, uṣṇāṅgatwa, matibhrama, kāntihāni, kaṇṭhashoṣa, mukhashoṣa, alpashukratā, tiktāsyatā, amlavakratā, swedasrāva, aṅgapākatā, klama, haritavarṇatā, atṛpti, pītagātratā, raktasrāva, aṅgadaraṇa, lohagandhāsyatā, daurgandhya, pītamūtratā, arati, pītaviṭkatā, pītāvalokana, pītanetratā, pītadantatā, shītecchā, pītanakhatā, tejodweṣa, alpanidratā, kopa, gātrasāda, bhinnaviṭkatā, andhatā, uṣṇamūtratā, uṣṇamalatā, tamodarshana, pītamaṇḍala darshana and niḥsahatwa (115–121).

कफस्य विंशतिः प्रोक्ता रोगास्तन्द्रातिनिद्रता । गौरवं मुखमाधुर्यं मुखलेपः प्रसेकता ॥ १२२ ॥
श्वेतावलोकनं श्वेतविट्कत्वं श्वेतमूत्रता । श्वेताङ्गवर्णता शैत्यमुष्णेच्छा तिक्तकामिता ॥ १२३ ॥
मलाधिक्यं च शुक्रस्य बाहुल्यं बहुमूत्रता । आलस्यं मन्दबुद्धित्वं तृप्तिर्घर्घरवाक्यता ॥ १२४ ॥
अचैतन्यं च गदिता विंशतिः श्लेष्मजा गदाः ।

Kapharogas are twenty–tandrā, atinidrā, gauravam, mukhamādhurya, mukhalepa, prasekatā, shwetāvalokanam, shwetaviṭkatā, śwetamūtratā, shwetāṅgavarṇatā, shaitya, uṣṇecchā, tiktakāmitā, malādhikya, shukrabāhulya, bahumūtratā, ālasya, mandabuddhi, tṛptī, ghurghuravākyatā and acaitanya (122–124).

रक्तस्य च दश प्रोक्ता व्याधयस्तेषु गौरवम् ॥ १२५ ॥
रक्तमण्डलता रक्तनेत्रत्वं रक्तमूत्रता । रक्तनिष्ठीवनं रक्तपिडकानां च दर्शनम् ॥ १२६ ॥
औष्ण्यं च पूतिगन्धत्वं पीडा पाकश्च जायते ।

Rakta rogas are ten–gaurava, raktamaṇḍalatā, raktanetratwa, raktamūtratā, raktaniṣṭhīvana, raktapiḍaka, auṣṇya, pūtigandhatā, pīḍā and pāka (125–126).

चतुःसप्ततिसंख्याका मुखरोगास्तथोदिताः ॥ १२७ ॥
तेष्वोष्ठरोगा गणिता एकादशमिता बुधैः । वातपित्तकफैस्त्रेधा त्रिदोषैरसृजा तथा ॥ १२८ ॥
क्षतं मांसार्बुदं चैव खण्डोष्ठं च जलार्बुदम् । मेदोऽर्बुदं चार्बुदं च रोगा एकादश स्मृताः ॥ १२९ ॥
दन्तरोगा दशाख्याता दालानः कृमिदन्तकः । दन्तहर्षः करालश्च दन्तचालश्च शर्करा ॥ १३० ॥
अधिदन्तः श्यावदन्तो दन्तभेदः कपालिका । तथा त्रयोदशमिता दन्तमूलामयाः स्मृताः ॥ १३१ ॥
शीतादोपकुशौ द्वौ तु दन्तविद्रधिपुप्पुटौ । अधिमांसो विदर्भश्च महासौषिरसौषिरौ ॥ १३२ ॥
तेष्वेव गतयः पञ्च वातात्पित्तात्कफादपि । सन्निपातादृतिश्चान्या रक्तनाडी च पञ्चमी ॥ १३३ ॥

Mukha rogas (diseases of the mouth) are totally seventy four; of them oṣṭharogas (diseases of the lips) are eleven–vātaja, pittaja, tridoṣaja, raktaja, māṃsārbuda, khaṇḍoṣṭa, jalārbuda, medorbuda and arbuda; dantarogas (disorders of the teeth) are ten–dālāna, kṛmidanta, dantaharṣa, karāladanta, dantachala, dantasharkarā, adhidanta, shyāvadanta, dantabheda, kapālikā; dantamūlarogas (disorders of the socket of the teeth) are thirteen–shītāda, upakusha, dantavidradhi, dantapupputa, adhimāṃsa, vidarbha, mahāsaushira, saushira, vātaja danta nāḍī, pittaja danta nāḍī, kaphaja danta nāḍī, sannipātaja danta nāḍī, and raktaja danta nāḍī (127–133).

तथा जिह्वामयाः षट् स्युर्वातपित्तकफैस्त्रिधा । अलासश्च चतुर्थः स्यादधिजिह्वा च पञ्चमी ॥ १३४ ॥
षष्ठी चैवोपजिह्वा स्यात्—

Jihwā rogas (disorders of the tongue) are six–vātaja, pittaja, kaphaja, alāsa, adhijihwā and upajihwā, the sixth (134).

तथाष्टौ तालुजा गदाः ।
अर्बुदं तालुपिडका कच्छपी तालुसंहतिः ॥ १३५ ॥
गलशुण्डी तालुशोषस्तालुपाकश्च पुप्पुटः । गलरोगास्तथाख्याता अष्टादशमिता बुधैः ॥ १३६ ॥

Tālurogas (disorders of the palate) are eight–arbuda, tālupiḍakā, kacchapī, tālusaṃhati, galashuṇḍī, tālushoṣa, tālupāka and tālupupputa (135–136).

वातरोहिणिका पूर्वं द्वितीया पित्तरोहिणी । कफरोहिणिका प्रोक्ता त्रिदोषैरपि रोहिणी ॥ १३७ ॥
मेदोरोहिणिका वृन्दो गलौघो गलविद्रधिः । स्वरहा तुण्डिकेरी च शतघ्नी शालुकोऽर्बुदम् ॥ १३८ ॥
गिलायुर्वलयश्चापि वाताद्गण्डः कफात्तथा । मेदोगण्डस्तथैव स्यादित्यष्टादश कण्ठजाः ॥ १३९ ॥

Galarogas (diseases of the throaṭ) are eighteen–vātarohiṇī, pittarohiṇī, kapharohiṇī, tridoṣajarohiṇī, medorohiṇī vṛnda, galavidradhi, swarahā, tuṇḍikerī, shataghnī, shālukā, arbuda, gilāyu, vātaja gaṇḍa, kapha gaṇḍa and medo gaṇḍa (137–139).

मुखान्तःसंभवा रोगा अष्टौ ख्याता महर्षिभिः । मुखपाको भवेद्वातात्पित्तात्तद्वत्कफादपि ॥ १४० ॥
रक्ताच्च सन्निपाताच्च पूत्यास्योर्ध्वगदादपि । अर्बुदं चेति मुखजाश्चतुःसप्ततिरामयाः ॥ १४१ ॥

Mukhāntargata rogas (disorders of the mouth cavity) are eight—mukhapākās, vātaja, pittaja, sannipātaja, pūtyāsya, ūrdhwa, gada and arbuda. All these together make up seventy four (140–141).

कर्णरोगाः समाख्याता अष्टादशमिता बुधैः । वातात्पित्तात्कफाद्रक्तात्सन्निपाताच्च विद्रधिः ॥१४२॥
शोथोऽर्बुदं पूतिकर्णः कर्णार्शः कर्णहल्लिका । बाधिर्यं तन्त्रिका कण्डूः शष्कुली कृमिकर्णकः ॥१४३॥
कर्णनादः प्रतीनाह इत्यष्टादश कर्णजाः । कर्णपालीसमुद्भूता रोगाः सप्त इहोदिताः ॥ १४४ ॥
उत्पातः पालिशोषश्च विदारी दुःखवर्धनः । परिपोटश्च लेही च पिप्पली चेति संस्कृताः ॥ १४५ ॥
कर्णमूलामयाः पञ्च वातात्पित्तात्कफादपि ।
सन्निपाताच्च रक्ताच्च—

Karṇa rogas (diseases of the ears) are eighteen–vātaja, pittaja, kaphaja, raktaja, sannipātaja, vidradhi, shotha, arbuda, pūtikarṇa, karṇārshas, karṇahallikā, bādhirya, tantrikā, kaṇḍū, shaṣkulī, kṛmikarṇa, karṇanāda and pratīnāha. Karṇapālī rogas (diseases of pinna) are–utpāta, pālishoṣa, vidārī, dukhavardhana, paripoṭa, lehī and pippalī. Karṇamūla rogas (disorders of the root of the ear) are five–vātaja, pittaja, kaphaja, sannipātaja and raktaja (142–146).

तथा नासाभवा गदाः ॥ १४६ ॥
अष्टादशैव संख्याताः प्रतिश्यायास्तु तेष्वपि । वातात्पित्तात्कफाद्रक्तात्सन्निपातेन पञ्चमः ॥ १४७ ॥
अपीनसः पूतिनासो नासार्शो भ्रंशथुः क्षवः । नासानाहः पूतिरक्तमर्बुदं दुष्टपीनसम् ॥ १४८ ॥
नासाशोषो घ्राणपाकः पूयस्रावश्च दीप्तकः ।

Nāsā rogas (diseases of the nose) are also eighteen–five types of pratishyāya-vātaja, pittaja, kaphaja, raktaja, sannipātaja; apīnasa, pūtināsā, nāsārshas, bhraṃshathu, kshava, nāsānāha, pūtirakta, arbuda, duṣṭapīnasa, nāsāshoṣa, ghrāṇapāka, pūtisrāva and dīpti (146–149).

तथा दश शिरोरोगा वातेनार्धावभेदकः ॥ १४९ ॥
शिरस्तापश्च वातेन पित्तपीडा तृतीयका । चतुर्थी कफजा पीडा रक्तजा सन्निपातजा ॥ १५० ॥
सूर्यावर्ताच्छिरःकम्पात्क्रिमिभिः शङ्खकेन च । तथा कपालरोगाः स्युर्नव तेषूपशीर्षकम् ॥ १५१ ॥
अरुंषिका विद्रधिश्च दारुणं पिडिकाऽर्बुदम् । इन्द्रलुप्तं च खलतिः पलितं चेति ते नव ॥ १५२ ॥

Shirorogas (diseases of the head) are ten–vātaja ardhāvabheda, five shirobhitāpa–vātaja, pittaja, kaphaja, raktaja, sannipātaja; sūryāvarta, shirakampa, kṛmija, shiroroga and shaṅkhaka. Kapālarogas (diseases of the skull) are nine-upashīrṣaka, arunṣikā, vidradhi, dāruṇa, piḍikā, arbuda, indralupta, khalita and palita (149–152).

तथा नेत्रभवाः ख्याताश्चतुर्नवतिरामयाः । तेषु वर्त्मगदाः प्रोक्ताश्चतुर्विंशतिसंज्ञकाः ॥ १५३ ॥
कृच्छ्रोन्मीलः पक्ष्मपातः कफोत्क्लिष्टश्च लोहितः । अरुन्निमेषः कथितो रक्तोत्क्लिष्टः कुकूणकः ॥१५४॥
पक्ष्मार्शः पक्ष्मरोधश्च पित्तोत्क्लिष्टश्च पोथकी । क्लिष्टवर्त्मा च बहलः पक्ष्मोत्संगस्तथार्बुदम् ॥१५५॥
कुम्भिका सिकतावर्त्म लगणोऽञ्जननामिका । कर्दमः श्याववर्त्मा च बिसवर्त्मा तथाऽलजी ॥१५६॥
उत्क्लिष्टवर्त्मेति गदा प्रोक्ता वर्त्मसमुद्भवाः । नेत्रसंधिसमुद्भूता नव रोगाः प्रकीर्तिताः ॥ १५७ ॥
जलस्रावः कफस्रावो रक्तस्रावश्च पर्वणी । पूयस्रावः क्रिमिग्रन्थिरुपनाहस्तथाऽलजी ॥ १५८ ॥
पूयालस इति प्रोक्ता रोगा नयनसंधिजाः । तथा शुक्लगता रोगा बुधैः प्रोक्तास्त्रयोदश ॥ १५९ ॥
सिरोत्पातः सिराहर्षः सिराजालश्च शुक्तिका । शुक्लार्म चाधिमांसार्म प्रस्तार्यर्म च पिष्टकः ॥ १६० ॥
शिरायाश्चिप्पिटं चैव कफग्रथितकोऽर्जुनः । स्नाय्वर्म शोणितार्म स्यादिति शुक्लगता गदा ॥ १६१ ॥
तथा कृष्णसमुद्भूताः पञ्च रोगा प्रकीर्तिताः । शुद्धशुक्रं शिराशुक्रं क्षतशुक्रं तथाऽजका ॥ १६२ ॥
शिरासंगश्च सर्वेऽपि प्रोक्ता कृष्णगता गदाः । काचं तु षड्विधं ज्ञेयं वातात्पित्तात्कफादपि ॥ १६३ ॥
सन्निपाताच्च रक्ताच्च षष्ठं संसर्गसंभवम् । तिमिराणि षडेव स्युर्वातपित्तकफैस्त्रिधा ॥१६४॥
संसर्गेण च रक्तेन षष्ठं स्यात्संनिपाततः । लिङ्गनाशः सप्तधा स्याद्वातात्पित्तात्कफेन च ॥ १६५ ॥
त्रिदोषैरुपसर्गेण संसर्गेणासृजा तथा । अष्टधा दृष्टिरोगाः स्युस्तेषु पित्तविदग्धकम् ॥ १६६ ॥
अम्लपित्तविदग्धं च तथैवोष्णविदग्धकम् । नकुलान्ध्यं धूसरान्ध्यं रात्र्यान्ध्यं ह्रस्वदृष्टिकः ॥१६७॥
गम्भीरदृष्टिरित्येते रोगा दृष्टागता मताः । (चत्वारश्चाधिमन्थाः स्युर्वातपित्तकफास्रतः ॥ १६८ ॥)
अभिष्यन्दाश्च चत्वारो रक्ताद्दोषैस्त्रिभिस्त्रिधा । सर्वाक्षिरोगाश्चाष्टौ स्युस्तेषु वातविपर्ययः ॥१६९॥
अल्पशोफोऽन्यतोवातस्तथा पाकात्ययः स्मृतः । शुष्काक्षिपाकश्च तथा शोफोऽध्युषित एव च ॥१७०॥
हताधिमन्थ इत्येते रोगाः सर्वाक्षिसंभवाः ।

Netra rogas (diseases of the eyes) are totally nintyfour–of them those of the vartma (disorders of the lids) are twenty four–kṛcchronmīla, pakshmapāta, kaphotkliṣṭa, lohita, arunnimeṣa, raktotkliṣṭa, kukūṇaka, pakshmārshas, pakshmarodha, pittotkliṣṭa, pothakī, kliṣṭavartma, bahala, pakshmotsaṅga, arbuda, kumbhikā, sikatāvartma, lagaṇa, añjananāmikā, kardama, shyāvavartma, bisavartma, alajī and utkliṣṭavartma; netrasandhi rogas (disorders of the joints) are nine–jalasrāva, kaphasrāva, raktasrāva, parvaṇi, pūyasrāva, kṛmigranthi, upanāha, alaji, pūyālasa; shuklagatarogas (disorders of the sclera) are thirteen—sirotpāta, sirāharṣa, sirājāla, shuklikā, shuklārma, adhimāṃsārma, prastāryarma, piṣṭaka, śirajachippiṭa, kaphagranthi, arjuna, snāyvarma and shoṇatārma; kṛṣṇa gata rogas (disorders of the cornea) are five—shuddha shukra, śirāshukra, kshatashukra, ajaka and śirāsaṅga; kācha rogas (disorders of the lens) are six—vātaja, pittaja, kaphaja, sannipātaja, raktaja and saṃsargaja. Timira rogas (disorders of vision) are six–vātaja, pittaja, kaphaja saṃsargaja, raktaja and sannipātaja; liṅganāsha rogas (vision defects) are seven–vātaja, pittaja, kaphaja, tridoṣaja, upasargaja, saṃsargaja and asṛja; dṛṣṭimaṇḍala rogas (disorders of retina) are eight—pittavidagdha, amlapittavidagdha, ūṣṇavidagdha, nakulāndhya, dhūsarāndhya, rātryāndha, hraswadṛṣṭi and gambhīradṛṣṭika. The four adhimanthas–vātaja, pittaja, kaphaja, asṛja; the four abhiṣyandas—raktaja, vātaja, pittaja and kaphaja. Sarvākshirogas (disorders affecting the entire eye) are also eight–vātaviparyaya, alpashopha, anyatovāta, pākātyaya, shuṣkākshi pāka, shopha, adhyuṣita and hatādhimantha (153–170).

पुंस्त्वदोषास्तु पञ्चैव प्रोक्तास्तत्रेर्ष्यकः स्मृतः ॥ १७१ ॥
आसेक्यश्चैव कुम्भीकः सुगन्धिः षण्ढसंज्ञकः । शुक्रदोषास्तथाष्टौ स्युर्वातात्पित्तात्कफेन च ॥ १७२ ॥
कुणपं चास्रपित्ताभ्या पूयाभं श्लेष्मपित्ततः । क्षीणं च वातपित्ताभ्यां ग्रन्थिलं श्लेष्मवाततः ॥ १७३॥
मलाभं संनिपाताच्च शुक्रदोषा इतीरिताः ।

Puṃsthwa rogas (diseases of male sexuality, impotence) are five–irṣyaka, āsekya, kumbhīka, sugandhi and ṣaṇḍa; shukra doṣas (disorders of semen) are eight–vātaja, pittaja, kaphaja, kuṇapagandhi from asrapitta, pūyābha from shleṣmapitta, kshīṇa from vātapitta, granthila from shleṣmavāta and malābha from sannipāta (171–173).

अथ स्त्रीरोगनामानि प्रोच्यन्ते पूर्वशास्त्रतः ॥ १७४ ॥
अष्टावार्तवदोषाः स्युर्वातपित्तकफैस्त्रिधा । पूयाभं कुणपं ग्रन्थि क्षीणं मलसमं तथा ॥ १७५ ॥
तथा च रक्तप्रदरं चतुर्विधमुदाहृतम् । वातपित्तकथैस्त्रेधा चतुर्थं संनिपाततः ॥ १७६ ॥
विंशतिर्योनिरोगाः स्युर्वातात्पित्तात्कफादपि । संनिपाताच्च रक्ताच्च लोहितक्षयतस्तथा ॥ १७७ ॥
शुष्का च वामिनी चैव खण्डितान्तर्मुखी तथा । सूचिमुखी विप्लुता च पुत्रघ्नी च परिप्लुता ॥१७८॥
उपप्लुता प्राक्चरणा महायोनिश्च कर्णिनी । स्यान्नन्दा चातिचरणा योनिरोगा इतीरिताः ॥ १७९ ॥
चतुर्विधं योनिकन्दं वातपित्तकफैस्त्रिधा । चतुर्थं संनिपातेन तथाष्टौ गर्भजा गदाः ॥ १८० ॥
उपविष्टकगर्भः स्यात्तथा नागोदरः स्मृतः । मक्कल्लो मूढगर्भश्च विष्कम्भो गूढगर्भकः ॥ १८१ ॥
जरायुदोषो गर्भस्य पातश्चाष्टमकः स्मृतः ।

Strī rogas (diseases of women) as known to ancients are eight; ārtava doṣas (menstrual disorders)—vātaja, pittaja, kaphaja, pūyābha, kuṇapa, granthi, kshīṇa and malasama; rakta pradara is four—vātaja, pittaja, kaphaja and fourth from sannipāta. Yoni rogas (diseases of vaginal tract) are twenty—vātaja, pittaja, kaphaja, sannipātaja, raktaja, that due to raktakshaya, shuṣka, vāminī, khaṇḍitā, antarmukhī, sūchīmukhī, viplutā, putraghnī, pariplutā, upaplutā, prākcharaṇā, mahāyonī, karṇinī, nandā and aticharaṇā; yonikanda (tumours of the vagina) are four—vātaja, pittaja, kaphaja and sannipātaja. Garbhāshaya rogas (diseases of the uterus) are eight—upaviṣṭakagarbha, nāgodara, makkalla, mūḍhagarbha, viṣkambha, gūḍha garbha, jarāyudoṣa and the eighth garbhapāta (174–181).

पञ्चैव स्तनरोगाः स्युर्वातात्पित्तात्कफादपि ॥ १८२ ॥
संनिपातात्क्षताच्चैव तथा स्तन्योद्भवा गदाः । बालरोगेषु कथिताः स्त्रीदोषाश्च त्रयः स्मृताः ॥१८३॥
अदक्षपुरुषोत्पन्नः सपत्नीविहितस्तथा । दैवाज्जातस्तृतीयस्तु तथा ये सूतिकागदाः ॥ १८४ ॥
ज्वरादयश्चिकित्स्यास्ते यथादोषं यथाबलम् ।

Stana rogas (diseases of the breasts) are five—vātaja, pittaja, kaphaja, sannipātaja and kshataja. Stanya rogas (disorders of breast milk) will be described under bālarogas; strīdoṣas (mental disorders of women) are three, adaksha-puruṣotpanna, sapatnivihita and devaja. Sūtikā rogas (purpural disorders) are the usual jwaras (fevers) etc., due to doṣas and severity which need treatment (182–184).

द्वाविंशतिर्बालरोगास्तेषु क्षीरालसास्त्रयः ॥ १८५ ॥
वातात्पित्तात्कफाच्चैव दन्तोद्भेदश्चतुर्थकः । दन्तघातो दन्तशब्दोऽकालदन्तोऽहिपूतनम् ॥ १८६ ॥
मुखपाको मुखस्रावो गुदपाकोपशीर्षकौ । पार्श्वारुणस्तालुकण्टो विच्छिन्नं पारिगर्भिकः ॥ १८७ ॥
दौर्बल्यं गात्रशोषश्च शय्यामूत्रं कुकूणकः । रोदनं चाजगल्ली स्यादिति द्वाविंशतिः स्मृताः ॥१८८॥
तथा बालग्रहाः ख्याता द्वादशैव मुनीश्वरैः । स्कन्दग्रहो विशाखः स्यात्स्वग्रहश्च पितृग्रहः ॥१८९॥
नैगमेयग्रहस्तद्वच्छकुनिः शीतपूतना । मुखमण्डितिका तद्वत्पूतना चान्धपूतना ॥ १९० ॥
रेवती चैव संख्याता तथा स्याच्छुष्करेवती ।

Bāla rogas (diseases of children) are twenty two, of which three from bad milk—vātaja, pittaja, kaphaja, dantodbheda, dantaghāta, dantashabda, akāla-danta, ahipūtana, mukhapāka, mukhasrāva, gudapāka, upashīrṣaka, pārsh-wāruṇa, tālukanṭaka, vicchinna, pārigarbhika, daurbalya, gātrashoṣa, shayyā-mūtra, kukūṇaka, rodana and ajagallī. Bālagrahas (seizures by evil spirits) enumerated by the sages are twelve—skandagraha, vishākha, swagraha, pitṛgraha, naigameyagraha, shakunigraha, shītapūtanā graha, mukhamaṇḍitikā, pūtanā, andhapūtanā, revatī, and shuṣka revatī graha (185–190).

तथा चरणभेदास्तु वातरक्तादिकाश्च ये ॥ १९१ ॥
द्विचत्वारिंशदुक्तास्ते रोगेष्वेव मुनीश्वरैः । द्विषष्टिर्दोषभेदाः स्युः संनिपातादिकाश्च ये ॥ १९२ ॥
तेऽपि रोगेषु गणिताः पृथक्प्रोक्ता न ते क्वचित् ।

Pāda rogas (diseases of the foot) are forty-two as described previously under vātarakta etc.

Sixty two are the disorders of doṣas (tridoṣas) from the permutation and combinations of their increase or decrease and the sixty third is from the combination of all the three of them in their normalcy. These are not enumerated here even though counted as diseases (191–192)

हीनमिथ्यातियोगेन भेदैः पञ्चदशोदिताः ॥ १९३ ॥
पञ्चकर्मभवा रोगा रोगेष्वेव प्रकीर्तिताः । स्नेहस्वेदौ तथा धूमो गण्डूषोऽञ्जनतर्पणे ॥ १९४ ॥
पीडा अष्टादशैतज्जास्ताश्च रोगेषु लक्षिताः ।

Pañchakarmaja rogas (diseases arising from bad therapies) are in total fifteen; three (hīna, mithyā, and ati) from each of the five karmas. Sneha, sweda, dhūma, gaṇḍūṣa, añjana, tarpaṇa also cause eighteen diseases by their hīna, mithyā and ati yogas (193–194).

शीतोपद्रव एकः स्यादेकश्चोष्णोद्भवो मतः ॥ १९५ ॥
शल्योपद्रव एकश्च क्षाराच्चैकः स्मृतस्तथा ।

Upadravas (minor diseases) are four—first that arising from cold, second from heat, third from shalya (foreign body) and the fourth from kshāra (alkali, cautery etc.) (195).

स्थावरं जङ्गमं चैव कृत्रिमं च त्रिधा विषम् ॥ १९६ ॥
तेषां च कालकूटाद्यैर्नवधा स्थावरं विषम् । जङ्गमं बहुधा प्रोक्तं तत्र लूता भुजङ्गमाः ॥ १९७ ॥
वृश्चिका मूषिकाः कीटाः प्रत्येकं ते चतुर्विधाः । दंष्ट्राविषं नखविषं वालशृङ्गास्थिभिस्तथा ॥१९८॥
मूत्रात्पुरीषाच्छुक्राच्च दृष्टेर्निश्वासतस्तथा । लालायाः स्पर्शतस्तद्वत्तथा शङ्काविषं मतम् ॥ १९९ ॥
कृत्रिमं द्विविधं प्रोक्तं गरदूषीविभेदतः । सप्तधातुविषं ज्ञेयं तथा सप्तोपधातुजम् ॥ २०० ॥
तथैवोपविषेभ्यश्च जातं सप्तविधं मतम् । दुष्टनीरविषं चैकं तथैकं दिग्धजं विषम् ॥ २०१ ॥
कपिकच्छूभवा कण्डूर्दुष्टनीरभवा तथा । तथा सूरण कण्डूश्च शोथो भल्लातजस्तथा ॥ २०२ ॥
मदश्चतुर्विधश्चान्यः पूगभङ्गाक्षकोद्रवैः । चतुर्विधोऽन्यो द्रव्याणां फलत्वङ्मूलपत्रजः ॥ २०३ ॥

Viṣarogas (poisons) are three—those produced by sthāvara viṣa (herbs, metals, minerals), jaṅgama viṣa (animal poisons) and kṛtrima (homicidal poisons). Of them, diseases of sthāvara viṣa are nine as from kālakūṭa etc. jaṅgama is of many varieties such as from lūtā (spiders), bhujaṅga (snakes), vṛśchika (scorpion), mūṣikā (mice) and kīṭa (insects) each of four kinds; poisoning occurs from daṃṣtra (teeth), nakha (claws), bāla (hairs), śṛṅga (horns), asthi (bones), mūtra (urine), purīṣa (faeces), shukra (semen), dṛṣṭi (sight), niśwāsa (respiration), lālā (saliva),. sparsha (touch) and shaṅkā viṣa (pseudo poisoning, poisoning fright). Kṛtrima viṣa (homicidal poisoning) is of two kinds, viz., gara and dūṣī viṣa; Dhātuja and upadhātuja viṣas (poisons from the metals and minerals) are seven each. Like wise seven are the diseases from upaviṣas; disease arising from drinking of polluted water, disease produced by poisoned weapons—are one each.

Kaṇḍū (itching) are those produced by kapikacchu, polluted and poisoned water, sūraṇakanda and shotha produced by bhallātaka.

Mada (intoxication) are four—one each from consuming of pūga, bhaṅga, aksha and kodrava, like wise are from consuming phala (fruit), twak (bark), mūla (root) and patra (leaves) of poisonous plants) (196-203).

इति प्रसिद्धा गणिता ये किलोपद्रवा भुवि । असंख्याश्चापरे धातुमूलजीवादिसंभवाः ॥ २०४ ॥

Thus are enumerated the diseases which are popularly known, innumerable are the diseases which are produced by various other causes, such as dhātu (metals and minerals), mūla (roots), jīva (animals) etc. (204).

इति श्रीदामोदरसूनुना शार्ङ्गधरेण विरचितायां शार्ङ्गधरसंहितायां निदानरोगगणनाध्यायः ॥

Thus ends the seventh chapter.

इति शार्ङ्गधरसंहितायां पूर्वखण्डः समाप्तः ।

Here ends the first section of Śārṅgadhara Saṃhitā.

MADHYAMA KHAṆḌA

(Second Section)

प्रथमोऽध्यायः

CHAPTER I

अथ स्वरसाध्यायः

Swarasa Adhyāya

अथातः स्वरसः कल्कः क्वाथश्च हिमफाण्टकौ । ज्ञेयाः कषायाः पञ्चैते लघवः स्युर्यथोत्तरम् ॥ १ ॥

Swarasa (fresh juice), kalka (wet bolus), qwātha (decoction), hima (cold infusion), phāṇṭa (hot infusion)—are called the pañcha kaṣāyas, the succeeding ones are laghu (easily digestible) than the preceding (1).

आहतात्तत्क्षणाकृष्टाद्द्रव्यात्क्षुण्णात्समुद्धरेत् । वस्त्रनिष्पीडितो यः स रसः स्वरस उच्यते ॥ २ ॥

The juice extracted from a fresh green drug by pounding it and squeezing through cloth, is called swarasa (pure juice, native juice, extract) (2).

कुडवं चूर्णितं द्रव्यं क्षिप्तं च द्विगुणे जले । अहोरात्र-स्थितं तस्माद्भवेद्वा रसः उत्तमः ॥ ३ ॥

One kuḍava of powder of a dry drug put in twice its quantity of water, kept over for a day and night, then filtered is also a good swarasa (3).

आदाय शुष्कद्रव्यं वा स्वरसानामसंभवे । जलेऽष्टगुणिते साध्यं पादशिष्टं च गृह्यते ॥ ४ ॥

In case of drugs which are very dry and which do not give out any juice, boiling them in eight times their quantity of water and reducing to a quarter can also be used as swarasa (4).

स्वरसस्य गुरुत्वाच्च पलमर्धं प्रयोजयेत् । निशोषितं चाग्निसिद्धं पलमात्रं रसं पिबेत् ॥ ५ ॥

Swarasa (pure juice) being guru (hard to digest), its dose should be half pala per time and one pala if it is extracted after boiling (5).

प्रक्षेपप्रमाणम्—

मधु श्वेता गुडं क्षारान् जीरकं लवणं तथा । घृतं तैलं च चूर्णादीन्कोलमात्रान्द्रसे क्षिपेत् ॥ ६ ॥

Madhu (honey), sharkarā (sugar), guḍa (jaggery), kshāra (alkalies), jīrāka, lavaṇa, ghṛta (ghee), taila (oil) or any powder if required to be added should be one kola each in quantity (6).

अमृतास्वरसः—

स यथा-अमृताया रसः क्षौद्रयुक्तः सर्वप्रमेहजित् । हरिद्राचूर्णयुक्तो वा रसो धात्र्याः समाक्षिकः ॥ ७ ॥

The swarasa of amṛtā along with honey cures all kinds of prameha (polyuria); likewise is the juice of dhātrī mixed with powder of haridrā or honey (7).

रक्तपित्तादिषु वासकादिस्वरसः—

वासकः स्वरसः पेयो मधुना रक्तपित्तजित् । ज्वरकासक्षयहरः कामलाश्लेष्मपित्तहा ॥ ८ ॥

Swarasa of vāsaka taken with honey relieves raktapitta (purpura), jwara (fever), kāsa (cough), kshaya (consumption), kāmalā (jaundice) and mitigates kapha and pitta (8).

त्रिफलाया रसः क्षौद्रयुक्तो दार्वीरसोऽथ वा । निम्बस्य वा गुडूच्या वा पीतो जयति कामलाम् ॥९॥

Swarasa of triphalā, dārvī, nimba or guḍuchī taken with honey cures kāmalā (jaundice) (9).

विषमज्वरे तुलसीद्रोणपुष्पीस्वरसौ—

पीतो मरिचचूर्णेन तुलसीपत्रजो रसः । द्रोणपुष्पीरसो वापि निहन्ति विषमज्वरान् ॥ १० ॥

Swarasa of leaves of tulasī or droṇapuṣpī taken along with powder of maricha cures viṣama jwaras (intermittent fevers) (10).

रक्तातिसारे जम्ब्वादिस्वरसः—

जम्ब्वाम्रामलकीनां च पल्लवोत्थो रसो जयेत् । मध्वाज्यक्षीरसंयुक्तो रक्तातीसारमुल्बणम् ॥ ११ ॥

Swarasa of the tender leaves of jambu, āmra, āmalaka taken with honey, ghee and milk relieves even severe raktātisāra (bloody diarrhoea) (11).

बब्बूल-स्योनाक-कुटजस्वरसाः—

स्थूलबब्बूलिकापत्ररसः पानाद्व्यपोहति । सर्वातिसारान्स्योनाककुटजत्वग्रसोऽथवा ॥ १२ ॥

Swarasa of leaves of sthūla babbūla or the extract of bark of syonāka and kuṭaja cures all kinds of atisāras (diarrhoeas) (12).

प्रतिश्यायै-आर्द्रकस्वरसः—

आर्द्रकस्वरसः क्षौद्रयुक्तो वृषणवातनुत् । श्वासकासारुचीर्हन्ति प्रतिश्यायं व्यपोहति ॥ १३ ॥

Rasa of ārdraka mixed with honey relieves vṛṣaṇa vāta (orchitis), śwāsa (dyspnoea), kāsa (cough), aruchi (loss of taste) and pratishyāya (rhinitis) (13).

पार्श्वादिशूलेषु-बीजपूरस्वरसः—

बीजपूररसः पानान्मधुक्षारयुतो जयेत् । पार्श्वहृद्बस्तिशूलानि कोष्ठवायुं च दारुणम् ॥ १४ ॥

Swarasa of bījapūra taken with honey and kshāras (alkalies) relieves pain of the pārshva (flanks), hṛt (heart), basti (bladder) and koṣṭhavāta (tympanitis) however severe (14).

पित्तशूले-शतावरीस्वरसः—

शतावर्याश्च मधुना पित्तशूलहरो रसः । निशाचूर्णयुतः कन्यारसः प्लीहापचीहरः ॥ १५ ॥

Swarasa of shatāvarī taken with honey relieves pittashūla (colic due to pitta), rasa of kanyā with powder of nishā relieves plīhā (splenic disorders) and apachī (scrofula) (15).

अथालम्बुषास्वरस अपच्यादौ—

अलम्बुषायाः स्वरसः पीतो द्विपलमात्रया । अपचीगण्डमालानां कामलायाश्च नाशनः ॥ १६ ॥

Swarasa of alambuṣā two palas—relieves apachī, gaṇḍamālā (scrofula, lymphadenoma) and kāmalā (jaundice) (16).

मुण्डीस्वरसः-सूर्यावर्तार्धशीर्षव्यथादौ—

रसो मुण्ड्याः सकोष्णो वा मरिचैरेव धूलितः । जयेत्सप्तदिनाभ्यासात्सूर्यावर्तार्धभेदकौ ॥ १७ ॥

Swarasa of muṇḍī, warmed and taken with powder of maricha, relieves sūryāvarta (migraine) and ardhāvabheda (hemicrania) within seven days (17).

अथोन्मादादौ-ब्राह्मयादिस्वरसः—

ब्राह्मीकूष्माण्डषड्ग्रन्थाशङ्खिनीस्वरसाः पृथक् । मधुकुष्ठयुताः पीताः सर्वोन्मादापहारिणः ॥ १८ ॥

Swarasa of brāhmī, kūṣmāṇḍa, ṣaḍgrantha or shaṅkhinī taken with powder of kuṣṭha and honey relieves all varieties of unmāda (insanity) (18).

कोद्रवमदे—कूष्माण्डस्वरसः—

कूष्माण्डकस्य स्वरसो गुडेन सह योजितः । दुष्टकोद्रवसंजातमदं पानाद्व्यपोहति ॥ १९ ॥

Swarasa of kūṣmāṇḍa taken with guḍa (jaggery) relieves the intoxication of kodrava (19).

गाङ्गेरुकीस्वरसमाह व्रणे—

खड्गादिच्छिन्नगात्रस्य तत्कालं पूरितो व्रणः । गाङ्गेरुकीमूलरसैर्जायते गतवेदनः ॥ २० ॥

Swarasa of roots of gāṅgerukī poured over an ulcer caused by a sharp weapon relieves the pain immediately and helps healing (20).

पुटपाकविधिः—

पुटपाकस्य कल्कस्य स्वरसो गृह्यते यतः । अतस्तु पुटपाकानां युक्तिरत्रोच्यते मया ॥ २१ ॥

Further on I will describe the *puṭapāka vidhi* since the juices taken out by this method is also considered as swarasa (21).

पुटपाकस्य मात्रेयं लेपस्याङ्गारवर्णता । लेपं च द्व्यङ्गुलं स्थूलं कुर्याद्वाङ्गुष्ठमात्रकम् ॥ २२ ॥

A ball of mud holding within it the kalka (paste) of drugs is put into fire and removed when it has become red hot. The thickness of the layer of mud should be two aṅgulis (fingers) or two aṅguṣṭhas (thumbs) (22).

काश्मरीवटजम्ब्वादिपत्रैर्वेष्टनमुत्तमम् । पलमात्रो रसो ग्राह्यः कर्षमात्रं मधु क्षिपेत् ॥ २३ ॥
कल्कचूर्णद्रवाद्यास्तु देयाः स्वरसवद्बुधैः ।

It is better to wrap the paste of drugs with leaves of kāshmarī, vaṭa, jambu, etc. The juice should be taken in dose of one pala to which is added one karṣa of honey and the proportion of kalka (paste), chūrṇa (powders) or other liquids if to be added shall be the same as described earlier under swarasa (23½).

कुटजपुटपाक अतिसारे—

स यथा—तत्कालाकृष्टकुटजत्वचं तण्डुलवारिणा ॥ २४ ॥
पिष्टां चतुष्पलमितां जम्बूपल्लववेष्टिताम् । सूत्रेण बद्धां गोधूमपिष्टेन परिवेष्टिताम् ॥ २५ ॥
लिप्तां च घनपङ्केन गोमयैर्वह्निना दहेत् । अङ्गारवर्णां च मृदं दृष्ट्वा वह्नेः समुद्धरेत् ॥ २६ ॥
ततो रसं गृहीत्वा च शीतं क्षौद्रयुतं पिबेत् । जयेत्सर्वानतीसारान्दुस्तरान्सुचिरोत्थितान् ॥२७॥

Four palas of fresh bark of kuṭaja made into a thick paste with taṇḍulodaka (rice-wash) is wrapped with tender leaves of jambu, tied with thread over this ball. One layer each of paste of godhūma and mud is made, later slightly dried in sun, put into the fire of cowdung heaps. When the layer of mud becomes red hot the ball is taken out, layers removed and juice of the drug inside is squeezed out. This juice administered with honey cures all varieties of atisāra (diarrhoeas) however severe or longstanding (24–27).

कण्डितं तण्डुलपलं जलेऽष्टगुणिते क्षिपेत् । भावयित्वा जलं ग्राह्यं देयं सर्वत्र कर्मसु ॥ २८ ॥

Taṇḍula jala (rice-wash) is obtained by soaking and squeezing one pala of broken rice in eight times its quantity of water (28).

अतीसारे—अरलुपुटपाकः—

अरलुत्वक्कृतश्चैव पुटपाकोऽग्निदीपनः । मधुमोचरसाभ्यां च युक्तः सर्वातिसारजित् ॥ २९ ॥

Puṭapāka rasa of the bark of aralu mixed with honey and mocharasa is dīpana (improves digestion) and cures all atisāras (diarrhoeas) (29).

सर्वातीसारे-तित्तिरपुटपाकः—

न्यग्रोधादेश्च कल्केन पूरयेद्गौरतित्तिरेः । निरन्त्रमुदरं सम्यक्पुटपाकेन तत्पचेत् ॥ ३० ॥
तत्कल्कस्य रसः क्षौद्रयुक्तः सर्वातिसारनुत् ।

Paste of the leaves of nyagrodha is to be filled into the abdomen of a yellow tittira bird whose internal organs have been removed. It is then subjected to puṭapāka. The juice taken out later and used with honey relieves all varieties of atisāra (diarrhoea) (30½).

अतीसारविशेषे दाडिमीपुटपाकमाह—

पुटपाकेन विपचेत्सुपक्वं दाडिमीफलम् ॥ ३१ ॥
तद्रसो मधुसंयुक्तः सर्वातीसारनाशनः ।

A ripe fruit of dāḍima is subjected to puṭapāka and its juice used with honey relieves all atisāras (31).

अथ बीजपूरादिपुटपाकश्छर्द्याम्—

बीजपूराम्रजम्बूनां पल्लवानि जटाः पृथक् ॥ ३२ ॥
विपचेत्पुटपाकेन क्षौद्रयुक्तश्च तद्रसः । छर्दिं निवारयेद्घोरां सर्वदोषसमुद्भवाम् ॥ ३३ ॥

Puṭapāka rasa of tender leaves and roots of bījapūra, āmra, jambu taken with honey relieves even severe vomitings due to increase of all the tridoṣas (32–33).

रक्तपित्तादौ—वासापुटपाकमाह—

पिष्टानां वृषपत्राणां पुटपाकरसो हिमः । मधुयुक्तो जयेद्रक्तपित्तकासज्वरक्षयान् ॥ ३४ ॥

Juice of leaves of vṛṣa (vāsaka) with honey relieves raktapitta (purpura), kāsa (cough), jwara (fever) and kshaya (consumption) (34).

अथ कण्टकारीपुटपाकः कासश्वासादौ—

पचेत्क्षुद्रां सपञ्चाङ्गां पुटपाकेन तद्रसः । पिप्पलीचूर्णसंयुक्तः कासश्वासकफापहः ॥ ३५ ॥

The entire plant of kshudrā (kaṇṭakārī) is subjected to puṭapāka, juice from it taken with powder of pippalī is good for kāsa, śwāsa and kapha (35).

अथ बिभीतकपुटपाकः कासादौ—

बिभीतकफलं किंचिद्घृतेनाभ्यज्य लेपयेत् । गोधूमपिष्टेनाङ्गारैर्विपचेत्पुटपाकवत् ॥ ३६ ॥
ततः पक्वं समुद्धृत्य त्वचं तस्य मुखे क्षिपेत् । कासश्वासप्रतिश्यायस्वरभङ्गाञ्जयेत्ततः ॥ ३७ ॥

Vibhītakī is smeared with little ghee, given a covering of the paste of godhūma and cooked as a puṭapāka. Its outer rind thus cooked, held in the mouth relieves kāsa (cough), śwāsa (dyspnoea), pratishyāya (running in the nose) and swarabhaṅga (loss of voice, hoarseness) (36–37)

अथ शुण्ठीपुटपाक आमातीसारादौ—

चूर्णं किंचिद्घृताभ्यक्तं शुण्ठ्या एरण्डजैर्दलैः । वेष्टितं पुटपाकेन विपचेन्मन्दवह्निना ॥ ३८ ॥
तत उद्धृत्य तच्चूर्णं ग्राह्यं प्रातः सितान्वितम् । तेन यान्ति शमं पीडा आमातीसारसंभवाः ॥ ३९ ॥

Powder of shuṇṭhī mixed with a little quantity of ghee, rolled inside the leaves of eraṇḍa and subjected to puṭapāka in mild fire. This chūrṇa taken in the morning with equal quantity of sugar relieves troubles of āmatisāra (dirrhoea due to indigestion) (38–39).

अथ शुण्ठीपुटपाकः आमवातादौ—

शुण्ठीकल्कं विनिक्षिप्य रसैरेरण्डमूलजैः । विपचेत्पुटपाकेन तद्रसः क्षौद्रसंयुतः ॥ ४० ॥
आमवातसमुद्भूतां पीडां जयति दुस्तराम् ।

Paste of shunṭhī with juice of erandamūla is subjected to puṭapāka. This juice taken with honey relieves the troubles of āmavāta (rheumatism) however severe ($40\frac{1}{2}$).

सूरणपुटपाकः अर्शोरोगे—

सौरणं कन्दमादाय पुटपाकेन पाचयेत् ॥ ४१ ॥
सतैललवणस्तस्य रसश्चार्शोविकारनुत् ।

Puṭapāka rasa of sūraṇakanda taken with taila (oil) and lavaṇa (salt) relieves arshas (haemorrhoids) (41).

अथ मृगशृङ्गपुटपाकः शूलादौ—

शरावसंपुटे दग्धं शृङ्गं हरिणजं पिबेत् ॥ ४२ ॥
गव्येन सर्पिषा युक्तं हृच्छूलं नाशयेद्‌ध्रुवम् ।

Pieces of stag's horn are put inside two earthen saucers sealed with mud and subjected to puṭapāka. This used with cow's ghee relieves hṛtshūla (heart pain) quickly (42).

इति श्रीशार्ङ्गधरसंहितायां चिकित्सास्थाने स्वरसादिकल्पनाध्यायः ॥ १ ॥

Thus ends the first chapter.

द्वितीयोऽध्यायः

CHAPTER 2

Qwātha Kalpanā (Decoctions, Infusions)

पानीयं षोडशगुणं क्षुण्णे द्रव्यपले क्षिपेत् । मृत्पात्रे क्वाथयेद्ग्राह्यमष्टमांशावशेषितम् ॥ १ ॥
तज्जलं पाययेद्धीमान्कोष्णं मृद्वग्निसाधितम् । शृतः क्वाथः कषायश्च निर्यूहः स निगद्यते ॥ २ ॥
आहाररसपाके च संजाते द्विपलोन्मितम् । वृद्धवैद्योपदेशेन पिबेत्क्वाथं सुपाचितम् ॥ ३ ॥

One pala of coarsely powdered drug is boiled with 16 parts of water in an earthen pot, over a mild fire till the liquid is reduced to 1/8 of the original quantity. This liquid is known as shṛta, qwātha, kaṣāya or niryūha (decoction). Ancient physicians advise its administration after the digestion of food in doses of 2 palas, per time, slightly warmed (1–3).

क्वाथे क्षिपेत्सितामंशैश्चतुर्थाष्टमषोडशैः । वातपित्तकफातङ्के विपरीतं मधु स्मृतम् ॥ ४ ॥

Sugar may be added to the decoction in doses of 1/4, 1/8 and 1/16 part respectively for vāta, pitta and kapha disorders; if honey is to be added it should be in the reverse order of proportion (4).

जीरकं गुग्गुलं क्षारं लवणं च शिलाजतु । हिङ्गु त्रिकटुकं चैव क्काथे शाणोन्मितं क्षिपेत् ॥ ५ ॥

Jīraka, guggulu, kshāra, lavaṇa, shilājatu, hiṅgu or trikaṭu are to be added in proportion of one shāṇa each (5).

क्षीरं घृतं गुडं तैलं मूत्रं चान्यद्द्रवं तथा । कल्कं चूर्णादिकं क्काथे निक्षिपेत्कर्षसंमितम् ॥ ६ ॥

Milk, ghee, jaggery, oil, cow's urine or any other liquid, kalka (paste) or powder are to be added in doses of one karṣa each (6).

(अपिधानमुखे पात्रे जलं दुर्जरतां व्रजेत् । तस्मादावरणं त्यक्त्वा क्काथादीनां विनिश्चयः ॥७॥)

The earthen pot should not be covered with a lid while preparing the decoction; by doing so the decoction will not become easily digestible (7).

सर्वज्वरे गुडूच्यादिक्काथः—

स यथा—गुडूचीधान्यकारिष्टरक्तचन्दनपद्मकैः । गुडूच्यादिगणक्काथः सर्वज्वरहरः स्मृतः ॥ ८ ॥
दीपनो दाहहृल्लासतृष्णाछर्द्यरुचीर्जयेत् ।

Qwātha of guḍūchi, dhānyaka, ariṣṭa, raktachandana and padmaka (gudūchyādi gaṇa qwātha) cures all varieties of fevers, is dīpana (stomachic) and relieves dāha (burning sensation), hṛllāsa (nausea), tṛṣnā (thirst), chardi (vomiting) and aruchi (anorexia) (8).

नागरं देवकाष्ठं च धान्यकं बृहतीद्वयम् । दद्यात्पाचनकं पूर्वं ज्वरितानां ज्वरापहम् ॥
क्षुद्रा किराततिक्तं च शुण्ठी छिन्ना च पौष्करम् । कषाय एषां शमयेत्पीतश्चाष्टविधं ज्वरम् ॥
गुडूचीपिप्पलीमूलनागरैः पाचनं स्मृतम् ॥ ९ ॥
दद्याद्वातज्वरे पूर्णालङ्घे सप्तमवासरे । शालिपर्णी बला द्राक्षा गुडूची सारिवा तथा ॥ १० ॥
आसां क्काथं पिबेत्कोष्णं तीव्रवातज्वरच्छिदम् । काश्मरीसारिवाद्राक्षात्रायमाणामृताभवः ॥ ११ ॥
कषायः सगुडः पीतो वातज्वरविनाशनः । कट्फलेन्द्रयवापाठातिक्तामुस्तैः श्रृतं जलम् ॥ १२ ॥
पाचनं दशमेऽह्नि स्यात्तीव्रे पित्तज्वरे नृणाम् । पर्पटो वासकस्तिक्ता कैरातो धन्वयासकः ॥ १३ ॥
प्रियङ्गुश्च कृतः क्काथ एषां शर्करया युतः । पिपासादाहपित्तास्रयुतं पित्तज्वरं जयेत् ॥ १४ ॥
द्राक्षा हरीतकी मुस्तं कटुकी कृतमालकः । पर्पटश्च कृतः क्काथ एषां पित्तज्वरापहः ॥ १५ ॥
तृण्मूर्च्छादाहपित्तास्रक्शमनो भेदनः स्मृतः । (एकः पर्पटकः श्रेष्ठः पित्तज्वरविनाशनः ॥ १६ ॥
(किं पुनर्यदि युज्येत चन्दनोशीरवालकैः ।)

Qwātha of nāgara, devakāṣṭha, dhānyaka, two bṛhatis, is pāchana (digestive), and relieves jwaras (fevers) if given in the early stages (8½).

Qwātha of kṣhudrā (kaṇṭakāri), kirātatiktā, shuṇṭhī, chinnā and puṣkaramūla—mitigates all the eight kinds of jwaras.

Qwātha of guḍūchi, pippalimūla and nāgara is pāchana (digestive) and so can be given on the seventh day of vāta jwara (9).

Qwātha of shāliparṇī, balā, drākshā, guḍūchī and sārivā taken warm cures severe vāta jwaras (10).

Qwātha of kāshmarī, sārivā, drākshā, trayamāṇā and amṛtā—taken with jaggery cures vāta jwara (11).

Qwātha of kaṭphala, indrayava, pāṭhā, tiktā, mustā is given as a pāchana (digestive) on the tenth day of severe pittajwara (12).

Qwātha of parpaṭa, vāsaka, tiktā, kirāta, dhanwayāsaka and priyaṅgu-taken with sugar relieves pipāsā (thirst), dāha (burning sensation) and pitta-jwara associated with rakta pitta (13).

Qwātha of drākshā, harītakī, mustā, kaṭukī, kṛtamālaka and parpaṭa-relieves pittajwara (fevers), tṛṭ (thirst), mūrchā (faint), dāha (burning), raktapitta and acts as a bhedana (purgative) (15).

Qwātha of parpaṭaka alone is capable of curing pittajwara, what to tell, when it is taken along with chandana, ushīra and vālaka (cures it more efficiently) (16).

अथ बीजपूरादिः श्लेष्मज्वरे—

बीजपूरशिफापथ्यानागरग्रन्थिकैः शृतम् ॥ १७ ॥
सक्षारं पाचनं श्लेष्मज्वरे द्वादशवासरे ।

Qwātha of roots of bījapūra, pathyā, nāgara, and granthika taken with kshāra is a pāchana (digestive) and useful in kapha jwara (phlegmatic fevers) of twelve days (17–18).

कफज्वरे—भूनिम्बादिक्काथः—

भूनिम्बनिम्बपिप्पल्यः शठी शुण्ठी शतावरी ॥ १८ ॥
गुडूची बृहती चेति क्काथो हन्यात्कफज्वरम् । पटोलत्रिफलातिक्ताशठीवासामृताभवः ॥ १९ ॥
क्काथो मधुयुतः पीतो हन्यात्कफकृतं ज्वरम् ।

Qwātha of bhūnimba, nimba, pippalī, shaṭhī, shuṇṭhī, shatāvarī, guḍūchī and bṛhatī cures kapha jwaras (phlegmatic fevers). Qwātha of paṭola, triphalā, tiktā, shaṭhī, vasā and amṛtā—taken with honey cures kapha jwara (18–20).

वातपित्तज्वरे—पञ्चभद्रक्काथः—

पर्पटाब्दामृताविश्वकैरातैः साधितं जलम् ॥ २० ॥
पञ्चभद्रमिदं ज्ञेयं वातपित्तज्वरापहम् ।

Qwātha prepared out of parpaṭa, abda, amṛtā, vishwa and kirāta—is known as *pañcha bhadra qwātha.* It relieves vāta-pitta jwara (20–21).

कफवातज्वरादौ लघुक्षुद्रादिक्वाथः—

क्षुद्राशुण्ठीगुडूचीनां कषायः पौष्करस्य च ॥ २१ ॥
कफवाताधिके पेयो ज्वरे वापि त्रिदोषजे। कासश्वासारुचिहरे पार्श्वशूलविनाशनः ॥ २२ ॥

Qwātha of kshudrā, shuṇṭhī, guḍūchī and puṣkara is beneficial in kapha-vāta-jwara and even tridoṣaja jwara (fevers), kāsa (cough), śwāsa (dyspnoea), aruchi (anorexia) and pārshwa shūla (pain in the flanks) (21-22).

वातकफज्वरादौ आरग्वधादिक्वाथः—

आरग्वधकणामूलमुस्तातिक्ताभयाकृतः। क्वाथः शमयति क्षिप्रं ज्वरं वातकफोद्भवम् ॥ २३ ॥
आमशूलप्रशमनो भेदी दीपनपाचनः।

Qwātha of āragwadha, kaṇāmūla, mustā, tiktā and abhayā relieves vāta-kapha-jwara (fevers) and āmashūla (colic due to indigestion) quickly and acts as bhedī (laxative), dīpana and pāchana (carminative and digestive) (23–24).

पित्तश्लेष्मज्वरे—अमृताष्टकम्—

अमृतारिष्टकटुकामुस्तेन्द्रयवनागरैः ॥ २४ ॥
पटोलचन्दनाभ्यां च पिप्पलीचूर्णयुक्शृतम्। अमृताष्टकमेतच्च पित्तश्लेष्मज्वरापहम् ॥ २५ ॥
छर्द्यरोचकहृल्लासदाहतृष्णाविनाशनम्।

Qwātha of amṛtā, ariṣṭa, kaṭuka, mustā, indrayava, nāgara, paṭola and chandana is known as *Amṛtāṣṭaka qwātha.* Taken with the powder of pippalī it is beneficial for pitta shleṣma jwara (fevers), chardi (vomiting), arochaka (anorexia), hṛllāsa (nausea), dāha (burning) and tṛṣṇā (thirst) (24–25).

(पटोलं चन्दनं मूर्वातिक्तापाठामृतागणः ॥ २६ ॥
पित्तश्लेष्मज्वरच्छर्दिदाहकण्डूविषापहः।

सर्वज्वरादौ—कण्टकारिक्वाथः—

कण्टकारिद्वयं शुण्ठी धान्यकं सुरदारु च ॥ २७ ॥
एभिः शृतं पाचनं स्यात्सर्वज्वरविनाशनम्।

Qwātha of paṭola, chandana, mūrvā, tiktā, pāṭhā and amṛtā relieves pitta shleṣma jwara (fevers), chardi (vomiting), dāha (burning), kaṇḍū (itching) and viṣa (poisoning).

Qwātha of the two kaṇṭakārīs, shuṇṭhī, dhānyaka and suradāru is pāchana (digestive) and cures all types of jwara (fevers) (26–28).

अथ दशमूलक्वाथः वातश्लेष्मज्वरे—

शालिपर्णीपृष्टिपर्णीबृहतीद्वयगोक्षुरैः ॥ २८ ॥
बिल्वाग्निमन्थस्योनाककाश्मरीपाटलायुतैः। दशमूलमिति ख्यातं कथितं तज्जलं पिबेत् ॥ २९ ॥
पिप्पलीचूर्णसंयुक्तं वातश्लेष्मज्वरापहम्। सन्निपातज्वरहरं सूतिकादोषनाशनम् ॥ ३० ॥
शोषशैत्यभ्रमस्वेदकासश्वासविकारनुत्। हृत्कण्ठग्रहपार्श्वार्तितन्द्रामस्तकशूलहृत् ॥ ३१ ॥

Qwātha of shāliparṇī, pṛṣṭhīparṇī, the two bṛhatis, gokshura, bilwa, agnimantha, syonāka, kāshmarī and pāṭalā is known as *Dashamūla qwātha.* Taken with powder of pippalī it relieves vāta shleṣma jwara, sannipāta jwara (toxic fevers), sūtika doṣa (post-natal disorders), shoṣa (consumption), shaitya (coldness), bhrama (giddiness), sweda (perspiration), kāsa (cough), śwāsa (dyspnoea), disorders of hṛdaya (heart) and kaṇṭha (throat); pārshwā rti (pain of the flanks), tandrā (drowsiness) and mastaka shūla (headache) (28–31).

अथाभयादिक्वाथस्त्रिदोषादौ—

अभयामुस्तधान्याकरक्तचन्दनपद्मकैः । वासकेन्द्रयवोशीरगुडूचीकृतमालकैः ॥ ३२ ॥
पाठानागरतिक्ताभिः पिप्पलीचूर्णयुक्शृतम् । पिबेत्रिदोषज्वरजितिपिपासाकासदाहनुत् ॥ ३३ ॥
प्रलापश्वासतन्द्राघ्नं दीपनं पाचनं परम् । विण्मूत्रानिलविष्टम्भवमिशोषारुचिं जयेत् ॥ ३४ ॥

Qwātha of abhayā, musta, dhānyaka, raktachandana, padmaka, vāsaka, indrayava, ushīra, guḍūchī, kṛtamālaka, pāṭhā, nāgara and tiktā—taken with powder of pippalī relieves tridoṣaja jwara (fevers), pipāsā (thirst), kāsa (cough), dāha (burning), pralāpa (delirium), śwāsa (dyspnoea), tandrā (stupor), viṣṭambha of purīṣa, mūtra and anila (obstruction of faeces, urine and flatus), vami (vomiting), shoṣa (consumption), aruchi (anorexia) and is a good dīpana pāchana (carminative, digestive) (32–34).

(पिप्पलीपिप्पलीमूलचव्यचितकनागरैः । वचासातिविषाजाजीपाठावत्सकरेणुकैः ॥ ३५ ॥)
किराततिक्तकं मूर्वा सर्षपा मरिचानि च । कटुकं पुष्करं भार्ङ्गी विडङ्गं कर्कटाह्वयम् ॥ ३६ ॥
अर्कमूलं बृहत्सिंही श्रेयसी सदुरालभा । दीप्यकं चाजमोदा च शुकनासादिहिङ्गुभिः ॥ ३७ ॥
एतानि समभागानि गणोऽष्टविंशको मतः । कषायमुपभुञ्जीत वातश्लेष्मज्वरापहम् ॥ ३८ ॥
हन्ति वातं तथा शीतं छेदजं प्रबलं कफम् । प्रलापं चातिनिद्रां च रोमहर्षारुची तथा ॥ ३९ ॥
महावातेऽपतन्त्रे च सर्वगात्रे च शून्यताम् । अयं सर्वज्वरान्हन्ति सन्निपातांस्त्रयोदश ॥ ४० ॥

Qwātha of equal parts of pippalī, pippalīmūla, chavya, chitraka, nāgara, vachā, ativiṣā, ajajī, pāṭhā, vatsaka, reṇuka, kirātatiktā, mūrvā, sarṣapa, maricha, kaṭuka, puṣkara, bhārṅgī, viḍaṅga, karkaṭa, arkamūla, bṛhatsiṃhī, shreyasī, durālabha, dīpyaka, ajamodā, shukanāśa and hiṅgu—is known as *Aṣṭa viṃshaka gaṇa qwātha.* It relieves vāta sleṣma jwara (fevers), mitigates vāta, shīta (coldness) produced by excessive sweating, pralāpa (delirium), atinidrā (excess sleep), romaharṣa (horripilations), aruchi (anorexia), mahāvāta (tetanus), apatantra (tetanus), shūnya gātra (unconciousness) and all kinds of fevers including thirteen types of sannipāta jwaras (toxic fevers) (35–40).

अथ सन्निपातज्वरे अष्टादशाङ्गक्काथः—

कैरातकटुकीमुस्ताधान्येन्द्रयवनागरैः। दशमूलमहादारुगजपिप्पलिकायुतैः ॥ ४१ ॥
कृतः कषायः पार्श्वार्तिसन्निपातज्वरं जयेत्। कासश्वासवमीहिक्कातन्द्राहृद्ग्रहनाशनः ॥ ४२ ॥

Qwātha of kirāta, kaṭukī, mustā, dhānya, indrayava, nāgara, dashamūlas mahādāru and gajapippalī—made into decoction relieves pārshwārti (pain in the flanks), sannipāta jwaras (toxic fever), kāsa (cough), śwāsa (dyspnoea), vami (vomiting), hikkā (hiccough), tandrā (drowsiness) and hṛdgraha (pain in the precordium) (41–42).

त्रिदोषजज्वरादौ कट्फलादिक्काथः—

कट्फलाम्बुदभार्ङ्गीभिर्धान्यरोहिषपर्पटैः। वचाहरीतकीशृङ्गीदेवदारुमहौषधैः ॥ ४३ ॥
हिक्कां कासज्वरं हन्ति श्वासश्लेष्मगलग्रहान्। क्काथो जीर्णज्वरं हन्ति गुडूच्याः पिप्पलीयुतः ॥ ४४ ॥

Qwātha of kaṭphala, ambuda, bhārṅgī, dhānya, rohiṣa, parpaṭa, vachā, harītakī, śṛṅgī, devadāru and mahauṣadha—relieves kāsa (cough), jwara (fever), śwāsa (dyspnoea), sleṣma and galagraha (pain in the throat).

Qwātha of guḍūchī taken with pippalī powder cures jīrna jwara (chronic fever) (43–44).

तथा पर्पटजः क्काथः पित्तज्वरहरः परः। किं पुनर्यदि युज्येत चन्दनोदीच्यनागरैः ॥ ४५ ॥

Qwātha of parpaṭa cures pitta jwara (bilious fevers) what to say if it is taken along with chandana, udīchya and nāgara (definitely cures pitta jwara) (45).

अथ निदिग्धिकादिर्जीर्णज्वरे—

निदिग्धिकामृताशुण्ठीकषायं पाययेद्भिषक्। पिप्पलीचूर्णसंयुक्तं श्वासकासार्दितापहम् ॥ ४६ ॥
पीनसारुचिवैस्वर्यशूलाजीर्णज्वरच्छिदम्।

Qwātha of nidigdhika, amṛtā and shunṭhī—taken with powder of pippalī relieves śwāsa (dyspnoea), kāsa (cough), ardita (facial paralysis), pīnasa (rhinitis), aruchi (loss of taste), vaiswarya (defective speech), shūla (colic), jīrṇa jwara (chronic fevers) (46–47).

(देवदारु वचा कुष्ठं पिप्पली विश्वभेषजम् ॥ ४७ ॥
कट्फलं मुस्तभूनिम्बतिक्तधान्या हरीतकी। गजकृष्णा च दुःस्पर्शा गोक्षुरुर्धन्वयासकम् ॥ ४८ ॥
बृहत्यतिविषा छिन्ना कर्कटं कृष्णजीरकम्। क्काथमष्टावशेषं तु प्रसूतां पाययेत्स्त्रियम् ॥ ४९ ॥
शूलकासज्वरश्वासमूर्च्छाकम्पशिरोर्तिजित्।)

Qwātha of devadāru, vachā, kuṣṭha, pippalī, vishwabheṣaja, kaṭphala, musta, bhūnimba, tikta, dhānya, harītakī, gajakṛṣnā, duḥsparshā, gokshura, dhanvayāsaka, bṛhatī, ativiṣā, chinnā, karkaṭa and kṛṣṇa jīraka—decoction of these reduced to one eighth part, if administered to woman who has delivered relieves shūla (colic), kāsa (cough), jwara (fever), śwāsa (dyspnoea), mūrchā (fainting), kampa (tremors) and shirorti (headache) (47–50).

इदानीं विषमज्वरनाशनार्थं योगपञ्चकमाह—

क्षुद्राधान्यकशुण्ठीभिर्गुडूचीमुस्तपद्मकैः ॥ ५० ॥
रक्तचन्दनभूनिम्बपटोलवृषपौष्करैः । कटुकेन्द्रयवाऽरिष्टभार्ङ्गीपर्पटकैः समैः ॥ ५१ ॥
क्वाथं प्रातर्निषेवेत सर्वशीतज्वरच्छिदम् ।

Qwātha of equal parts of kshudrā, dhānyaka, shuṇṭhī, guḍūchī, musta, padmaka, raktachandana, bhūnimba, paṭola, vṛṣa, puṣkara, indrayava, ariṣṭa, bhārṅgī and parpaṭaka—taken in the early morning cures all shīta-jwaras (fevers with rigours) (50–52).

मुस्तक्षुद्रामृताशुण्ठीधात्रीक्वाथः समाक्षिकः ॥ ५२ ॥
पिप्पलीचूर्णसंयुक्तो विषमज्वरनाशनः ।

Qwātha of musta, kshudrā, amṛtā, shuṇṭhī and dhātrī—mixed with honey and powdered pippalī cures viṣama jwaras (intermittent fevers) (53).

पटोलेन्द्रयवादारुत्रिफलामुस्तगोस्तनैः ॥ ५३ ॥
मधुकामृतवासानां क्वाथं क्षौद्रयुतं पिबेत् । संतते सतते चैव द्वितीयकतृतीयके ॥ ५४ ॥
ऐकाहिके वा विषमे दाहपूर्वे नवज्वरे ।

Qwātha of paṭola, indrayava, dāru, triphalā, musta, gostana (drākshā), madhuka, amṛtā and vasā—decoction taken with honey relieves santata, satata, dwitīyaka, tritīyaka and ekāhika varieties of viṣama jwara and dāha pūrvanava jwara (fevers which start suddenly with high temperature) (54–55).

पटोलत्रिफलानिम्बद्राक्षाशम्याकवासकैः ॥ ५५ ॥
क्वाथः सितामधुयुतो जयेदैकाहिकं ज्वरम् ।

Qwātha of paṭola, triphalā, nimba, drākshā, shamyāka (āragwadha) and vāsaka—taken with honey and sugar relieves ekāhika jwara (daily remittent fever) (55–56).

अथ गुडूच्यादिस्तृतीयकज्वरे—

गुडूचीधान्यमुस्ताभिश्चन्दनोशीरनागरैः ॥ ५६ ॥
कृतं क्वाथं पिबेत्क्षौद्रसितायुक्तं ज्वरातुरः । तृतीयज्वरनाशाय तृष्णादाहनिवारणम् ॥ ५७ ॥

Qwātha of guḍūchī, dhānya, musta, chandana, ushīra and nāgara taken with honey and sugar cures tritīyaka jwara, tṛṣṇā (thirst) and dāha (burning) (56–57).

अथ देवदार्वादि चातुर्थिकज्वरे—

देवदारुशिवावासाशालिपर्णीमहौषधैः । धात्रीयुतं शृतं शीतं दद्यान्मधुसितायुतम् ॥ ५८ ॥
चातुर्थिकज्वरे श्वासे कासे मन्दानले तथा ।

Qwātha of devadāru, shivā, vāsā, shāliparṇī, mahauṣadhi and dhātrī taken with honey and sugar relieves chaturthaka jwara (quartan fevers), śwāsa (dyspnoea), kāsa (cough) and mandānala (dyspepsia) (58–59).

अथ बृहद्गुडूच्यादि ज्वरातीसारे—

गुडूचीधान्यकोशीरशुण्ठीवालकपर्पटैः ॥ ५९ ॥
बिल्वप्रतिविषापाठारक्तचन्दनवत्सकैः । किरातमुस्तेन्द्रयवैः क्वथितं शिशिरं पिबेत् ॥ ६० ॥
सक्षौद्रं रक्तपित्तघ्नं ज्वरातीसारनाशनम् ।

Qwātha of guḍūchī, dhānyaka, ushīra, shuṇṭhī, vālaka, parpaṭa, bilwa, prativiṣa, pāṭhā, raktachandana, vatsaka, kirāta, musta and indrayava—taken cold with honey relieves raktapitta (purpura) and jwarātisāra (fever with diarrhoea) (59–61).

अथ नागरादिक्काथो ज्वरातीसारे—

नागरं कुटजो मुस्तममृतातिविषा तथा ॥ ६१ ॥
एभिः कृतं पिबेत्काथं ज्वरातीसारनाशनम् ।

Qwātha of nāgara, kuṭaja, musta, amṛtā and ativiṣā relieves jwarātisāra fevers accompanied by diarrhoea) (61–62).

अथ धान्यपञ्चकक्काथ आमशूलादौ—

धान्यवालकबिल्वाब्दनागरैः साधितं जलम् ॥ ६२ ॥
आमशूलहरं ग्राही दीपनं पाचनं परम् ।

Qwātha of dhānya, vālaka, bilwa, abda and nāgara relieves āmashūla (colic due to indigestion), is grāhī (stops diarrhoea) and dīpana-pāchana (digestive and carminative) (62–63).

धान्यनागरक्काथः पाचने—

धान्यनागरजः क्काथः पाचनो दीपनस्तथा ॥ ६३ ॥
एरण्डमूलयुक्तश्च जयेदामानिलव्यथाम् ।

Qwātha of dhānya and nāgara is carminative and digestive, with eraṇḍa-mūla it relieves troubles of āmānila (rheumatism) (63–64).

अथ वत्सकादिक्काथः सामरक्तातीसारे—

वत्सकातिविषाबिल्वमुस्तवालकजः शृतः ॥ ६४ ॥
अतीसारं जयेत्सामं चिरजं रक्तशूलजित् ।

Qwātha of vatsaka, ativiṣā, bilwa, musta and vālaka relieves āma atisāra (diarrhoea due to indigestion) and pain due to raktātisāra (bloody diarrhoea) (64-65).

अथ कुटजाष्टकं आमरक्तशूलादौ—

कुटजातिविषापाठाधातकीलोध्रमुस्तकैः ॥ ६५ ॥

ह्रीबेरदाडिमयुतैः कृतः क्वाथः समाक्षिकः । पेयो मोचरसेनैव कुटजाष्टकसंज्ञकः ॥ ६६ ॥

अतीसाराञ्जयेद्दाहरक्तशूलामदुस्तरान् ।

Qwātha of kuṭaja, ativiṣā, pāṭhā, dhātakī, lodhra, musta, hrībera and dāḍima is known as *kuṭajāṣṭaka qwātha*—taken with honey and mocharasa it relieves atisāra (diarrhoea) and āmashūla (pain in the abdomen due to indigestion) (65-67).

अथ ह्रीबेरादिक्वाथोऽतीसारे—

ह्रीबेरधातकीलोध्रपाठालज्जालुवत्सकैः ॥ ६७ ॥

धान्यकातिविषामुस्तागुडूचीबिल्वनागरैः । कृतः कषायः शमयेदतीसारं चिरोत्थितम् ॥ ६८ ॥

अरोचकामशूलास्रज्वरघ्नः पाचनः स्मृतः ।

Qwātha of hrībera, dhātakī, lodhra, pāṭhā, lajjālu, vatsaka, dhānyaka, ativiṣā, musta, guḍūchī, bilva and nāgara cures even chronic atisāras (diarrhoeas), arochaka (anorexia), āmashūla (colic), raktashūla (pain of bloody diarrhoeas), jwara (fevers) and is a pāchana (digestive) (67-79).

अथ धातक्यादि क्वाथः बालातीसारे—

धातकीबिल्वरोध्राणि वालकं गजपिप्पली ॥ ६९ ॥

एभिः कृतं श्रृतं शीतं शिशुभ्यः क्षौद्रसंयुतम् । प्रदद्यादवलेहं वा सर्वातीसारशान्तये ॥ ७० ॥

Qwātha of dhātakī, bilwa, rodhra, vālaka and gajapippalī, cooled and given to children with honey relieves all types of atisāras (diarrhoeas) (69-70).

अथ शालिपर्ण्यादिक्वाथो ग्रहण्यां—

शालिपर्णीबलाबिल्वधान्यशुण्ठीकृतः श्रृतः । आध्मानशूलसहितां वातजां ग्रहणीं जयेत् ॥ ७१ ॥

गुडूच्यतिविषाशुण्ठीमुस्तैः क्वाथः कृतो जयेत् । आमानुषक्तां ग्रहणीं ग्राही पाचनदीपनः ॥ ७२ ॥

Qwātha of shāliparṇī, balā, bilwa, dhānya and shuṇṭhī relieves vātaja grahaṇī (sprue) accompanied with ādhmāna (tympanitis) and shūla (colic).

Qwātha of guḍūchī, ativiṣā, shuṇṭhī and musta—relieves āmaja grahaṇī (sprue) and is a grāhī (water absorbant), pāchana (digestive) and dīpana (carminative) (71-72).

अथ इन्द्रयवादिक्वाथः सर्वातीसारे—

यवधान्यपटोलानां क्वाथः सक्षौद्रशर्करः । योज्यः सर्वातिसारेषु बिल्वाम्रास्थिभवस्तथा ॥ ७३ ॥

Qwātha of yava (indrayava), dhānya and paṭola—taken with honey and sugar is useful in all types of atisāra (diarrhoeas); like wise is the qwātha of bilwa and āmrāsthi (pulp of mango seed) (73).

अथ फलादिकाथः कृमिरोगे—

त्रिफला देवदारुश्च मुस्ता मूषककर्णिका । शिग्रूरेतैः कृतः काथः पिप्पलीचूर्णसंयुतः ॥ ७४ ॥
विडङ्गचूर्णयुक्तश्च कृमिघ्नः क्रिमिरोगहा । फलत्रिकामृतातिक्तानिम्बकैरातवासकैः ॥ ७५ ॥
जयेन्मधुयुतः काथः कामलां पाण्डुतां तथा ।

Qwātha of triphalā, devadāru, mustā, mūṣakakarṇī and shīgru taken with powder of pippalī and viḍaṅga is good krimighna (anthelmentic) and cures parasitic diseases (74–75).

Qwātha of triphalā, amṛtā, tiktā, nimba kirāta and vāsaka—decoction taken with honey relieves kāmalā (jaundice) and pāṇḍu (anaemia).

अथ पुनर्नवादिकाथः पाण्डुशोथादौ—

पुनर्नवाभयानिम्बदार्वीतिक्तापटोलकैः ॥ ७६ ॥
गुडूचीनागरयुतैः काथो गोमूत्रसंयुतः । पाण्डुकासोदरश्वासशूलसर्वाङ्गशोथहा ॥ ७७ ॥

Qwātha of punarnavā, abhayā, nimba, dārvī, tiktā, paṭola, guḍūchī and nāgara taken with cow's urine relieves pāṇḍu (anaemia), kāsa (cough), udara (enlargment of abdomen), śwāsa (dyspnoea), shūla (colic) and sarvāṅga shotha (general anasarca) (76–77).

अथ वासादिकाथः रक्तपित्तादौ—

वासाद्राक्षाभयाकाथः पीतः सक्षौद्रशर्करः । निहन्ति रक्तपित्तार्तिश्वासकासान्सुदारुणान् ॥ ७८ ॥

Qwātha of vasā, drākshā and abhayā—taken with honey and sugar cures raktapitta (purpura), śwāsa (dyspnoea) and kāsa (cough) though severe (78).

रक्तपित्तं क्षयं कासं श्लेष्मपित्तज्वरं तथा । केवलो वासककाथः पीतः क्षौद्रेण नाशयेत् ॥ ७९ ॥

Qwātha of vasā alone taken with honey is capable of curing raktapitta (purpura), kshaya (consumption), kāsa (cough) and shleṣma pitta jwara (fever due to kapha and pitta) (79).

कासे योगद्वयमाह

वासाक्षुद्रामृताकाथः क्षौद्रेण ज्वरकासहा । कासघ्नः पिप्पलीचूर्णयुक्तः क्षुद्राश्टतस्तथा ॥८०॥

Qwātha of vasā, kshudrā and amṛtā—taken with honey relieves jwara and kāsa; even so decoction of kshudrā taken with powder of pippalī relieves kāsa (cough) (80).

अथ श्वासकासादौ क्षुद्रक्वाथः—

क्षुद्राकुलत्थवासाभिर्नागरेण च साधितः । क्वाथः पौष्करचूर्णाढ्यः श्वासकासौ निवारयेत् ॥८१॥

Qwātha of kshudrā, kulattha, vasā and nāgara—taken with powder of puṣkaramūla relieves śwāsa (dyspnoea) and kāsa (cough) (81).

अथ हिक्कायां रेणुकादिक्वाथः—

रेणुकापिप्पलीक्वाथो हिङ्गुकल्केन संयुतः । पानादेव हि पञ्चापि हिक्का नाशयति क्षणात् ॥ ८२ ॥

Qwātha of reṇukā and pippali taken with hiṅgu relieves all the five kinds of hikkā (hiccough) immediately (82).

बिल्वत्वचो गुडूच्या वा क्वाथः क्षौद्रेण संयुतः । जयेत्त्रिदोषजां छर्दिं पर्पटः पित्तजां तथा ॥ ८३ ॥

Qwātha of bark of bilwa or guḍūchi taken with honey relieves chardi (vomiting) due to increase of tridoṣas; qwātha of parpaṭa relieves pittaja chardi (vomiting due to increase of pitta) (83).

अथ गृध्रस्यां योगद्वयमाह—

हिङ्गुपुष्करचूर्णाढ्यं दशमूलश्टतं जयेत् । गृध्रसीं केवलः क्वाथः शेफालीपत्रजस्तथा ॥ ८४ ॥

Qwātha of dashamūla taken with hiṅgu and puṣkaramūla powder cures gṛdhrasī (sciatica); like wise is the qwātha of shephālī leaves (84).

रास्नापञ्चकं सप्तधातुगतवाते—

रास्नामृतामहादारुनागरैरण्डजैः श्टतम् । सप्तधातुगते वाते सामे सर्वाङ्गजे पिबेत् ॥ ८५ ॥

Qwātha of rāsnā, amṛtā, mahādāru, nāgara and eraṇḍa is beneficial in vāta disorders of all the seven dhātus and āma accumulation in the entire body (85).

अथ रास्नासप्तकं जङ्घावातादौ—

रास्ना गोक्षुरकैरण्डदेवदारु पुनर्नवा । गुडूच्यारग्वधश्चैव क्वाथमेषां विपाचयेत् ॥ ८६ ॥
शुण्ठीचूर्णेन संयुक्तं पिबेज्जङ्घाकटिग्रहे । पार्श्वपृष्ठोरुपीडायामामवाते सुदुस्तरे ॥ ८७ ॥

Qwātha of rāsnā, gokshura, eraṇḍa, devadāru, punarnavā, guḍūchi and āragwadha—taken with powder of shuṇṭhī can cure pain in jaṅghā (calves), kaṭi (waist), pārshwa (flanks), pṛṣṭha (back), uru (thighs) and sever āmavāta (rheumatism) (86–87).

महारास्नादियोगः सर्ववातरोगे—

रास्ना द्विगुणभागा स्यादेकभागास्ततः परे । धन्वयासबलैरण्डदेवदारुशठीवचाः ॥ ८८ ॥
वासको नागरं पथ्या चव्या मुस्ता पुनर्नवा । गुडूची वृद्धदारुश्च शतपुष्पा च गोक्षुरः ॥ ८९ ॥
अश्वगन्धा प्रतिविषा कृतमालः शतावरी । कृष्णा सहचरश्चैव धान्यकं बृहतीद्वयम् ॥ ९० ॥
एभिः कृतं पिबेत्क्वाथं शुण्ठीचूर्णेन संयुतम् । कृष्णाचूर्णेन वा योगराजगुग्गुलुनाथवा ॥ ९१ ॥

अजमोदादिना वापि तैलेनैरण्डजेन वा । सर्वाङ्गकम्पे कुब्जत्वे पक्षाघातेऽपबाहुके ॥ ९२ ॥
गृध्रस्यामामवाते च श्लीपदे चापतानके । अन्त्रवृद्धौ तथाध्माने जङ्घाजानुगतेऽर्दिते ॥ ९३ ॥
शुक्रामये मेढ्ररोगे वन्ध्यायोन्यामयेषु च । महारास्नादिराख्यातो ब्रह्मणा गर्भकारणम् ॥ ९४ ॥

Dhanwayāsava, balā, eraṇḍa, devadāru, shaṭhī, vachā, vāsaka, nāgara, pathyā, chavyā, mustā, punarnavā, guḍūchī, vṛddhadāru, shatapuṣpā, gokshura, ashwagandhā, prativiṣā, kṛtamāla, shatāvarī, kṛṣṇā, sahachara, dhānyaka, the two bṛhatis—together making up one part and two parts of rāsnā (double the total quantity) are taken and decoction prepared. This known as *Mahā Rāsnādi Qwātha*, expounded by Brahma; taken with powder of shunṭhī, kṛṣṇā, yogarājaguggula, ajamodādi chūrṇa, castor oil, is highly effective in sarvāṅga kampa (tremors of the whole body), kubjatwa (hunch back, kyphosis), pakshāghāta (hemiplegia), apabāhuka (shoulder–hand syndrome), gṛdhrasī (sciatica), āmavāta (rheumatism), shlīpada (filariasis), apatānaka (tetanus), antravṛddhi (hernia), ādhmāna (tympanitis), pain in jaṅghā (calves), jānu (knee); ardita (facial palsy), shukrāmaya (disorders of sperm), medraroga (diseases of penis), vandhyā (sterility), yoniroga (diseases of vagina) and is a garbhakara (helps conception) (88–94).

एरण्डसप्तकं स्तनादिगतवाते—

एरण्डो बीजपूरश्च गोक्षुरो बृहतीद्वयम् । अश्मभेदस्तथा बिल्व पतन्मूलैः कृतः श्रृतः ॥ ९५ ॥
एरण्डतैलहिङ्ग्वाढ्यः सयवक्षारसैन्धवः । स्तनस्कन्धकटीमेढ्रहृदयोत्थां व्यथां जयेत् ॥ ९६ ॥

Qwāṭha of the roots of eraṇḍa, bījapūra, gokshura, the two bṛhatis, ashmabheda, and bilwa—taken with castor oil, hiṅgu, yavakshāra and saindhava relieves the pain of stana (chest), skandha (neck), kaṭi (waist), medra (penis) and hṛdaya (heart) (95–96).

नागरादिर्वातशूलादौ—

नागरैरण्डजः क्वाथः क्वाथो इन्द्रयवस्य च । हिङ्गुसौवर्चलोपेतो वातशूलनिवारणः ॥ ९७ ॥

Qwātha of nāgara and eraṇḍa or of indrayava taken with hiṅgu and sauvarchalā relieves vātashūla (colic due to vāta vṛddhi) (97).

पित्तशूले त्रिफलादिक्वाथः

त्रिफलारग्वधक्वाथः शर्कराक्षौद्रसंयुतः । रक्तपित्तहरो दाहपित्तशूलनिवारणः ॥ ९८ ॥

Qwātha of triphalā and āragwadha taken with sugar and honey cures raktapitta (purpura), dāha (burning), pittashūla (colic due to increase of pitta) (98).

कफशूलादौ एरण्डक्वाथः

एरण्डमूलं द्विपलं जलेऽष्टगुणिते पचेत् । तत्क्वाथो यावशूकाढ्यः पार्श्वहृत्कफशूलहा ॥ ९९ ॥

Qwātha prepared with two palas of roots of eraṇḍa and eight times its quantity of water, taken mixed with yavashūka (barley husk) relieves pārshwashūla (pain in the flanks), hṛtshūla (precordial pain) and kaphashūla (pain due to increase of kapha) (99).

हृद्रोगादौ दशमूलक्वाथः

दशमूलकृतः क्वाथः सयवक्षारसैन्धवः । हृद्रोगगुल्मशूलानि कासं श्वासं च नाशयेत् ॥ १०० ॥

Qwātha of dashamūla taken with yavakshāra and saindhava relieves hṛdroga (heart troubles), gulma (abdominal tumors), shūla (colic), kāsa (cough) and śwāsa (dyspnoea) (100).

हरीतक्यादि मूत्रकृच्छ्रादौ—

हरीतकीदुरालम्भाकृतमालकगोक्षुरैः । पाषाणभेदसहितैः क्वाथो माक्षिकसंयुतः ॥ १०१ ॥
विबन्धे मूत्रकृच्छ्रे च सदाहे सरुजे हितः ।

Qwātha of harītakī, durālabhā, kṛtamāla, gokshura and pāṣāṇabheda taken with honey is beneficial in cases of vibandha (constipation), mūtrakṛchra (dysurea) associated with burning and pain (101–102).

वीरतर्वादिगणः—

वीरतरुर्वृक्षवन्दा काशः सहचरत्रयम् ॥ १०२ ॥
कुशद्वयं नलो गुन्द्रा बकपुष्पोऽग्निमन्थकः । मूर्वा पाषाणभेदश्च स्योनाको गोक्षुरस्तथा ॥ १०३ ॥
अपामार्गश्च कमलं ब्राह्मी चेति गणो वरः । वीरतर्वादिरित्युक्तः शर्कराश्मरिकृच्छ्रहा ॥ १०४ ॥
मूत्राघातं वायुरोगान्नाशयेन्निखिलानपि ।

Qwātha prepared from vīrataru, vṛkshavandā, kāsha, the three sahacharas, the two kushas, nala, gundrā, bakapuṣpā, agnimantha, mūrvā, pāṣāṇabheda, syonāka, gokshura, apāmārga, kamala and brāhmī—known as *vīratarvādi gaṇa qwātha* cures, sharkarā, ashmarī (renal calculii), mūtrakṛchra (dysurea), mūtrāghāta (suppression of urine) and all kinds of vātarogas (nervous disorders) (102–105).

मूत्रकृच्छ्रे एलादिक्वाथः—

एलामधुकगोकण्टरेणुकैरण्डवासकाः ॥ १०५ ॥
कृष्णाश्मभेदसहिताः क्वाथ एषां सुसाधितः । शिलाजतुयुतः पेयः शर्कराश्मरिकृच्छ्रहा ॥ १०६ ॥

Qwātha of elā, madhuka, gokaṇṭa, reṇuka, eraṇḍa, vāsaka, kṛṣṇā and ashmabheda—taken mixed with shilājatu relieves sharkarā-ashmarī (renal calculii) and mūtra kṛchra (dysurea) (105–106).

समूलगोक्षुरक्वाथः सितामाक्षिकसंयुतः । नाशयेन्मूत्रकृच्छ्राणि तथा चोष्णसमीरणम् ॥ १०७ ॥

Qwātha of entire plant of gokshura taken with sugar and honey relieves mūtrakṛchra (dysurea) and uṣṇavāta (burning micturition) (107).

अथ प्रमेहे वरादिक्वाथः—

वरादार्व्यब्ददारूणां क्वाथः क्षौद्रेणं मेहहा । वत्सकत्रिफला दार्वी मुस्तको बीजकस्तथा ॥ १०८ ॥

Qwātha of varā (triphala) dārvī, abda, dāru—taken with honey relieves pramehas (diabetes), like wise is the decoction of vatsaka, triphalā, dārvī, musta and bījaka (108).

फलत्रिकादिः प्रमेहे—

फलत्रिकाब्ददार्वीणां विशालायाः शृतं पिबेत् । निशाकल्कयुतं सर्वप्रमेहविनिवृत्तये ॥ १०९ ॥

Qwātha of triphalā, abda, dārvī and vishālā—taken with paste of nishā is beneficial in all types of prameha (polyurea) (109).

दार्व्यादिक्वाथः प्रदरे—

दार्वी रसाञ्जनं मुस्तं भल्लातः श्रीफलं वृषः । कैरातश्च पिबेदेषां क्वाथं शीतं समाक्षिकम् ॥ ११० ॥
जयेत्सशूलं प्रदरं पीतश्वेतासितारुणम् ।

Qwātha of dārvī, rasāñjana, musta, bhallāta, shrīphala, vṛṣa and kirāta taken cold, mixed with honey, relieves pradara of all kinds (vaginal discharges, yellow, white, black or red) accompanied with pain (110–111).

न्यग्रोधादिक्वाथः योनिरोगव्रणादौ—

न्यग्रोधप्लक्षकोशाम्रवेतसा बदरी तुणिः ॥ १११ ॥
मधुयष्टी प्रियालश्च लोध्रद्वयमुदुम्बरः । पिप्पलश्च मधूकश्च तथा पारिसपिप्पलः ॥ ११२ ॥
सल्लकी तिन्दुकी जम्बूद्वयमाम्रतरुः शिवा । कदम्बककुभौ चैव भल्लातकफलानि च ॥ ११३ ॥
न्यग्रोधादिगणक्वाथं यथालाभं च कारयेत् । अयं क्वाथो महाग्राही व्रण्यो भग्नं च साधयेत् ॥११४॥
योनिदोषहरो दाहमेदोमेहविषापहः ।

Qwātha of bark of nyagrodha, plaksha, koshāmra, vetasa, badarī, tuṇī, madhuyaṣṭī, priyāla, the two lodhras, udumbara, pippala, madhūka, pārisapippala, sallakī, tindukī, two jambūs, āmra, shivā, kadamba, kakubha and fruits of bhallataka known as *nyagrodhādi gaṇa qwātha* is a powerful grāhī (water absorbant), cures vraṇa (ulcers), bhaṅga (fractures) diseases of uterus and vagina, dāha (burning sensation), medas (obesity), prameha (diabetes) and viṣas (poisons) (111–115).

अथ मेदोदोषे योगत्रयं—

बिल्वोऽग्निमन्थः स्योनाकः काश्मरी पाटला तथा ॥ ११५ ॥

क्वाथ एषां जयेन्मेदोदोषं क्षौद्रेण संयुतः । क्षौद्रेण त्रिफलाक्वाथः पीतो मेदोहरः स्मृतः ॥ ११६ ॥
शीतीभूतं तथोष्णाम्बु मेदोहृत्क्षौद्रसंयुतम् ।

Qwātha of bilwa, agnimantha, syonāka, kāshmarī, and pāṭalā—taken with honey relieves obesity; like wise is the decoction of triphalā taken with honey and warm water (115–117).

उदररोगे चव्यादिक्वाथः—

चव्यचित्रकविश्वानां साधितो देवदारुणा ॥ ११७ ॥
क्वाथस्त्रिवृच्चूर्णयुतो गोमूत्रेणोदराञ्जयेत् ।

Qwātha of chavya, chitraka, vishwā and dāru mixed with powder of trivṛt and taken with cow's urine relieves udara roga (abdominal enlargements). (118).

शोथोदरे पुनर्नवादिक्वाथः—

पुनर्नवामृतादारुपथ्यानागरसाधितः ॥ ११८ ॥
गोमूत्रगुग्गुलुयुतः क्वाथः शोथोदरापहः ।

Qwātha of punarnavā, amṛtā, dāru, pathyā and taken with cow's urine and guggulu relieves shotha (anasrca) and udara (abdominal enlargement).

पथ्यादिक्वाथः यकृत्प्लीहगुल्मोदरे—

पथ्यारोहितकक्वाथं यवक्षारकणायुतम् ॥ ११९ ॥
पिबेत्प्रातर्यकृत्प्लीहगुल्मोदरनिवृत्तये ।

Qwātha of pathyā and rohitaka mixed with yavakshāra and powder of kaṇā taken in the morning relieves diseases of spleen, liver, gulma (abdominal tumors) and udara (abdominal enlargements) (119–120).

शोथे पुनर्नवादिक्वाथः—

पुनर्नवा दारुनिशा निशा शुण्ठी हरीतकी ॥ १२० ॥
गुडूची चित्रको भार्ङ्गी देवदारु च तैः शृतः । पाणिपादोदरमुखप्राप्तं शोफं निवारयेत् ॥ १२१ ॥

Qwātha of punarnavā, dārunishā, nishā, shunṭhī, harītakī, guḍūchī, chitraka, bhārṅgī and devadāru relieves shopha (oedema) of the limbs, abdomen and face (120–121).

वृषणशोथे त्रिफलादिः—

फलत्रिकोद्भवं क्वाथं गोमूत्रेणैव पाययेत् । वातश्लेष्मकृतं हन्ति शोथं वृषणसंभवम् ॥ १२२ ॥

Qwātha of triphalā taken with cow's urine relieves vṛṣaṇa shotha (oedema of the scrotum) due to vāta-kapha vṛddhi (122).

रास्नादिः अन्त्रवृद्धौ—

रास्नामृताबलायष्टीगोकण्टैरण्डजः शृतः । एरण्डतैलसंयुक्तो वृद्धिमन्त्रभवां जयेत् ॥ १२३ ॥

Qwātha of rāsnā, amṛtā, balā, yaṣṭhī, gokaṇṭa, and eraṇḍa taken with castor oil relieves āntra vṛddhi (hernia—scrotal or inguinal) (123).

काञ्चनारक्वाथः गण्डमालायां—

काञ्चनारत्वचः क्वाथः शुण्ठीचूर्णेन नाशयेत् । गण्डमालां तथा क्वाथः क्षौद्रेण वरुणत्वचः ॥ १२४ ॥

Qwātha of bark of kāñchanāra taken with the powder of shunṭhī relieves gaṇḍamālā (enlarged glands in the neck); like wise is the qwātha of the bark of varuṇa taken with honey (124).

अथ शाखोटक्वाथः श्लीपदे मेदोरोगे च—

शाखोटवल्कलक्वाथं गोमूत्रेण युतं पिबेत् । श्लीपदानां विनाशाय मेदोदोषनिवृत्तये ॥ १२५ ॥

Qwātha of bark of shākhoṭaka with cow's urine relieves shlīpada (filariasis) and medo doṣa (obesity) (125).

पुनर्नवावरुणयोः क्वाथोऽन्तर्विद्रधिं जयेत् । तथा शिग्रुभवः क्वाथो हिङ्गुसैन्धवसंयुतः ॥ १२६ ॥

Qwātha of punarnavā and varuṇa taken relieves antarvidradhi (internal abscesses) like wise the decoction of bark of shigru taken with hiṅgu and saindhava (126).

अपरमपि विद्रधौ वरुणादिकयोगमाह—

वरुणादिगणक्वाथमपक्वे मध्यविद्रधौ । ऊषकादिरजोयुक्तं पिबेच्छमनहेतवे ॥ १२७ ॥

Qwātha of varuṇādi gaṇa taken with powder of ūṣakādi gaṇa is beneficial in the early and ripening stages of vidradhi (abscess) (127).

वरुणो बकपुष्पश्च बिल्वापामार्गचित्रकाः । अग्निमन्थद्वयं शिग्रुद्वयं च बृहतीद्वयम् ॥ १२८ ॥
सौरेयकत्रयं मूर्वा मेषश्रृङ्गी किराततकः । अजश्रृङ्गी च बिम्बी च करञ्जश्च शतावरी ॥ १२९ ॥
वरुणादिगणक्वाथः कफमेदोहरः स्मृतः । हन्ति गुल्मं शिरःशूलं तथाभ्यन्तरविद्रधीन् ॥ १३० ॥

Varuṇa, bakapuṣpa, bilwa, apāmārga, chitraka, the two agnimanthas, the two shigrus, two bṛhatis, the three saireyaka, mūrvā, meṣasṛṅgi, kirātaka, ajashṛṅgi, bimbī, karañja and shatāvarī—all these together known as *varuṇādi gaṇa*, Made into a decoction it relieves disorders of kapha, medas (fat), gulma (abdominal tumor), shiraḥ shūla (headache) and abhyantara vidradhi (internal abscesses) (128–130).

खदिरादिर्भगन्दरे—

खदिरत्रिफलाक्वाथो महिषीघृतसंयुतः । विडङ्गचूर्णयुक्तश्च भगन्दरविनाशनः ॥ १३१ ॥

Qwātha of khadira and triphalā along with buffaloe's ghee and powder of viḍaṅga cures bhagandara (fistula in ano) (131).

पटोलादिः उपदंशरोगे—

पटोलत्रिफलानिम्बकिराततखदिरासनैः । क्वाथः पीतो जयेत्सर्वानुपदंशान्सगुग्गुलुः ॥ १३२ ॥

Qwātha of paṭola, triphalā, nimba, kirāta, khadira and asana, with powder of guggulu relieves all types of upadaṃsha (syphilis) (132).

अमृतादिर्वातरक्ते—

अमृतैरण्डवासानां क्वाथ एरण्डतैलयुक् । पीतः सर्वाङ्गसंचारि वातरक्तं जयेद्ध्रुवम् ॥ १३३ ॥

Qwātha of amṛtā, eraṇḍa, vasā taken with castor oil relieves vātarakta (gout) moving of all over the body quickly (133).

अथ पटोलादिक्वाथो वातरक्ते—

पटोलं त्रिफला तिक्ता गुडूची च शतावरी । एतत्क्वाथो जयेत्पीतो वातास्रं दाहसंयुतम् ॥ १३४ ॥

Qwātha of paṭola, triphalā, tiktā, guḍūchī, shatāvarī—relieves vātarakta (gout) accompanied with burning sensation (134).

श्वेतकुष्ठे बाकुचीक्वाथः—

क्वाथोऽवल्गुजचूर्णाढ्यो धात्रीखदिरसारयोः । जयेत्सुशीलितो नित्यं श्वित्रं पथ्याशिनां नृणाम् ॥१३५॥

Qwātha of powder of avalguja, dhātrī, and khadirasāra can cure shwitra (leucoderma) of persons who adhere to the instructions of the physician (135).

रक्तकुष्ठादौ लघुमञ्जिष्ठादिक्वाथः—

मञ्जिष्ठा त्रिफला तिक्ता वचा दारुनिशामृता । निम्बश्चैषां कृतः क्वाथो वातरक्तविनाशनः ॥ १३६ ॥
पामाकपालिकाकुष्ठरक्तमण्डलजिन्मतः ।

Qwātha of mañjiṣṭhā, triphalā, tiktā, vachā, dārunishā, amṛtā and nimba relieves vātarakta (gout), pāmā (scabies), kapālakuṣṭha and raktamaṇḍala (varieties of leprosy) (136–137).

बृहन्मञ्जिष्ठादिः सर्वकुष्ठे—

मञ्जिष्ठामुस्तकुटजगुडूचीकुष्ठनागरैः ॥ १३७ ॥
भार्ङ्गीक्षुद्रावचानिम्बनिशाद्वयफलत्रिकैः । पटोलकटुकीमूर्वाविडङ्गासनचित्रकैः ॥ १३८ ॥
शतावरीत्रायमाणाकृष्णेन्द्रयववासकैः । भृङ्गराजमहादारुपाठाखदिरचन्दनैः ॥ १३९ ॥
त्रिवृद्वरुणकैरातबाकुचीकृतमालकैः । शाखोटकमहानिम्बकरञ्जातिविषाजलैः ॥ १४० ॥
इन्द्रवारुणिकानन्तासारिवापर्पटैः समैः । एभिः कृतं पिबेत्क्वाथं कणागुग्गुलसंयुतम् ॥ १४१ ॥
अष्टादशसु कुष्ठेषु वातरक्तार्दिते तथा । उपदंशे श्लीपदे च प्रसुप्तौ पक्षघातके ॥ १४२ ॥
मेदोदोषे नेत्ररोगे मञ्जिष्ठादिः प्रशस्यते ।

Qwātha of mañjiṣṭhā, musta, kuṭaja, guḍūchī, kuṣṭha, nāgara, bhārṅgī, kshudrā, vacha, nimba, two nishās, triphalā, paṭola, kaṭukī, mūrvā, viḍaṅga, asana, chitraka, shatāvarī, trāyamāṇā, kṛṣṇa indrayava, vāsaka, bhṛṅgarāja, mahādāru, pāṭhā, khadira, chandana, trivṛt, varuṇa, kirāta, bakuchī, kṛtamālaka, shākhoṭaka, mahānimba, karañja, ativiṣā, jala, indravāruṇī, anantā, sārivā and parpaṭa—taken with powder of kaṇā and guggulu is known as *bṛhan mañjiṣṭhādi qwātha.* It is beneficial in the eighteen kinds of kuṣṭha (leprosy), vātarakta (gout), ardita (facial paralysis), upadaṃsha (veneral diseases), shlīpada (filariasis), supti (numbness), pakshāghāta (hemiplegia), medodoṣa (obesity) and netraroga (eye disease) (137-143).

पथ्यादिषडङ्गक्वाथः शिरोरोगे—

नेत्ररोगादौ च—

पथ्याक्षधात्रीभूनिम्बैर्निशानिम्बामृतायुतैः ॥ १४३ ॥
कृतः क्वाथः षडङ्गोऽयं सगुडः शीर्षशूलहृत् । भ्रूशङ्खकर्णशूलानि तथार्धशिरसो रुजम् ॥ १४४ ॥
सूर्यावर्तं शङ्खकं च दन्तपातं च तद्रुजम् । नक्तान्ध्यं पटलं शुक्रं चक्षुःपीडां व्यपोहति ॥ १४५ ॥

Qwātha of pathyā, aksha, dhātrī, bhūnimba, nishā, nimba and amṛtā taken with jaggery relieves headaches, pain in the eye brows, temples, ear, hemicrania, sūryāvarta (migraine), shaṃkhaka (temporal headache), pain due to teeth falling out; eye diseases like naktāndhya (night blindness), paṭala (pannus), shukra (corneal ulcers and pain in the eyes) (143-145).

अथ वासादिर्नेत्ररोगे—

वासाविश्वामृतादार्वीरक्तचन्दनचित्रकैः । भूनिम्बनिम्बकटुकापटोलत्रिफलाम्बुदैः ॥ १४१ ॥
यवकालिङ्गकुटजैः क्वाथः सर्वाक्षिरोगहा । वैस्वर्यं पीनसं श्वासं नाशयेदुरसः क्षतम् ॥ १४७ ॥

Qwātha of vasā, viśwā, amṛtā, dārvī, raktachandana, chitraka, bhūnimba, nimba, kaṭuka, paṭola, triphalā, ambuda, yava, kāliṅga and kuṭaja cures all eye diseases, vaiswarya (disorders of voice), pīnasa (coryza), śwāsa (dyspnoea) and urakshata (ulcers inside the lungs) (146-147).

अथामृतादिर्नेत्ररोगे—

अमृतात्रिफलाक्वाथः पिप्पलीचूर्णसंयुतः । सक्षौद्रः शीलितो नित्यं सर्वनेत्रव्यथां जयेत् ॥ १४८ ॥

Qwātha of amṛtā and triphalā taken with powder of pippalī and honey relieves all eye diseases (148).

पञ्चवल्कलक्वाथो व्रणक्षालनादौ—

अश्वत्थोदुम्बरप्लक्षवटवेतसजं शृतम् । व्रणशोथोपदंशानां नाशनं क्षालनात्स्मृतम् ॥ १४९ ॥

Qwātha of ashwatha, udumbara, plaksha, vaṭa and vetas—used externally as a wash heals vraṇa (ulcers), shotha (oedema) and upadaṁsha (venereal ulcers (149).

प्रमथ्या प्रोच्यते द्रव्यपलात्कल्कीकृताच्छृतात् । तोयेऽष्टगुणिते तस्याः पानमाहुः पलद्वयम् ॥१५०॥

One pala of drug boiled in eight parts of water and reduced to quarter is called *pramathyā.* It's dosage is two palas (150).

सा यथा—मुस्तकेन्द्रयवैः सिद्धा प्रमथ्या ह्रिपलोन्मिता । सुशीता मधुसंयुक्ता रक्तातीसारनाशिनी ॥१५१॥

Mustaka and indrayava made into a pramathyā and taken cold mixed with honey relieves raktātisara (diarrhoea accompanied with blood) (151).

इदानीं यवागूपरिभाषामाह—

साध्यं चतुष्पलं द्रव्यं चतुःषष्टिपलेऽम्बुनि । तत्क्वाथेनार्धशिष्टेन यवागूं साधयेद्घनाम् ॥ १५२ ॥

Four palas of drug is boiled in sixtyfour palas of water and reduced to half. In this decoction broken grains are added and thick gruel (porridge) prepared. This is called *yavāgū* (152).

सा यथा—आम्राम्रातकजम्बूत्वक्कषाये विपचेद्बुधः । यवागूं शालिभिर्युक्तां तां भुक्त्वा ग्रहणीं जयेत् ॥१५३॥

An yavāgū prepared with barks of āmra, āmrātaka, jambū and broken rice relieves grahaṇī (sprue) (153).

संप्रति यूषमाह—

कल्कद्रव्यपलं शुण्ठी पिप्पली चार्धकार्षिकी । वारिप्रस्थेन विपचेत्स द्रवो यूष उच्यते ॥ १५४ ॥

One pala of the drug with powders of shunṭhī and pippalī each half karṣa boiled in one prastha of water becomes a yūṣa (154).

सप्तमुष्टियूषः

स यथा—कुलत्थयवकोलैश्च मुद्गैर्मूलकशुण्ठकैः । शुण्ठीधान्याकयुक्तैश्च यूषः श्लेष्मानिलापहः ॥ १५५ ॥
सप्तमुष्टिक इत्येष सन्निपातज्वरापहः । आमवातहरः कण्ठहृद्वक्त्राणां च विशोधनः ॥ १५६ ॥

Yūṣa prepared with kulattha, yava, kola, mudga, mūlakashunṭhaka, shunṭhī, and dhānyaka cures diseases due to shleṣma and vāta. This is known as *sapta muṣṭika yūṣa* relieves sannipāta jwaras (toxic fevers), āmavāta (rheumatism) and clears the throat and mouth (155–156).

इदानीं पानादिकल्पनामाह—

क्षुण्णं द्रव्यपलं साध्यं चतुःषष्टिपले जले । अर्धशिष्टं च तद्देयं पाने भक्तादिसंविधौ ॥ १५७ ॥

One pala of drug boiled in sixtyfour palas of water and reduced to half the quantity is called *pānīya jala* and used as a drink (157).

षडङ्गपानम्

सा यथा—उशीरपर्पटोदीच्यमुस्तनागरचन्दनैः । जलं शृतं हिमं पेयं पिपासाज्वरनाशनम् ॥ १५८ ॥

Pānīya prepared with ushīra, parpaṭa, udīchya, musta, nāgara and chandana and taken cold is beneficial in cases of pipāsā (thirst) and jwara (fevers) (158).

ज्वरादौ उष्णोदकविधिं दर्शयन्नाह—

अष्टमेनांशशेषेण चतुर्थेनार्धकेन वा । अथवा क्वथनेनैव सिद्धमुष्णोदकं वदेत् ॥ १५९ ॥
श्लेष्मामवातमेदोघ्नं बस्तिशोधनदीपनम् । कासश्वासज्वरहरं पीतमुष्णोदकं निशि ॥ १६० ॥

Reduction of water after boiling to 1/8, 1/4, or 1/2 its original quantity is called *'uṣṇodaka'*-taken at bed time it relieves kapha, vāta, āma, medas and acts as bastishodhana (clears urinary bladder) and dīpana (carminative) cures kāsa (cough), śwāsa (dyspnoea), and jwara (fevers) (159–160).

इदानीं क्षीरपाकविधिमाह—

क्षीरमष्टगुणं द्रव्यात्क्षीरान्नीरं चतुर्गुणम् । क्षीरावशेषं तत्पीतं शूलमामोद्भवं जयेत् ॥ १६१ ॥

One part of drug, eight parts of cow's milk, thirty two parts of water boiled together and reduced to the quantity equivalent of milk (i.e., one eighth) is known as *kshīra pāka*. It relieves abdominal pain due to accumulation of āma (undigested matter) (161).

पञ्चमूलपयः

(सर्वज्वराणां जीर्णानां क्षीरं भैषज्यमुत्तमम् । श्वासात्कासाच्छिरः शूलात्पार्श्वशूलात्सपीनसात् ॥१६२॥
मुच्यते ज्वरितः पीत्वा पञ्चमूलीशृतं पयः ।

Kṣīra (milk) is the best medicine for all types of chronic fevers.

Kshīrapāka prepared out of pañchamūlas relieves śwāsa (dyspnoea), kāsa (cough), shirashūla (headache), pārshwashūla (pain in the flanks), pīnasa (coryza) and jwara (fever) (162–163).

त्रिकण्टकपयः

त्रिकण्टकबलाव्याघ्रीगुडनागरसाधितम् ॥ १६३ ॥
वर्चोमूत्रविबन्धघ्नं कफज्वरहरं पयः ।)

Kshīrapāka of trikaṇṭaka, balā, vyāghri, guḍa and nāgara relieves constipation, difficulty of micturition and kapha jwaras (163–164).

संप्रति यवागूप्रभृतिकान्नप्रक्रियामाह—

अथान्नप्रक्रियात्रैव प्रोच्यते नातिविस्तरात् ॥ १६४ ॥
यवागूः षड्गुणजले सिद्धा स्यात्कृशरा घना । तण्डुलैर्मुद्गमाषैश्च तिलैर्वा साधिता हिता ॥ १६५ ॥
यवागूर्ग्राहिणी बल्या तर्पणी वातनाशिनी ।

Herein is described in brief the annaprakriyā (preparation of rice puddings).

One part of corn-flour such as of tandula (rice), mugda (green gram), māṣa (black gram) or tila (sesame) boiled in six parts of water and prepared into thin paste is called 'kṛsharā' such a preparation is grāhī (stops loose motion), balya (strengthening), tarpaṇa (nourishing) and vātanāshinī (relieves vāta) (164–166).

अथ विलेपीविवरणं दर्शयन्नाह—

विलेपी घनसिक्था स्यात्सिद्धा नीरे चतुर्गुणे ॥ १६६ ॥
तर्पणी बृंहणी हृद्या मधुरा पित्तनाशिनी ।

Pudding prepared with one part of grain and four parts of water cooked into a thick paste is vilepī. It is tarpaṇa (satiating), bṛṃhaṇa (strengthening), hṛdya (good for heart), madhura (delicious) and pittanāshana (166-167).

इदानीं पेयायूषावप्याह—

द्रवाधिका स्वल्पसिक्था चतुर्दशगुणे जले ॥ १६७ ॥
सिद्धा पेया बुधैर्ज्ञेया यूषः किंचिद्घनस्ततः । पेया लघुतरा ज्ञेया ग्राहिणी धातुपुष्टिदा ॥ १६८ ॥
यूषो बल्यस्ततः कण्ठ्यो लघुपाकः कफापहः ।

One part of grain and fourteen parts of water, slightly boiled into watery consistence is known as '*yūṣa*'. This is quickly digestable, grāhī (stops loose motions), nourishes the tissues, balya (strengthening), kaṇṭhya (good for throat) and kaphahara (167–169).

इदानीं भक्तविधिमाह—

जले चतुर्दशगुणे तण्डुलानां चतुष्पलम् ॥ १६९ ॥
विपचेत्स्रावयेन्मण्डं स भक्तो मधुरो लघुः ।

Four palas of rice and fourteen parts of water are boiled together and the fluid drained out while boiling gives 'bhakta' (cooked rice meal). This is madhura (sweet) and laghu (easily digestable) (169–170).

अधुना शुद्धमण्डमाह—

नीरे चतुर्दशगुणे सिद्धो मण्डस्त्वसिक्थकः ॥ १७० ॥
शुण्ठीसैन्धवसंयुक्तः पाचनो दीपनः स्मृतः ।

One part of rice and fourteen parts of water are boiled together. The fluid (without grains) emerging thereby is called *maṇḍa.* This fluid mixed with powder of shuṇṭhī and saindhava is a good dīpana–pāchana (digestive and carminative) (170–171).

अथाष्टगुणमण्डमाह—

धान्यत्रिकटुसिन्धूत्थमुद्गतण्डुलयोजितः ॥ १७१ ॥
भृष्टश्च हिङ्गुतैलाभ्यां स मण्डोऽष्टगुणः स्मृतः । दीपनः प्राणदो बस्तिशोधनो रक्तवर्धनः ॥ १७२ ॥
ज्वरजित्सर्वदोषघ्नो मण्डोऽष्टगुण उच्यते ।

Maṇḍa prepared with dhānya, trikaṭu, saindhava, mudga and tandula,—and added with fried hiṅgu is *aṣṭa guṇa maṇḍa.* This acts as dīpana (carminative, prāṇada (restorative), bastishodhana (clears the urinary bladder), rakta vardhana, (improves blood), relieves jwara (fever) and all the three doṣas (171–173).

इदानीं वाट्यमण्डमाह—

सुकण्डितैस्तथा भृष्टैर्वाठ्यमण्डो यवैर्भवत् ॥ १७३ ॥
कफपित्तहरः कण्ठ्यो रक्तपित्तप्रसादनः ।

Maṇḍa prepared with broken and fried yava (barley) grain is kaphapittahara, kaṇṭhya (good for throat), raktapitta prasādana (relieves purpura) (173–174).

अथ लाजमण्डमाह—

लाजैर्वा तण्डुलैर्भृष्टैर्लाजमण्डः प्रकीर्तितः ॥ १७४ ॥
श्लेष्मपित्तहरो ग्राही पिपासाज्वरजिन्मतः ।

Maṇḍa prepared with lājā (parched rice) is sleṣmapittahara, grāhī (stops diarrhoea), relieves pipāsā (thirst) and jwara (fever) (174–175).

इति श्रीदामोदरसूनुना शार्ङ्गधरेण विरचितायां शार्ङ्गधरसंहितायां चिकित्सास्थाने
क्राथकल्पनाध्यायो द्वितीयः ॥ २ ॥

Thus ends the second chapter.

तृतीयोऽध्यायः

CHAPTER 3

Phāṇṭa Kalpanā (Infusions)

फाण्टकल्पना

क्षुण्णे द्रव्यपले सम्यग्जलमुष्णं विनिक्षिपेत् । मृत्पात्रे कुडवोन्मानं ततस्तु स्रावयेत्पटात् ॥ १ ॥
तस्य चूर्णद्रवः फाण्टस्तन्मानं द्विपलोन्मितम् । सितामधुगुडादींश्च क्राथवत्तत्र निक्षिपेत् ॥ २ ॥

One pala of a powdered drug and one kuḍava of hot water are kept in a mudpot, and filtered through cloth after some time. This liquid known as chūrṇa-drava or phāṇṭa (infusion) is administered in doses of two palas; honey, sugar or jaggery to be added shall be in the same proportion as that of qwātha.(1–2)

अथ बृहन्मधूकफाण्टः

स यथा–मधूकपुष्पं मधुकं चन्दनं सपरूषकम् । मृणालं कमलं लोध्रं कम्भारी नागकेशरम् ॥ ३ ॥
त्रिफला-सारिवा-द्राक्षा-लाजान्कोष्णजले क्षिपेत् । सितामधुयुतः पेयः फाण्टो ह्यसौ हिमोऽथवा ॥४॥
वातपित्तज्वरं दाहं तृष्णामूर्च्छारतिभ्रमान् । रक्तपित्तं मदं हन्यान्नात्र कार्या विचारणा ॥ ५ ॥

Infusion of madhūka puṣpa, madhuka, chandana, parūṣaka, mṛṇāla, kamala, lodhra, gambhārī, nāgakeśara, triphalā, sārivā, drākshā and lājā-taken either warm or cold, surely relieves without doubt, vātapitta jwara (fevers), dāha (buring), tṛṣṇā (thirst), mūrcchā (fainting), arati (restlessness), bhrama (giddiness), raktapitta (purpura) and mada (intoxication) (3–5).

अथाम्रादिफाण्टः ज्वरादौ

आम्रजम्बूकिसलयैर्वटशुङ्गप्ररोहकैः । उशीरेण कृतः फाण्टः सक्षौद्रो ज्वरनाशनः ॥ ६ ॥
पिपासाछर्द्यतीसारान्मूर्छां जयति दुस्तराम् ।

Infusion of tender leaves of āmra, jambū, buds of vaṭa and ushīra with honey relieves severe jwaras (fevers), pipāsā (thirst), chardi (vomiting). atisāra (diarrhoea) and mūrcchā (fainting) (6–7).

लघुमधूकपुष्पादिफाण्टो दाहपित्तादौ ।

मधूकपुष्पकम्भारीचन्दनोशीरधान्यकैः ॥ ७ ॥
द्राक्षया च कृतः फाण्टः शीतः शर्करया युतः । तृष्णापित्तहरः प्रोक्तो दाहमूर्च्छाभ्रमाञ्जयेत् ॥ ८ ॥

Infusion of madhūka puṣpa, gambhārī, chandana, ushīra, dhānyaka and drākshā along with sugar and taken cold relieves tṛṣṇā (thirst), pittahara (reduces pitta), dāha (burning), mūrcchā (fainting) and bhrama (giddiness) (7–8).

मन्थविधिः ।

मन्थोऽपि फाण्टभेदः स्यात्तेन चात्रैव कथ्यते । जले चतुःपले शीते क्षुण्णं द्रव्यपलं क्षिपेत् ॥ ९ ॥
मृत्पात्रे मन्थयेत्सम्यक्तस्माच्च द्विपलं पिबेत् ।

As *'mantha'* is also a kind of phāṇṭa it is described here itself. One pala of powdered drug is put in four palas of cold water and churned well in a pot for some time to a thick consistence. This liquid kuown as *mantha* should be administered in doses of two palas (9–10).

मदात्ययादौ खर्जूरादिमन्थः ।

खर्जूरदाडिमीद्राक्षातिन्तिडीकाम्लिकामलैः ॥ १० ॥
सपरूषैः कृतो मन्थः सर्वमद्यविकारनुत् ।

Mantha of kharjūra, dāḍima, drākshā, tintidīka, āmlikā, amalakī and parūṣaka relieves intoxication of all alcoholic drinks (10–11).

अथ मसूरादिमन्थः छर्द्याम्—

क्षौद्रयुक्ता मसूराणां सक्तवो दाडिमाम्भसा ॥ ११ ॥
मथिता वारयन्त्याशु छर्दिं दोषत्रयोद्भवाम् ।

Mantha of powder of masūra gram, juice of dāḍima and honey well churned and taken relieves chardi (vomiting) arising from aggravation of all the three doṣas (11–12).

तृष्णादाहादौ यवसक्तुमन्थः—

प्लावितैः शीतनीरेण सघृतैर्यवसक्तुभिः ॥ १२ ॥
नातिसान्द्रद्रवो मन्थस्तृष्णादाहास्रपित्तहा ।

Mantha of powder of yava, cold water and ghee—neither too thin or too thick and taken relieves tṛṣṇā (thirst), dāha (burning), and raktapitta (purpura).

इति श्रीदामोदरसूनुना शार्ङ्गधराचार्येण विरचितायां श्रीशार्ङ्गधरसंहितायां मध्यखण्डे फाण्टादिकल्पना नाम तृतीयोऽध्यायः ॥ ३ ॥

Thus ends the third chapter.

चतुर्थोऽध्यायः

CHAPTER 4

Hima Kalpanā (Cold Infusions)

अथ हिमकल्पनां निदर्शयन्नाह—

क्षुण्णं द्रव्यपलं सम्यक्षड्भिर्नीरपलैः प्लुतम् । निशोषितं हिमः स स्यात्तथा शीतकषायकः ॥१॥
तन्मानं फाण्टवज्ज्ञेयं सर्वत्रैवैष निश्चयः ।

One pala of powdered drug is put into eight palas of cold water and kept one night in a pot. It is filtered through cloth next morning and used in the same dosage as that of phāṇṭa. This is knwon as hima or shīta kaṣāya (cold extract) (1–2).

आम्रादिहिमो रक्तपित्ते—

आम्र-जम्बू च ककुभं चूर्णीकृत्य जले क्षिपेत् ॥ २ ॥
हिमं तस्य पिबेत्प्रातः सक्षौद्रं रक्तपित्तजित् ।

Powder of barks of āmra, jambu, and kakubha is kept in water over-night and taken the next morning mixed with honey relieves raktapitta (purpura) (2–3).

अथ मरीच्यादिहिमस्तृष्णादौ—

मरीचं मधुयष्टी च काकोदुम्बरपल्लवाः ॥ ३ ॥
नीलोत्पलं हिमस्तज्ज्ञस्तृष्णाछर्दिनिवारणः ।

Maricha, madhuyaṣṭī, buds of kākodumbara and petals of nīlotpala made into a cold extract relieves tṛṣṇā (thirst) and chardi (vomiting) ($3\frac{1}{2}$).

वातपित्तादौ नीलोत्पलादिहिमः—

नीलोत्पलं बला द्राक्षा मधूकं मधुकं तथा ॥ ४ ॥
उशीरं पद्मकं चैव काश्मरी च पुरुषकम् । एष शीतकषायश्च वातपित्तज्वराञ्जयेत् ॥ ५ ॥
सप्रलापभ्रमच्छर्दिमोहतृष्णानिवारणः ।

Hima of nīlotpala, balā, drākshā, madhūka, madhuka, ushīra, padmaka, kāshmarī and parūṣaka relieves vātapitta jwara (fevers) accompanied with pralāpa (delirium), bhrama (giddiness), chardi (vomiting), moha (delusion) and tṛṣṇā (thirst) (4–6).

गुडूचीहिमः जीर्णज्वरे—

अमृताया हिमः पेयो जीर्णज्वरहरः स्मृतः ॥ ६ ॥
वासायाश्च हिमः कासं रक्तपित्तज्वराञ्जयेत् ।

Hima of amṛtā relieves jīrṇajwara (chronic fevers) while that of vasā relieves raktapitta (purpura) and jwara (fevers) (6–7).

अथ धान्यादिहिमोऽन्तर्दाहादौ—

प्रातः सशर्करः पेयो हिमो धान्याकसंभवः ॥ ७ ॥
अन्तर्दाहं तथा तृष्णां जयेत्स्रोतोविशोधनः ।

Hima of dhānyaka taken with sugar relieves dāha (burning), tṛṣṇā (thirst) and clears the srotas (cell pores, channels, ducts etc.) (7–8).

अथ धान्याकादिर्हिमः रक्तपित्तादौ—

धान्याकधात्रीवासानां द्राक्षापर्पटयोर्हिमः ॥ ८ ॥
रक्तपित्तज्वरं दाहं तृष्णां शोषं च नाशयेत् ।

Hima of dhānyaka, dhātrī, vasā, drākshā and parpaṭa cures raktapitta (purpura), jwara (fever), dāha (burning), tṛṣṇā (thirst) and shoṣa (wasting).

इति श्रीदामोदरसूनुना श्रीशार्ङ्गधराचार्येण विरचितायां श्रीशार्ङ्गधरसंहितायां मध्यमखण्डे हिमकल्पना नाम चतुर्थोऽध्यायः ।

Thus ends the fourth chapter.

पञ्चमोऽध्यायः

CHAPTER 5

Kalka Kalpanā (wet pill or bolus)

अथेदानीं कल्ककल्पनां व्याख्यास्यामः—

द्रव्यमार्द्रं शिलापिष्टं शुष्कं वा सजलं भवेत् । प्रक्षेपावापकल्कास्ते तन्मानं कर्षसंमितम् ॥ १ ॥

A green drug or a dry drug converted into a paste by rubbing it on a stone with a little quantity of water added, is called 'kalka'. Its dose is one karṣa (1).

कल्के मधु घृतं तैलं देयं द्विगुणमात्रया । सितागुडं समं दद्याद्द्रवा देयाश्चतुर्गुणाः ॥ २ ॥

Honey, ghee and oil is added, if necessary, in double its quantity; sugar or jaggery in equal quantity and any liquid in four times the quantity of kalka (2).

वर्धमानपिप्पल्यः—

स यथा-त्रिवृद्ध्या पञ्चवृद्ध्या वा सप्तवृध्याथवा कणाः । पिबेत्पिष्ट्वा दशादिनं तास्तथैवापकर्षयेम् ॥३॥
एवं विंशद्दिनैः सिद्धं पिप्पलीवर्धमानकम् । अनेन पाण्डुवातास्रकासश्वासारुचिज्वराः ॥ ४ ॥
उदरार्शःक्षयश्लेष्मवाता नश्यन्त्युरोग्रहाः ।

Kalka of three pippalīs by count on the first day and increased in multiples of three pippaiīs each succeeding day upto ten days and then reduced by three each succeeding day for ten days—this recipe known as *"vardhamāna pippalī"* relieves pāṇḍu (anaemia), vātāsra (gout), kāsa (cough), śwāsa (dyspnoea), aruchi (loss of taste), jwara (fevers) udara (abdominal enlargement), arsha (piles), kshaya (consumption), urograha (chest pain) and diseases arising from sleṣma and vāta (3-5).

अथ निम्बकल्को व्रणच्छर्द्यादौ—

लेपान्निम्बदलैः कल्को व्रणशोधन रोपणः ॥ ५ ॥
भक्षणाच्छर्दिकुष्ठानि पित्तश्लेष्मकृमीञ्जयेत् ।

Kalka of tender leaves of nimba applied over wounds helps their healing, if taken internally relieves chhardi (vomiting), kuṣṭha (leprosy and other skin diseases and also diseases arising from pitta and sleṣma and kṛmi (5-6).

अथ महानिम्बकल्को गृध्रस्याम्—

महानिम्बजटाकल्को गृध्रसीनाशनः स्मृतः ॥ ६ ॥

Kalka of roots of mahānimba relieves gṛdhrasī (sciatica) (6).

अथ रसोनकल्कः वातरोगविषमज्वरादौ—

शुद्धः कल्को रसोनस्य तिलतैलेन मिश्रितः । वातरोगाञ्जयेत्तीव्रान्विषमज्वरनाशनः ॥ ७ ॥

Kalka of rasona added with tila taila (sesamum oil) relieves severe vāta-rogas (nervous diseases) and viṣama jwara (intermittent fevers) (7).

अथ द्वितीयरसोनकल्को वातव्याधौ—

पक्वकन्दरसोनस्य गुलिका निस्तुषीकृताः । पाटयित्वा च मध्यस्थं दूरीकुर्यात्तदङ्कुरम् ॥ ८ ॥
तदुग्रगन्धनाशाय रात्रौ तक्रे विनिक्षिपेत् । अपनीय च तन्मध्याच्छिलायां पेषयेत्ततः ॥ ९ ॥
तन्मध्ये पञ्चमांशेन चूर्णमेषां विनिक्षिपेत् । सौवर्चलं यवानीं च भर्जियं हिङ्गु सैन्धवम् ॥ १० ॥
कटुत्रिकं जीरकं च समभागानि चूर्णयेत् । एकीकृत्य ततः सर्वं कल्कं कर्षप्रमाणतः ॥ ११ ॥
खादेदग्निबलापेक्षी ऋतुदोषाद्यपेक्षया । अनुपानं ततः कुर्यादेरण्डश्रृतमन्वहम् ॥ १२ ॥
सर्वाङ्गैकाङ्गजं वातमर्दितं चापतन्त्रकम् । अपस्मारमथोन्मादमूरुस्तम्भं च गृध्रसीम् ॥ १३ ॥
उरः पृष्ठकटीपार्श्वकुक्षिपीडा क्रिमीञ्जयेत् । अजीर्णमातपं रोषमतिनीरं पयो गुडम् ॥ १४ ॥
रसोनमश्नन्पुरुषस्त्यजेदेतन्निरन्तरम् । मद्यं तथाम्लं च रसं सेवेत नित्यशः ॥ १५ ॥

Ripened *rasona* is taken, its husk and sprout removed from each pellicle of it and put in butter milk for a night to remove its strong smell. Next morning it is made into a paste. Sauvarchala, yavānī, fried hiṅgu, saindhava, trikaṭu and īraka—all equal quantities are powdered together and added to the paste of rasona in the proportion of one fifth its quantity. This kalka taken in doses of one karṣa daily followed by qwātha of eraṇḍamūla as anupāna relieves sarvāṅga uāta (nervous disorders affecting the entire body), ekāṅga vāta (affection of any one part of the body), ardita (facial palsy), apatantraka (tetanus), apasmāra (epilepsy), unmāda (insanity) urustambha (stiffness of leg), gṛdhrasī (sciatica), pain in uras (chest), pṛṣṭha (back), kaṭi (waist), pārshwa (flanks), kukshi (abdomen); and krimi. During this period the person should avoid ajīrṇa (indigestion), ātapa (sun), roṣa (anger), atinīra (too much of water drinking); paya (milk) and guḍa (jaggery) but use madya (alcoholic drinks), māṃsa (meat) and amla dravyas (sour things) every day (8–15).

पिप्पल्यादिकल्क उरुस्तम्भे—

पिप्पली पिप्पलीमूलं भल्लातकफलानि च । एतत्कल्कश्च सक्षौद्र उरुस्तम्भनिवारणः ॥ १६ ॥

Kalka of pippali, pippalīmūla and fruits of bhallātaka taken with honey relieves urustambha (stiffness of the thigh) (16).

अथ विष्णुक्रान्ताकल्कः परिणामशूले—

विष्णुक्रान्ताजटाकल्कः सिताक्षौद्रघृतैर्युतः । परिणामभवं शूलं नाशयेत्सप्तभिर्दिनैः ॥ १७ ॥

Kalka of roots of viṣṇukrānti with sugar, honey or ghee relieves pariṇāma shūla (colic due to peptic ulcer) within seven days (17).

अपरमपि परिणामशूलार्थं प्रयोगमाह—

शुण्ठीतिलगुडैः कल्को दुग्धेन सह योजयेत् । परिणामभवं शूलमामवातं च नाशयेत् ॥ १८ ॥

Kalka of shuṇṭhī, tila and jaggery taken with milk relieves pariṇāmashūla (peptic ulcers) and āmavāta (rheumatism) (18).

अथापामार्गकल्कः रक्तार्शसि—

अपामार्गस्य बीजानां कल्कस्तण्डुलवारिणा । पीतो रक्तार्शसां नाशं कुरुते नात्र संशयः ॥ १९ ॥

Kalka of seeds of apāmārga prepared with rice-wash relieves raktārshas (haemorrhoids) without doubt (19).

अथ बदरीमूलकल्कः रक्तातिसारे—

बदरीमूलकल्केन तिलकल्कश्च योजितः । मधुक्षीरयुतः कुर्याद्रक्तातीसारनाशनः ॥ २० ॥

Kalka of roots of badara and tila taken with honey and milk is beneficial in raktātisāra (bloody diarrhoea) (20).

रक्तक्षये लाक्षाकल्कः—

कूष्माण्डकरसोपेतां लाक्षां कर्षद्वयं पिबेत् । रक्तक्षयमुरोघातं क्षयरोगं च नाशयेत् ॥ २१ ॥

Two karṣas of lākshā taken with the juice of kūṣmāṇḍa is beneficial in loss of blood, uroghāta (chest injuries) and kshaya roga (consumption) (21).

अथ तण्डुलीयकल्कः रक्तप्रदरे—

तण्डुलीयजटाकल्कः सक्षौद्रः सरसाञ्जनः । तण्डुलोदकसंपीतो रक्तप्रदरनाशनः ॥ २२ ॥

Kalka of roots of taṇḍulīyaka and rasāñjana prepared with rice-wash and taken with honey relieves raktapradara (menorrhoegia) (22).

अथाङ्कोटककल्कोऽतीसारादौ—

अङ्कोटमूलकल्कश्च सक्षौद्रस्तण्डुलाम्बुना । अतीसारहरः प्रोक्तस्तथा विषहरः स्मृतः ॥ २३ ॥

Kalka of roots of aṅkoṭa prepared with rice-wash and taken with honey relieves atisāra (diarrhoea) and viṣa (poisons) (23).

वन्ध्याकर्कोटिकामूलं पाटलाया जटाऽथवा । घृतेन बिल्वमूलं वा द्विविधं नाशयेद्विषम् ॥ २४ ॥

Kalka or roots of vandhyākarkoṭikā or of roots of pāṭalā or of roots of bilwa taken with ghee relieves both varieties of (mineral and animal) poisons (24).

अथाभयादिकल्कः पाचनादौ—

अभयासैन्धवकणाशुण्ठीकल्कस्त्रिदोषहा । पथ्यासैन्धवशुण्डीभिः कल्को दीपनपाचनः ॥ २५ ॥

Kalka of abhayā, saindhava, kaṇā and shuṇṭhī alleviates the increase of tridoṣas; kalka of pathyā, saindhava and shuṇṭhī is dīpana-pāchana (carminative and digestive) (25).

अथ त्रिवृतादिकल्कः कृमिरोगे—

त्रिवृत्पलाशबीजानि पारसीकयमानिका । कम्पिल्लकं विडङ्गं च गुडश्च समभागिकम् ॥ २६ ॥
तक्रेण कल्कमेतेषां पिबेत् क्रिमिगणापहम् ।

Kalka, of trivṛt, palāshabīja, pārasīkayavānī, kampillaka, viḍaṅga and guḍa all equal parts taken with butter milk wards off all types of worms (26-27).

रक्तार्शसि तिलकल्क :—

नवनीततिलैः कल्को जेता रक्तार्शसां स्मृतः ॥ २७ ॥
नवनीतसितानागकेशरैश्चापि तद्विधः ।

Kalka of tila with butter or nāgakeshara and sugar cures raktārshas (haemorrhoids) (27–28).

संग्रहण्यां शुन्ठीकल्कः —

पीतो मसूरयूषेण कल्कः शुण्ठीशलाटुजः ॥ २८ ॥
जयेत्संग्रहणीं तद्वत्तक्रेण बृहतीभवः ।

Kalka of shunṭhī and shalāṭu (bilwa) taken with soup of masūra relieves saṅgrahaṇī (sprue); likewise is the kalka of bṛhatī taken with buttermilk (28).

इति श्रीदामोदरसूनुना श्रीशार्ङ्गधराचार्येण विरचितायां श्रीशार्ङ्गधरसंहितायां मध्यमखण्डे कल्ककल्पना नाम पञ्चमोऽध्यायः ।

Thus ends chapter five.

षष्ठोऽध्यायः

CHAPTER 6

Chūrṇa Kalpanā (Pulvis, Powders)

अत्यन्तशुष्कं यद्द्रव्यं सुपिष्टं वस्त्रगालितम् । तत्स्याच्चूर्णं रजः क्षोदस्तन्मात्रा कर्षसंमिता ॥ १ ॥

Nicely powdered dry drugs filtered through cloth is called chūrṇa, rajas or kshoda (pulvis, powder). It is administered in doses of one karṣa (1).

चूर्णे गुडादिमानकल्पना

चूर्णे गुडः समो देयः शर्करा द्विगुणा भवेत् । चूर्णेषु भर्जितं हिङ्गु देयं नोत्क्लेदकृद्भवेत् ॥ २ ॥
लिहेच्चूर्णं द्रवैः सर्वैर्घृताद्यैर्द्विगुणोन्मितैः । पिबेच्चतुर्गुणैरेव चूर्णमालोडितं द्रवैः ॥ ३ ॥

Jaggery, if, to be added to this powder should be equal in quantity, sugar double in quantity and fried hiṅgu only that much which shall not cause nausea. Chūrṇas are usually administered with equal quantities of ghee, honey or oil. If they are to be taken with decoctions, water, milk etc., such liquids should be four times the quantity of chūrṇa (2–3).

अथ चूर्णादीनामनुपानमात्रां दर्शयन्नाह—

चूर्णावलेहगुटिकाकल्कानामनुपानकम् । वातपित्तकफातङ्के त्रिद्व्येकपलमाहरेत् ॥ ४ ॥
यथा तैलं जले क्षिप्तं क्षणेनैव प्रसर्पति । अनुपानबलादङ्गे तथा सर्पति भेषजम् ॥ ५ ॥

Anupāna (vehicle for the medicine) for chūrṇa (pulvis), avaleha (confection), guṭikā (tablets), kalka (paste) should be three, two and one pala respectively for diseases of vāta, pitta and kapha; just as oil spreads quickly on water so also medicines spread inside the body by the strength of the vehicle (4–5).

अथ चूर्णार्थं भावनापरिमाणमाह—

द्रवेण यावता सम्यक्चूर्णं सर्वं प्लुतं भवेत् । भावनायाः प्रमाणं तु चूर्णे प्रोक्तं भिषग्वरैः ॥ ६ ॥

The quantity of any liquid which soaks the powder fully well is called bhāvanādrava (6).

अथामलक्यादिचूर्णं ज्वरादौ—

आमलं चित्रकं पथ्या पिप्पली सैन्धवस्तथा । चूर्णितोऽयं गणो ज्ञेयः सर्वज्वरविनाशनः ॥ ७ ॥
भेदी रुचिकरः श्लेष्मजेता दीपनपाचनः ।

Chūrṇa of āmalaka, chitraka, pathyā, pippalī and saindhava cures all varieties of jwaras (fevers) and acts as bhedana (purgative), ruchikara (appetiser), dīpana (carminative), pāchana (digestive) and kaphahara (7–8).

अथ पिप्पलीचूर्णं ज्वरे—

मधुना पिप्पलीचूर्णं लिहेत्कासज्वरापहम् ॥ ८ ॥
हिक्काश्वासहरं कण्ठ्यं प्लीहघ्नं बालकोचितम् ।

Chūrṇa of pippalī taken with honey relieves kāsa (cough), jwara (fevers), śwāsa (dyspnoea), hikkā (hiccough), kaṇṭhya (good for throst) and plīhaguṇa (relieves splenic enlargement) and specially suited for children (8–9).

मेहादिकेषु त्रिफलाचूर्णम्—

एका हरितकी योज्या द्वौ च योज्यौ बिभीतकौ ॥ ९ ॥
चत्वार्यामलकान्येवं त्रिफलैषा प्रकीर्तिता । त्रिफला मेहशोथघ्नी नाशयेद्विषमज्वरान् ॥ १० ॥
दीपनी श्लेष्मपित्तघ्नी कुष्ठहन्त्री रसायनी । सर्पिर्मधुभ्यां संयुक्ता सैव नेत्रामयाञ्जयेत् ॥ ११ ॥

One harītakī, two vibhītakī and four āmalaka—(parts by weight) together is called "*triphalā*". Powder of triphalā taken with honey and ghee relieves meha (polyurea), shotha (oedema), viṣamajwaras (remittent fevers), kuṣṭha (leprosy and other skin diseases), netrāmaya (eye diseases) and acts as dīpana (carminative), rasāyanī (tonic) and reduces kapha and pitta (9–11).

अथ त्र्यूषणचूर्णं दीपनादौ—

पिप्पली मरिचं शुण्ठी त्रिभिस्त्र्यूषणमुच्यते । दीपनं श्लेष्ममेदोघ्नं कुष्ठपीनसनाशनम् ॥ १२ ॥
जयेदरोचकं सामं मेहगुल्मगलामयान् ।

Pippalī, maricha and shunṭhī—together is known as "*tryūṣaṇa*". Powder of these acts as dīpana (carminative) decreases kapha and medas (fat) beneficial in kuṣṭha (leprosy and other skin diseases), pīnasa (rhinitis), arochaka (anorexia), āma (indigestion), meha (polyurea), gulma (abdominal tumors) and galāmaya (throat diseases) (12–13).

अथ पञ्चकोलमरुच्यादौ—

पिप्पलीचव्यविश्वाह्वापिप्पलीमूलचित्रकैः ॥ १३ ॥
पञ्चकोलमिति ख्यातं रुच्यं दीपनपाचनम् । अनाहप्लीहगुल्मघ्नं शूलश्लेष्मोदरापहम् ॥ १४ ॥

Pippalī, chavya, vishwā, pippalimūla and chitraka—together called *pañcha-kola* acts as ruchya (improves taste), dipana-pāchana (carminative and digestive) and relieves anāha (tympanitis), plīhā (splenic enlargement), gulma (abdominal tumors), shūla (colic) and sleṣmodara (enlargement of abdomen due to kaphavṛddhi) (13–14).

इदानीं त्रिगन्धचातुर्जातकचूर्णमाह—

त्रिगन्धमेलात्वक्पत्रैश्चतुर्जातं सकेशरैः । त्रिगन्धं सचतुर्जातं रूक्षोष्णं लघु पित्तकृत् ॥ १५ ॥
वर्ण्यं रुचिकरं तीक्ष्णं विषश्लेष्मामयाञ्जयेत् ।

Twak, patra and elā—together is tri-sugandha; with kesara they become chaturjātaka. Both these are rūksha (causing dryness), uṣṇa (causing heat), laghu (easily digestible), cause increase of pitta, varṇya (improves colour of the skin), ruchikara (improve taste), tikshṇa (penetrating) relieves diseases due to viṣa (poisons) and sleṣma (15–16).

अथ जीवनीयगणः—

काकोली क्षीरकाकोली जीवकर्षभकौ तथा ॥ १६ ॥
मेदा चान्या महामेदा जीवन्ती मधुकं तथा । मुद्गपर्णी माषपर्णी जीवनीयो गणस्त्वयम् ॥ १७ ॥
जीवनीयगणः स्वादुर्गर्भसंधानकृद्गुरुः । स्तन्यकृद्बृंहणो वृष्यः स्निग्धः शीतस्तृषापहः ॥ १८ ॥
रक्तपित्तं क्षयं शोषं ज्वरदाहानिलाञ्जयेत् ।

Kākolī, kshīrakākolī, jīvaka, ṛsabhaka, medā, mahāmedā, jīvantī, madhuka, mudgaparṇī, māṣaparṇī—are together known as jīvanīya gaṇa. This group possess swādu rasa (sweet taste) is guru (hard to digest), garbhasandhānakṛt (helps development of foetus), stanyakṛt (promotes breast milk), bṛmhaṇa (nourishes the body), vṛṣya (aphrodisiac),-snigdha (cause oilyness), shīta

(coolant), tṛṣāpaha (relieves thirst); cures raktapitta (purpura), kshaya (consumption), shoṣa (emaciation), jwara (fever), dāha (burning) and decreases vāta (16–19).

अथाष्टकवर्गः—

द्वे मेदे द्वे च काकोल्यौ जीवकर्षभकौ तथा ॥ १९ ॥
ऋद्धिवृद्धी च तैः सर्वैरष्टवर्ग उदाहृतः। अष्टवर्गो बुधैः प्रोक्तो जीवनीयसमो गुणैः ॥ २० ॥

The two medas, the two kākolīs, ṛṣabhaka, ṛddhi and vṛddhi together is known as *"aṣṭavarga"*. This group is similar in properties and actions with that of jīvanīya group (19–20).

अथ लवणपञ्चकं सृष्टविण्मूत्रादौ—

सिन्धु सौवर्चलं चैव बिडं सामुद्रिकं गडम्। एकद्वित्रिचतुष्पञ्चलवणानि क्रमाद्विदुः ॥ २१ ॥
तेषु मुख्यं सैन्धवं स्यादनुक्ते तत्प्रयोजयेत्। सैन्धवाद्यं रोमकान्तं ज्ञेयं लवणपञ्चकम् ॥ २२ ॥
मधुरं सृष्टविण्मूत्रं स्निग्धं सूक्ष्मं बलापहम्। वीर्योष्णं दीपनं तीक्ष्णं कफपित्तविवर्धनम् ॥ २३ ॥

Saindhava, sauvarchala, biḍa, sāmudra and gaḍa (romaka) are the five lavaṇas (salts). Of these saindhava is best and is to be used where-ever no specific salt is mentioned. Saindhava alone is counted as ekalavaṇa (single salt). Combination of saindhava and sauvarchala is lavaṇa dwaya (two sallts); saindhava, sauvarchala and biḍa is trilavaṇa (three salts); saindhava, sauvarcha, biḍa, and sāmudra as chaturlavaṇa (four salts); a combination of all the five is called pañcha lavaṇa (five salts). This combination acts as madhura (sweet), sṛṣṭaviṭmūtra (helps elimination of urine and faeces), snigdha (causes unctousness), sūkshma (enters into minute pores), balāpaha (reduces strength), uṣṇavīrya (heat producing), dīpana (carminative), tīkshṇa (penetrating), makes for increase of kapha and pitta (21–23).

अथ क्षारयोगं दर्शयन्नाह—

स्वर्जिका यावशूकश्च क्षारयुग्ममुदाहृतम्। ज्ञेयौ वह्निसमौ क्षारौ स्वर्जिकायावशूकजौ ॥ २४ ॥
क्षाराश्चान्येऽपि गुल्मार्शोग्रहणीरुच्छिदः सराः। पाचनाः कृमिपुंस्त्वघ्नाः शर्कराश्मरिनाशनाः ॥२५॥

Swarjikā and yavashūka are kshāras yugma (two alkalies) are similar to fire in action. These and other kshāras (alkalies) are helpful in gulma (abdominal tumors), arsha (piles), grahaṇī (sprue) and kṛmi (worms), sharkarā-ashmarī (urinary calculi) act as sara (laxative), pāchana (digestive) and puṃstwaghna (causes impotence) (24–25).

सुदर्शनचूर्णम्—

त्रिफला रजनीयुग्मं कण्टकारीयुगं शठी । त्रिकटु ग्रन्थिकं मूर्वागुडूची धन्वयासकः ॥ २६ ॥
कटुका पर्पटो मुस्तं त्रायमाणा च वालकम् । निम्बः पुष्करमूलं च मधुयष्टी च वत्सकम् ॥ २७ ॥
यमानीन्द्रयवो भार्ङ्गी शिग्रुबीजं सुराष्ट्रकम् । वचा त्वक्पद्मकोशीरं चन्दनातिविषाबलाः ॥ २८ ॥
शालिपर्णी पृश्निपर्णी विडङ्गं तगरं यथा । चित्रको देवदारुश्च चव्यं पत्रं पटोलजम् ॥ २९ ॥
जीवकर्षभकौ चैव लवङ्गं वंशलोचना । पुण्डरीकं च काकोली पत्रकं जातिपत्रकम् ॥ ३० ॥
तालीसपत्रं च तथा समभागानि चूर्णयेत् । सर्वचूर्णस्य चार्धांशं कैरातं निक्षिपेत्सुधीः ॥ ३१ ॥
एतत्सुदर्शनं नाम चूर्णं दोषत्रयापहम् । ज्वरांश्च निखिलान्हन्यान्नात्र कार्या विचारणा ॥ ३२ ॥
पृथग्द्वन्द्वागन्तुजांश्च धातुस्थान्विषमज्वरान् । संनिपातोद्भवांश्चापि मानसानपि नाशयेत् ॥ ३३ ॥
शीतज्वरैकाहिकादीन्मोहं तन्द्रां भ्रमं तृषाम् । श्वासं कासं च पाण्डुं च हृद्रोगं हन्ति कामलाम् ॥३४॥
त्रिकपृष्ठकटीजानुपार्श्वशूलनिवारणम् । शीताम्बुना पिबेद्धीमान्सर्वज्वरनिवृत्तये ॥ ३५ ॥
सुदर्शनं यथा चक्रं दानवानां विनाशनम् । तद्वज्ज्वराणां सर्वेषामिदं चूर्णं प्रणाशनम् ॥ ३६ ॥

Triphalā, the two rajanīs, the two kaṇṭakārīs, shaṭhi, trikaṭu, granthika, mūrvā, guḍūchi, dhanvayāsaka, kaṭukā, parpaṭā, musta, trāyamāṇā, vālaka, nimba, puṣkaramūla, madhuyaṣṭhi, vatsaka, yamānī, indrayava, shigrubīja, saurāṣṭrakam, vachā, twak, padmaka, ushīra, chandana, ativiṣā, balā, shāliparṇi, pṛshnīparṇī, viḍaṅga, tagara, chitraka, devadāru, chavya, paṭola-patra, jīvaka, ṛṣabhaka, lavaṅga, vaṃśalochana, puṇḍarīka, kākolī, patra, jātīpatra and tālīsapatra—all equal parts are powdered and to it is added half the total quantity of powder of kirātatiktā, mixed well and used. This recipe known as '*Sudarshana Chūrṇa*' cures all types of fevers without any doubt. Fevers due to any one, two or all the three doṣas, āgantu jwara, dhātughāta jwara, viṣama-jwara, sannipātajwara, mānasika jwara, shītajwara, ekāhika jwara etc. moha, tandrā, bhrama, tṛṣā, śwāsa, pāṇḍu, hṛdroga, kāmalā, pain of joints, waist, back, knee, flanks are all relieved by this. Taken with cold water it cures all fevers just like the Sudarshana Chakra (of Lord Viṣṇu) destroys all the demons (26–36).

अथ ज्वरे पिप्पलीचूर्णम्—

कासश्वासज्वरहरी त्रिफला पिप्पलीयुता । चूर्णिता मधुना लीढा भेदिनी चाग्निबोधिनी ॥ ३७ ॥

Chūrṇa of triphalā and pippalī taken with honey relieves kāsa (cough), śwāsa (dyspnoea), jwara (fevers) and acts as bhedinī (purgative) and agnibodhinī (carminative) (37).

अथ कट्फलादिचूर्णं ज्वरादौ—

कट्फलं मुस्तकं तिक्ता शठी शृङ्गी च पौष्करम् । चूर्णमेषां च मधुना शृङ्गबेररसेन वा ॥ ३८ ॥
लेह्यं ज्वरहरं कण्ठ्यं कासश्वासारुचीर्जयेत् । वायुशूलं तथा छर्दिं क्षयं चैव व्यपोहति ॥ ३९ ॥

Chūrṇa of kaṭphala, mustā, tiktā, shaṭhi, shṛṅgī and puṣkara taken with honey or juice of shṛṅgavera (green ginger) is good for throat, relieves fevers, kāsa (cough), śwāsa (dyspnoea), aruchi (anorexia), vāyu (flatus), chardi (vomiting), shūla (colic) and kshaya (consumption) (38–39).

अथ बृहत्कट्फलादिचूर्णं—

कट्फलं पौष्करं शृङ्गी मुस्ता त्रिकटुकं शठी । समस्तान्येकशो वापि सूक्ष्मचूर्णानि कारयेत् ॥ ४० ॥
आर्द्रकस्वरसक्षौद्रैर्लिह्यात्कफविनाशनम् । शूलानिलारुचिच्छर्दिकासश्वासक्षयापहम् ॥ ४१ ॥

Chūrṇa of kaṭphala, puṣkara, shṛṅgī, mustā, trikaṭu and shaṭhī—taken with honey and ginger juice relieves kapha, shūla (colic), vāta aruchi (anorexia), chardi (vomiting), kāsa (cough), śwāsa (dyspnoea), and kshaya (consumption) (40–41).

कट्फलं पौष्करं कृष्णा शृङ्गी च मधुना सह । श्वासकासज्वरहरः श्रेष्ठो लेहः कफान्तकृत् ॥ ४२ ॥

Chūrṇa of kaṭphala, puṣkara, kṛṣṇā and śṛṅgi, taken with honey removes kapha effectively and relieves śwāsa (dyspnoea), kāsa (cough) and jwara (fevers) (42).

शृङ्गीचूर्णम्—

शृङ्गीं प्रतिविषां कृष्णां चूर्णितां मधुना लिहेत् । शिशोः कासज्वरच्छर्दिशान्त्यै वा केवलां विषाम् ॥४३॥

Chūrṇa of śṛṅgi, prativiṣā and kṛṣṇā given with honey to children relieves kāsa (cough), jwara (fever), chardi (vomiting). Viṣā (ativiṣā) alone can also be given likewise (43).

यवक्षारादिचूर्णम्—

(यवक्षारविषाशृङ्गीमागधीपौष्करोद्भवम् । चूर्णं क्षौद्रयुतं लीढं पञ्चकासाञ्जयेच्छिशोः ॥ ४४ ॥)

Chūrṇa of yavakshāra, viṣā, śṛṅgi, māgadhī, and puṣkara given with honey relieves the five kinds of kāsa (cough) of children (44).

अतीसारे शुण्ठ्यादिचूर्णमाह—

शुण्ठीप्रतिविषाहिङ्गुमुस्ताकुटजचित्रकैः । चूर्णमुष्णाम्बुना पीतमामातीसारनाशनम् ॥ ४५ ॥

Chūrṇa of shunṭhī, prativiṣā, hiṅgu, mustā, kuṭaja and chitraka taken with warm water relieves āmātisāra (early stage of diarrhoea) (45).

अथ हरीतक्यादिचूर्णमामातीसारादौ—

हरीतकी प्रतिविषा सिन्धु सौवर्चलं वचा । हिङ्गु चेति कृतं चूर्णं पिबेदुष्णेन वारिणा ॥ ४६ ॥
आमातीसारशमनं ग्राहि चाग्निप्रबोधनम् ।

Chūrṇa of harītakī, prativiṣā, saindhava, sauvarchala, vachā and hiṅgu taken with warm water relieves āmātisāra (early stage of diarrhoea), is grāhī (water absorbant) and agniprabodhana (carminative) (46–47).

लघुगङ्गाधरचूर्णम्—

मुस्तमिन्द्रयवं बिल्वं लोध्रं मोचरसं तथा ॥ ४७ ॥
धातकीं चूर्णयेत्तक्रगुडाभ्यां पाययेत्सुधीः । सर्वातीसारशमनं निरुणद्धि प्रवाहिकाम् ॥ ४८ ॥
लघुगङ्गाधरं नाम चूर्णं संग्राहकं परम् ।

Chūrṇa of mustā, indrayava, bilwa, lodhra, mocharasa and dhātakī taken with buttermilk and jaggery stops all varieties of atisāra (diarrhoea) and pravāhikā (dysentery). Known as *Laghu Gaṅgādhara Chūrṇa,* it is a good saṅgrāhaka (anti diarrhoeal) (48–49).

अथ वृद्धगङ्गाधरचूर्णम्—

मुस्तारलुकशुण्ठीभिर्धातकीलोध्रवालकैः ॥ ४९ ॥
बिल्वमोचरसाभ्यां च पाठेन्द्रयववत्सकैः । आम्रबीजं प्रतिविषा लज्जालुरिति चूर्णितम् ॥ ५० ॥
क्षौद्रतण्डुलपानीयैः पीतैर्याति प्रवाहिका । सर्वातिसारग्रहणी प्रशमं याति वेगतः ॥ ५१ ॥
वृद्धगङ्गाधरं चूर्णं सरिद्वेगस्य रोधकम् ।

Chūrṇa of mustā, araluka, shuṇṭhī, dhātakī, lodhra, vālaka, āmrabīja, prativiṣā and lajjālu—taken with honey and rice-wash quickly, relieves all varieties of pravāhikā (dysentery), atisāra (diarrhoea), grahaṇī (sprue). Known as *Vṛddha Gaṅgādhara Chūrṇa,* it stops atisāra (diarrhoeas) like a dam across the river (49–52).

अथाजमोदादिचूर्णमतीसारे—

अजमोदा मोचरसं सशृङ्गबेरं सधातकी कुसुमम् । गोदधिमथितयुक्तं गंगामपि वाहिनीं रुंध्यात् ॥५२॥

Chūrṇa of ajamodā, mocharasa, shṛṅgavera, and dhātakī-kusuma taken with buttermilk prepared from cow's milk can even stop the flow of river Gaṅgā (can stop severe diarrhoeas) (52).

मरिचादिचूर्णं—

तक्रेण यः पिबेन्नित्यं चूर्णं मरिचसंभवम् ।
चित्रसौवर्चलोपेतं ग्रहणी तस्य नश्यति । उदरप्लीहमन्दाग्निगुल्मार्शोनाशनं भवेत् ॥ ५३ ॥

He who takes every day the chūrṇa of maricha, chitraka and sauvarchala shall get rid of grahaṇī (sprue), udara (enlargement of abdomen), plīhā (splenic enlargement), mandāgni (dyspepsia), gulma (abdominal tumor) and arshas (piles) (53).

अथ कपित्थाष्टकं चूर्णं ग्रहण्यादौ—

अष्टौ भागाः कपित्थस्य षड्भागा शर्करा मता । दाडिमं तिन्तिडीकं च श्रीफलं धातकी तथा ॥५४॥
अजमोदा पिप्पली च प्रत्येकं स्युस्त्रिभागिकाः । मरिचं जीरकं धान्यं ग्रन्थिकं वालकं तथा ॥ ५५ ॥
सौवर्चलं यमानी च चातुर्जातं सचित्रकम् । नागरं चैकभागाः स्युः प्रत्येकं सूक्ष्मचूर्णितम् ॥ ५६ ॥
कपित्थाष्टकसंज्ञं स्याच्चूर्णमेतद्गलामयान् । अतीसारं क्षयं गुल्मं ग्रहणीं च व्यपोहति ॥ ५७ ॥

Eight parts of kapittha, six parts of sugar, three parts each of dāḍima, tintidīka, srīphala, dhātakī, ajamodā and pippali and one part of each of maricha, jīraka, dhānya, granthika, vālaka, sauvarchala yavānī, chāturjātakas, chitraka and nāgara—are powdered nicely. This recipe known as *Kapitthāṣṭaka Chūrṇa* is beneficial in diseases of the throat, atisāra (diarrhoea), kshaya (consumption), gulma (tumors of the abdomen) and grahaṇī (sprue) (54–57).

दाडिमाष्टकम्—

दाडिमी द्विपला ग्राह्या खण्डाद्दशपलानि च । त्रिगन्धस्य पलं चैकं त्रिकटु स्यात्पलत्रयम् ॥ ५८ ॥
एतदेकीकृतं सर्वं चूर्णं स्याद्दाडिमाष्टकम् । रुचिकृद्दीपनं कण्ठ्यं ग्राहि कासज्वरापहम् ॥ ५९ ॥

Two palas of dāḍima, ten palas of sugar candy, one pala of trisugandhas, three palas of trikaṭu—put together and nicely powdered becomes *Dāḍimāṣṭ aka Chūrṇa.* This recipe improves taste, digestion, good for throat, stops loose motions and relieves kāsa (cough) and jwara (fevers) (58–59).

अथ बृहद्दाडिमाष्टकं अतीसारादौ—

दाडिमस्य पलान्यष्टौ शर्करायाः पलाष्टकम् । पिप्पली पिप्पलीमूलं यमानी मरिचं तथा ॥ ६० ॥
धान्यकं जीरकं शुण्ठी प्रत्येकं पलसंमितम् । कर्षमात्रा तुगाक्षीरी त्वक्पत्रैलाश्च केशरम् ॥ ६१ ॥
प्रत्येकं कोलमात्राः स्युस्तच्चूर्णं दाडिमाष्टकम् । अतीसारं क्षयं गुल्मं ग्रहणीं च गलग्रहम् ॥ ६२ ॥
मन्दाग्निं पीनसं कासं चूर्णमेतद्व्यपोहति ।

Eight palas each of dāḍima and sugar, one pala each of pippalī, pippalīmūla yavānī, maricha, dhānyaka, jīraka and shunṭhī, one karṣa of tugākshīrī; and one kola each of twak, patra, elā and keśara—the powder of all these known as *Dāḍimāṣṭaka Chūrṇa (second)* relieves atisāra (diarrhoea), kshaya (consumption), gulma (abdominal tumors), grahaṇī (sprue), galagraha (pain in the throat), mandāgni (dyspnoea), pīnasa (rhinitis) and kāsa (cough) (60–63).

पिप्पल्यादिचूर्णम्—

(पिप्पली बृहती व्याघ्री यवक्षारकलिङ्गकाः ॥ ६३ ॥
चित्रकं सारिवा पाठा शठी लवणपञ्चकम् । तच्चूर्णं पाययेद्दध्ना सुरयोष्णाम्बुनापि वा ॥ ६४ ॥
मारुतग्रहणीदोषशमनं परमं हितम् ।)

Chūrṇa of pippalī, bṛhatī, vyāghrī, yavakshāra, kaliṅgakā, chitraka, sārivā, pāṭhā, shaṭhī and the five lavaṇas–taken with curds, fermented liquor or warm water relieves maruta grahaṇī (sprue) and is good for similar conditions (64–65).

अथ लवङ्गादिचूर्णं अरोचकादौ—

लवङ्गं शुद्धकर्पूरमेलात्वङ्नागकेशरम् ॥ ६५ ॥
जातीफलमुशीरं च नागरं कृष्णजीरकम् । कृष्णागरुस्तुगाक्षीरी मांसी नीलोत्पलं कणा ॥ ६६ ॥
चन्दनं तगरं वालं कङ्कोलं चेति चूर्णयेत् । समभागानि सर्वाणि सर्वेभ्योऽर्धा सिता भवेत् ॥ ६७ ॥
लवङ्गाद्यमिदं चूर्णं राजार्हं वह्निदीपनम् । रोपणं तर्पणं वृष्यं त्रिदोषघ्नं बलप्रदम् ॥ ६८ ॥
हृद्रोगं कण्ठरोगं च कासं हिक्कां च पीनसम् । यक्ष्माणं तमकं श्वासमतीसारंमुरःक्षतम् ॥ ६९ ॥
प्रमेहारुचिगुल्मादीन्ग्रहणीमपि नाशयेत् ।

Lavaṅga, shuddha karpūra, elā, twak, nāgakeśara, jātīphala, ushīra, nāgara, kṛṣṇa jīraka, kṛṣṇāgaru, tugākshīrī, māṃsī, nīlotpala, kaṇā, chandana, tagara, vāla, and kaṅkola—all equal parts are powdered and is added with half their total quantity of sugar. This recipe known as *Lavaṅgādi Chūrṇa*, suited for the princelymen, is dīpana (carminative), ropaṇa (heals ulcers), tarpaṇa (satisfies hunger), vṛṣya (aphrodisiac), tridoṣaghna (relieves the aggravated taidoṣas), balaprada (gives strength); cures hṛdroga (heart direases), kaṇṭharoga (throat diseases), kāsa (cough), hikkā (hiccough), pīnasa (rhinitis), yakshmā (consumption), tamaka śwāsa (bronchial asthma), atisāra (diarrhoeas), urakshata (injury to lungs), prameha (diabetes), aruchi (anorexia), gulma (abdominal tumor), and even grahaṇī (sprue) (66–69).

अथ जातीफलाद्यं चूर्णं ग्रहण्यादौ—

जातीफललवङ्गैलापत्रत्वङ्नागकेशरैः ॥ ७० ॥
कर्पूरचन्दनतिलैस्त्वक्क्षीरीतगरामलैः । तालीसपिप्पलीपथ्यास्थूलजीरकचित्रकैः ॥ ७१ ॥
शुण्ठीविडङ्गमरिचैः समभागविचूर्णितैः । यावन्त्येतानि सर्वाणि कुर्याद्भङ्गां च तावतीम् ॥ ७२ ॥
सर्वचूर्णसमा देया शर्करा च भिषग्वरैः । कर्षमात्रं ततः खादेन्मधुना प्लावितं सुधीः ॥ ७३ ॥
अस्य प्रभावाद्ग्रहणीकासश्वासारुचिक्षयाः । वातश्लेष्मप्रतिश्यायाः प्रशमं यान्ति वेगतः ॥ ७४ ॥

Jātīphala, lavaṅga, elā, patra, twak, nāgakeśara, karpūra, chandana, tila, twak-kshīrī, tagara, amala, tālīsa, pippalī, pathyā, sthūla jīraka, chitraka, shuṇṭhī, vidaṅga and maricha—all equal parts and bhaṅga equal to the total quantity of the above are powdered nicely and added with equal quantity of sugar. This recipe known as *jātīphalādi chūrṇa* if taken in doses of one karṣa, with honey, relieves quickly grahaṇī (sprue), kāsa (cough), śwāsa (dyspnoea), aruchi (anorexia), kshaya (consumption) and pratishyāya due to vāta kapha (rhinitis) (70–74).

अथ महाखाण्डवचूर्णमरुच्यादौ—

मरिचं नागपुष्पाणि तालीसं लवणानि च। प्रत्येकमेकभागाः स्युः पिप्पलीमूलचित्रकैः ॥ ७५ ॥
त्वक्कणा तिन्तिडीकं च जीरकं च द्विभागिकम्। धान्याम्लवेतसौ विश्वं भद्रैला बदराणि च ॥ ७६ ॥
अजमोदा जलधरः प्रत्येकं स्युस्त्रिभागिकाः। सर्वौषधिचतुर्थांशं दाडिमस्य पलं भवेत् ॥ ७७ ॥
द्रव्येभ्यो निखिलेभ्यश्च सिता देयार्धमात्रया। महाखाण्डवसंज्ञं स्याच्चूर्णमेतत्सुरोचनम् ॥ ७८ ॥
अग्निदीप्तिकरं हृद्यं कासातीसारनाशनम्। हृद्रोगकण्ठजठरमुखरोगप्रणाशनम् ॥ ७९ ॥
विषूचिकां तथाध्मानमर्शोगुल्मकृमीनपि। छर्दि पञ्चविधां श्वासं चूर्णमेतद्व्यपोहति ॥ ८० ॥

One part each of maricha, nāgapuṣpa, tālīsa, lavaṇas, two parts each of pippalīmūla, chitraka, twak, kaṇā, tintiḍīka, jīraka; three parts each of dhānyā, amlavetasa, viśwa, bhadrailā, badara, ajamodā, jaladhara; dāḍimaphala, four times the total quantity of all the above drugs and sugar half of the total quantity are powdered together nicely. This recipe known as *Mahā khāṇḍava chūrṇa* is a good rochana (appetiser), dīpana (carminative), hṛdya (good for heart), relieves kāsa (cough), atisāra (diarrhoea), diseases of hṛdaya (heart), kaṇṭha (throat), jaṭhara (stomach), mukha (mouth); viṣūchikā (vomiting and diarrhoea), ādhmāna (tympanitis), arshas (piles), gulma (abdominal tumors). Kṛmi (intestinal worms), chardi (vomiting) and five types of śwāsa (dyspnoea) (75-80).

अथ नारायणचूर्णमुदरादौ—

चित्रकं त्रिफला व्योषं जीरकं हपुषा वचा। यमानी पिप्पलीमूलं शतपुष्पाऽजगन्धिका ॥ ८१ ॥
अजमोदा शठी धान्यं विडङ्गं स्थूलजीरकम्। हेमाह्वा पौष्करं मूलं क्षारौ लवणपञ्चकम् ॥ ८२ ॥
कुष्ठं चेति समांशानि विशाला स्याद्द्विभागिका। त्रिवृत्त्रिभागा विज्ञेया दन्त्या भागत्रयं भवेत् ॥८३॥
चतुर्भागा शातला स्यात्सर्वाण्येकत्र चूर्णयेत्। पाचनस्नेहनाद्यैश्च स्निग्धकोष्ठस्य रोगिणः ॥ ८४ ॥
दद्याच्चूर्णं विरेकाय सर्वरोगप्रणाशनम्। हृद्रोगे पाण्डुरोगे च कासे श्वासे भगन्दरे ॥ ८५ ॥
मन्दाग्नौ च ज्वरे कुष्ठे ग्रहण्यां च गलग्रहे। दद्याद्युक्तानुपानेन तथाध्माने सुरादिभिः ॥ ८६ ॥
गुल्मे बदरनीरेण विड्भेदे दधिमस्तुना। उष्णाम्बुभिरजीर्णे च वृक्षाम्लैः परिकर्तिषु ॥ ८७ ॥
उष्ट्रीदुग्धेनोदरेषु तथा तक्रेण वा गवाम्। प्रसन्नया वातरोगे दाडिमाम्बुभिरर्शसि ॥ ८८ ॥
द्विविधे च विषे दद्याद्घृतेन विषनाशनम्। चूर्णं नारायणं नाम दुष्टरोगगणापहम् ॥ ८९ ॥

One part each of chitraka, triphalā, vyoṣā, jīraka, hapuṣā, vachā, yavānī, pippalīmūla, shatapuṣpā, ajamodā, shaṭhī, dhānya, viḍaṅga, sthūlajīraka, hemāhwā, puṣkaramūla, the two kshāras, the five lavaṇas and kuṣṭha two parts each of vishālā; three parts each of trivṛt and dantī; four parts of shātalā-all are powdered together nicely. This recipe known as *Nārāyaṇa Chūrṇa* acts as a purgative to cure all diseases. It is to be given after preparing the patient with snehana and pāchana drugs and with suitable anupāna (vehicle) in cases of hṛdroga (heart diseases), pāṇḍu (anaemia), kāsa (cough), śwāsa (dyspnoea), bhagandara (fistula-in-ano), agnimāndya (dyspepsia), jwara (fevers), kuṣṭha (leprosy and other skin disorders), grahaṇi (sprue), galagraha (throat disorders); with surā in cases of ādhmāna (tympanitis), with juice of badara in gulma (abdominal tumors), with dadhimastu (whey) in viḍbheda (diarrhoea); with hot water in ajīrṇa (indigestion); with juice of vṛkshāmla in parikārtika (pain in the rectum); in udara (enlargement of abdomen); with camel's milk or buttermilk prepared with cow's milk; with prasannā (distilled liquor) in vātarogas (nervous disorders); in arshas (piles) with juice of dāḍima and with ghee in both types of viṣa (poisons). A host of bad diseases shall be relieved by this (81– 9).

अथ हपुषाद्यं चूर्णमजीर्णोदरादौ—

हपुषा त्रिफला चैव त्रायमाणा च पिप्पली । हेमक्षीरी त्रिवृच्चैव शातला कटुका वचा ॥ ९० ॥
नीलिनी सैन्धवं कृष्णं लवणं चेति चूर्णयेत् । उष्णोदकेन मूत्रेण दाडिमत्रिफलारसैः ॥ ९१ ॥
तथा मांसरसेनापि यथायोग्यं पिबेन्नरः । अजीर्णे प्लीह्नि गुल्मेषु शोफार्शोविषमाग्निषु ॥ ९२ ॥
हलीमकामलापाण्डुकुष्ठाध्मानोदरेष्वपि ।

Hapuṣā, triphalā, trāyamāṇā, pippali, hemakshīrī, trivṛt, shātalā, kaṭukā, vachā, nīlinī, saindhava and kṛṣṇalavaṇa—all to be powdered nicely and taken with either warm water, cow's urine, juice of dāḍima, triphalā qwātha or meat soup, will prove beneficial in cases of ajīrṇa (indigestion), plihā (splenic enlargement), gulma (abdominal tumor), halīmaka (chlorosis), kāmalā (jaundice), pāṇḍu (anaemia), kuṣṭha (leprosy and other skin diseases), ādhmāna (tympanitis), and udara (abdominal enlargment) (90–93).

अथ पञ्चसमं चूर्णं शूलादौ—

शुण्ठी हरीतकी कृष्णा त्रिवृत्सौवर्चलं तथा ॥ ९३ ॥
समभागानि सर्वाणि सूक्ष्मचूर्णानि कारयेत् । ज्ञेयं पञ्चसमं चूर्णमेतच्छूलहरं परम् ॥ ९४ ॥
आध्मानजठरार्शोघ्नमामवातहरं स्मृतम् ।

Shuṇṭhī, harītakī, kṛṣṇā, trivṛt, sauvarchala—all equal parts powdered nicely is known as *Pañchasama Chūrṇa* relieves shūla (pain in the abdomen), ādhmāna (tympanitis), jaṭhara (enlargment of abdomen), arshas (haemorrhoids) and āmavāta (rheumatism) (93–95).

अथ नाराचचूर्णमाध्मानशूलादौ—

कर्षमात्रा भवेत्कृष्णा त्रिबृता स्यात्पलोन्मिता ॥ ९५ ॥
खण्डात्पलं च विज्ञेयं चूर्णमेकत्र कारयेत् । कर्षोन्मितं लिहेदेतत्क्षौद्रेणाध्माननाशनम् ॥ ९६ ॥
गाढविट्कोदरकफान्पित्तशूलं च नाशयेत् ।

One karṣa of pippalī, one pala each of trivṛt and sugar candy are powdered nicely and taken in doses of one karṣa with honey relieves ādhmāna (typanitis), gāḍhaviṭ (hard and constipated bowels), udara (abdominal enlargement), reduces kapha and pittashūla (colic due to pitta) (95–97).

अथ लवणत्रितयाद्यं चूर्णं यकृत्प्लीहशूलादौ—

लवणत्रितयं क्षारौ शतपुष्पाद्वयं वचा ॥ ९७ ॥
अजमोदाऽजगन्धा च हपुषा जीरकद्वयम् । मरिचं पिप्पलीमूलं पिप्पली गजपिप्पली ॥ ९८ ॥
हिङ्गुश्च हिङ्गुपत्री च शठी पाठोपकुञ्चिका । शुण्ठी चित्रकचव्यानि विडङ्गं चाम्लवेतसम् ॥ ९९ ॥
दाडिमं तिन्तिडीकं च त्रिवृद्दन्ती शतावरी । इन्द्रवारुणिका भार्ङ्गी देवदारु यवानिका ॥ १०० ॥
कुस्तुम्बुरुस्तुम्दुरूणि पौष्करं बदराणि च । शिवा चेति समांशानि चूर्णमेकत्र कारयेत् ॥ १०१ ॥
भावभेदार्द्रकरसैर्बीजपूररसैस्तथा । तत्पिबेत्सर्पिषा जीर्णमद्येनोष्णोदकेन वा ॥ १०२ ॥
कोलाम्भसा वा तक्रेण दुग्धेनौष्ट्रेण मस्तुना । यकृत्पृष्ठकटीशूलगुदकुक्षिहृदामयम् ॥ १०३ ॥
अर्शोविष्टम्भमन्दाग्निगुल्मप्लीहोदराणि च । हिक्काध्मानश्वासकासाञ्जयेदेतान्न संशयः ॥ १०४ ॥
एतैरेवौषधैः सम्यग्घृतं वा साधयेत्सुधीः ।

The three lavaṇas, the two kshāras, the two shatapuṣpas, vachā, ajamodā, ajagandhā, hapuṣā, the two jīrakas, maricha, pippalīmūla, pippalī, gajapippalī, hiṅgu, hiṅgupatrī, shaṭhī, pāṭhā, upakuñchikā, shuṇṭhī, chitraka, chavya, viḍaṅga, amlavetasa, dāḍima, tintidīka, trivṛt, dantī, shatāvarī, indravāruṇī, bhārṅgī, devadāru, yavānikā, kustumburu, tumburu, pauṣkara, badara and shivā—all equal parts are powdered nicely and given bhāvanā with (macerated with juice of) ārdraka and bījapūra and dried. This recipe taken with ghee, old wine, warm water, buttermilk, juice of kola, camel's milk, or whey of butter milk relieves yakṛt-plīhā (enlargement of liver and spleen), kaṭishūla (pain in the waist), diseases of guda (rectum), kukshi (abdomen), hṛd (heart), arshas (piles), viṣṭambha (constipation), mandāgni (dyspepsia), gulma (abdominal tumor), plīhā (splenic enlargement), udara (abdominal enlargement), hikkā (hiccough), ādhmāna (tympanitis), śwāsa (dyspnoea) and kāsa (cough). The above drugs may be prepared even as a ghṛta (medicated ghee) and used in these complaints (97–105).

अथ शूलादौ तुम्बुरादिचूर्णम्—

तुम्बुरूणि त्रिलवणं यमानी पुष्कराह्वयम् ॥ १०५ ॥
यवक्षाराभयाहिङ्गुविडङ्गानि समानि च । त्रिवृत्त्रिभागा विज्ञेया सूक्ष्मचूर्णानि कारयेत् ॥ १०६ ॥
पिबेदुष्णेन तोयेन यवक्काथेन वा पिबेत् । जयेत्सर्वाणि शूलानि गुल्माध्मानोदराणि च ॥ १०७ ॥

Tumburu, three lavaṇas, yavānī, puṣkara, yavakshāra, abhayā, hiṅgu and viḍaṅga—each one part and three parts of trivṛt are powdered nicely and with warm water or decoction of yava (barley water) relieves all types of shūla (abdominal pain), gulma (abdominal tumor), ādhmāna (tympanitis) and udara (abdominal enlargement) (105–107).

अथ चित्रकाद्यं चूर्णं मन्दाग्न्यादौ—

चित्रकं नागरं हिङ्गु पिप्पली पिप्पलीजटा । चव्याजमोदा मरिचं प्रत्येकं कर्षसंमितम् ॥ १०८ ॥
स्वर्जिका च यवक्षारः सिन्धु सौवर्चलं बिडम् । सामुद्रकं रोमकं च कोलमात्राणि कारयेत् ॥ १०९ ॥
एकीकृत्याखिलं चर्णं भावयेन्मातुलुङ्गजैः । रसैर्दाडिमजैर्वापि शोषयेदातपेन च ॥ ११० ॥
एतच्चूर्णं जयेद्गुल्मं ग्रहणीमामजां रुजम् । अग्निं च कुरुते दीप्तं रुचिकृत्कफनाशनम् ॥ १११ ॥

Chitraka, nāgara, hiṅgu, pippalī, pippalījaṭā, chavyā, ajamodā, maricha—each one karṣa, sarjikā, yavakshāra, saindhava, sauvarchala, biḍa, sāmudrika, romaka—each one kola are nicely powdered and given bhāvanā with juice of (maceracted with juices of) mātuluṅga or dāḍima and dried in sun. This recipe is beneficial in gulma (abdominal tumors), grahaṇī (sprue), āmaja ruja (abdominal pain due to indigestion) and acts as a dīpana (carminative), ruchikṛt (improves taste) and kaphanāshana (diminishes kapha) (108–111).

अथ वडवानलचूर्णं मन्दाग्न्यादौ—

सैन्धवं पिप्पलीमूलं पिप्पली चव्यचित्रकम् । शुण्ठी हरीतकी चेति क्रमवृद्धानि चूर्णयेत् ॥ ११२ ॥
वडवानलनामैतच्चूर्णं स्यादग्निदीपनम् ।

Saindhava, pippalīmūla, pippalī, chavya, shuṇṭhī and harītakī—each succeeding one taken in equally increased quantity of the preceding (viz. one part of saindhava, two of pippalīmūla; three of pippalī, four of chavya, five of chitraka, six of shuṇṭhī and seven of harītakī) are nicely powdered. This recipe known as *Baḍavānala Chūrṇa* is a good dīpana (carminative)(112–113).

अजमोदा विडङ्गानि सैन्धवं देवदारु च ॥ ११३ ॥
चित्रकः पिप्पलीमूलं शतपुष्पा च पिप्पली । मरिचं चेति कर्षांशं प्रत्येकं कारयेद्बुधः ॥ ११४ ॥
कर्षास्तु पञ्च पथ्याया दश स्युर्वृद्धदारुकात् । नागराच्च दशैव स्युः सर्वाण्येकत्र चूर्णयेत् ॥११५॥
पिबेत्कोष्णजलेनैव चूर्णं श्वयथुनाशनम् । आमवातरुजं हन्ति संधिपीडां च गृध्रसीम् ॥ ११६ ॥
कटिपृष्ठगुदस्थां च जङ्घयोश्च रुजां जयेत् । तूनीप्रतूनीविश्वाचीकफवातामयाञ्जयेत् ॥ ११७ ॥
समेन वा गुडेनास्य वटकान्कारयेद्भिषक् ।

Ajamodā, viḍaṅga, saindhava, devadāru, chitraka, pippalīmūla, shatapuṣpā, pippalī and maricha—each one karṣa; five karṣas of pathyā, ten karṣa of vṛddhadāru and nāgara—all are powderd nicely used with warm water it is beneficial in shotha (oedema), pain of āmavāta (rheumatism), sandhipīḍa (pain in the joints), gṛdhrasī (sciatica), pain in the waist, back, legs, and buttocks; tūṇī and pratitūnī (pain in the region of urinary bladdder), viśwāchī (painful arm) and other diseases of kapha and vata. This can be made into a pill adding equal quantity of jaggery (113–118).

श्वासादौ शुण्ठ्यादिचूर्णम्—

(शुण्ठी सौवर्चलं हिङ्गु दाडिमं चाम्लवेतसम् ॥ ११८ ॥
चूर्णमुष्णाम्बुना पेयं श्वासहृद्रोगशान्तये ।)

Shuṇṭhī, souvarchala, hiṅgu, dāḍima and amlavetasa–powder of these taken with water is beneficial in śwāsa (dyspnoea) and hṛdroga (heart disease) (118–119).

अथ हिंग्वादिचूर्णं शूलादौ—

हिङ्गु पाठाऽभया धान्यं दाडिमं चित्रकः शठी ॥ ११९ ॥
अजमोदा त्रिकटुकं हपुषा चाम्लवेतसम् । अजगन्धा तिन्तिडीकं जीरकं पौष्करं वचा ॥ १२० ॥
चव्यं क्षारद्वयं पञ्च लवणानि विचूर्णयेत् । प्राग्भोजनस्य मध्ये वा चूर्णमेतत्प्रयोजयेत् ॥ १२१ ॥
पिबेद्वा जीर्णमद्येन तक्रेणोष्णोदकेन वा । गुल्मे वातकफोद्भूते हृद्ग्रहेऽष्ठीलिकासु च ॥ १२२ ॥
हृद्वस्तिपार्श्वशूलेषु शूले च गुदयोनिजे । मूत्रकृच्छ्रे तथानाहे पाण्डुरोगेऽरुचौ तथा ॥ १२३ ॥
हिक्कायां यकृति प्लीह्नि श्वासे कासे गलग्रहे । ग्रहण्यर्शोविकारेषु चूर्णमेतत्प्रशस्यते ॥ १२४ ॥
भावितं मातुलुङ्गस्य बहुशः स्वरसेन वा । कुर्याच्च गुटिका बह्वीर्वातश्लेष्मामयापहाः ॥ १२५ ॥

Hiṅgu, pāṭhā, abhayā, dhānyā, dāḍima, chitraka, shaṭhī, ajamodā, trikaṭu, hapuṣā, amlavetasa, ajagandhā, tintidīka, pouṣkara, vachā, chavyā, the two kshāras and the five lavaṇas—all equal quantities are powdered nicely. Taken before or along with food or with old wine, buttermilk or water is beneficial in gulma (abdominal tumor) of vāta-kapha origin, hṛdgraha (precordial pain), asthīlā (prostatic enlargement), pain in the heart, urinary bladder, flanks, rectum, vagina; mūtrakṛcchra (dysuria), ānāha (abdominal enlargement), pāṇḍuroga (anaemia), aruchi (anorexia), hikka (hiccough), enlargement of yakṛt (liver), plīhā (spleen), kāsa (cough), śwāsa (dyspnoea), galagraha (pain in the throat), grahaṇī (sprue) and arshas (piles). It can be macerated with juice of matulunga several times, rolled into a pill of big size (of two shana quantity) and used in diseases arising from increase of vāta kapha (119–125).

अथ यमानीखाण्डवचूर्णमरोचकादौ—

यमानी दाडिमं शुण्ठी तिन्तिडीकाम्लवेतसौ । बदराम्लं च कुर्वीत चतुःशाणमितानि च ॥ १२६ ॥
सार्धद्विशाणं मरिचं पिप्पली दशशाणिका । त्वक्सौवर्चलधान्याकं जीरकं द्विद्विशाणकम् ॥१२७॥
चतुःषष्टिमितैः शाणैः शर्करामत्र योजयेत् । चूर्णितं सर्वमेकत्र यमानीखाण्डवाभिधम् ॥ १२८ ॥

चूर्णं जयेत्पाण्डुरोगं हृद्रोगं ग्रहणीं ज्वरम् । छर्दिशोषातिसारांश्च प्लीहानाहविबन्धताम् ॥ १२९ ॥
अरुचिं शूलमन्दाग्निमर्शोजिह्वागलामयान् ।

Yavānī, dāḍima, shuṇṭhī, tintiḍīka, amlavetasa, and badarāmla each four shāṇas, two and half shāṇas of maricha, ten shāṇas of pippalī, two shāṇas each of twak, dhānyaka and sixtyfour shāṇas of sugar are all powdered together. This recipe known as *Yavanī Khāṇḍava Chūrṇa* relieves pāṇḍuroga (anaemia), grahaṇī (sprue), jwara (fevers), chardi (vomiting), shoṣa (consumption), atisāra (diarrhoeas), plīhā (splenic enlargement), ānāha (abdominal enlargement), vibandha (constipation), aruchi (anorexia), shūla (colic), mandāgni (dyspepsia), arshas (piles), diseases of jihwā (tongue) and gala (throat) (126–130).

अथ तालीसादिचूर्णं अरोचकादौ—

तालीसं मरिचं शुण्ठी पिप्पली वंशरोचनम् ॥ १३० ॥
एकद्वित्रिचतुःपञ्चकर्षैर्भागान्प्रकल्पयेत् । एलात्वचोस्तु कर्षार्धं प्रत्येकं भागमाचरेत् ॥ १३१ ॥
द्वात्रिंशत्कर्षतुलिता प्रदेया शर्करा बुधैः । तालीसाद्यमिदं चूर्णं रोचनं पाचनं स्मृतम् ॥ १३२ ॥
कासश्वासज्वरहरं छर्द्यतीसारनाशनम् । शोषाध्मानहरं प्लीहाग्रहणीपाण्डुरोगजित् ॥ १३३ ॥
पक्त्वा वा शर्करां चूर्णं क्षिपेत्स्याद्गुटिका ततः ।

Tālīsa, maricha, shuṇṭhī, pippalī, vamshalochana—one, two, three, four and five karshas respectively, half karsha each of elā and twak, thirtytwo karshas of sugar are all powdered nicely. This recipe known as *Tālīsādi Chūrṇa* is rochana (appetiser), pāchana (digestive), relieves kāsa (cough), śwāsa (dyspnoea), jwara (fevers), chardi (vomiting), atisāra (diarrhoea), shoṣa (consumption), ādhmāna (tympanitis), plīhā (spleen enlargement), grahaṇī (sprue) and pāṇḍuroga (anaemia). This powder can be made into pills by cooking it with sugar (130–134).

सितोपला षोडश स्यादष्टौ स्याद्वंशरोचना ॥ १३४ ॥
पिप्पली स्याच्चतुष्कर्षा स्यादेला च द्विकार्षिकी । एकः कर्षस्त्वचः कार्यश्चूर्णयेत्सर्वमेकतः ॥ १३५ ॥
सितोपलादिकं चूर्णं मधुसर्पिर्युतं लिहेत् । श्वासकासक्षयहरं हस्तपादाङ्गदाहजित् ॥ १३६ ॥
मन्दाग्निं सुप्तजिह्वत्वं पार्श्वशूलमरोचकम् । ज्वरमूर्ध्वगतं रक्तं पित्तमाशु व्यपोहति ॥ १३७ ॥

Sixteen karṣas of sītopala, eight of vamshalochana, four of pippalī, two of elā and one of twak—are powdered together nicely. This recipe known as *Sitopalādi Chūrṇa* taken with honey and ghee relieves śwāsa (dyspnoea), kasa (cough), kshaya (consumption), burning sensation of palms, soles and body, mandāgni (dyspepsia), loss of taste in the tongue, parshwaślūa (pain in the flanks), arochaka (anorexia), jwara (fever), urdhwaga raktapitta (haemorrhagic purpura) (134–137)

अथ लवणभास्करचूर्णं ग्रहणीगुल्मादौ—

सामुद्रलवणं कार्यमष्टकर्षमितं बुधैः । पञ्च सौवर्चलं ग्राह्यं बिडं सैन्धवधान्यकात् ॥ १३८ ॥
पिप्पली पिप्पलीमूलं कृष्णजीरकपत्रकम् । नागकेशरतालीसमम्लवेतसकं तथा ॥ १३९ ॥
द्विकर्षमात्राण्येतानि प्रत्येकं कारयेद्बुधः । मरिचं जीरकं विश्वमेकैकं कर्षमात्रकम् ॥ १४० ॥
दाडिमं स्याच्चतुष्कर्षं त्वगेले चार्धकार्षिके । एतच्चूर्णीकृतं सर्वं लवणं भास्कराभिधम् ॥ १४१ ॥
शाणप्रमाणं देयं तु मस्तुतक्रसुरासवैः । वातश्लेष्मभवं गुल्मं प्लीहानमुदरं क्षयम् ॥ १४२ ॥
अर्शांसि ग्रहणीं कुष्ठं विबन्धं च भगन्दरम् । शोफं शूलं श्वासकासावामवातं च हृद्रुजम् ॥ १४३ ॥
मन्दाग्निं नाशयेदेतद्दीपनं पाचनं परम् । सर्वलोकहितार्थाय भास्करेणोदितं पुरा ॥ १४४ ॥

Eight karṣas of samudra lavaṇa, five of souvarçhala, two karṣas each of biḍa lavaṇa, saindhava lavaṇa, dhānyaka, pippalī, pippalīmūla, kṛṣṇa-jīrak, patra, nāgakesara, tālīsa, amlavetasa, one karsha each of maricha, jīraka, viśwā; four karṣas of dādima and half karṣa each of twak and elā all are nicely powdered. This recipe known as *Lavaṇa Bhāskara Chūrṇa* was formulated in the past by Bhāskara (Sun) for the benefit of the people. Given in doses of one shāṇa with whey, butter milk or wines relieves gulma of vāta kapha origin (abdominal tumers), plīhā (splenic enlargement), udara (enlargement of abdomen), kshaya (consumption), arshas (piles), grahaṇī (sprue), kuṣṭha (leprosy and other skin diseases), vibandha (constipation), bhagandara (fistula-in-ano), shopha (oedema), shūla (colic), śwāsa (dyspnoea), kāsa (cough), āmavāta (rheumatism), hṛdruja (cordiac pain), mandāgni (dyspepsia) and acts as a good dīpana (carminative) and pāchana (digestive) (138–144).

अथ एलादिचूर्णं छर्दिरोगे—

एलाप्रियङ्गुमुस्तानि कोलमज्जा च पिप्पली । श्रीचन्दनं तथा लाजा लवङ्गं नागकेशरम् ॥ १४५ ॥
एतच्चूर्णीकृतं सर्वं सिताक्षौद्रयुतं लिहेत् । वातपित्तकफोद्भूतां छर्दिं हन्त्यतिवेगतः ॥ १४६ ॥

Elā, priyaṅgu, musta, kolamajjā, pippalī, sṛchandana, lājā, lavaṅga, nagakesara—all equal parts are powdered nicely and given with sugar or honey relieves chardi (vomitting) arising from all the three doṣas quickly (145–146).

व्याघ्रीचूर्णम्—

(व्याघ्रीजीरकधात्रीणां चूर्णं मधुयुतं लिहेत् । ऊर्ध्ववातमहाश्वासतमकैर्मुच्यते क्षणात् ॥ १४७ ॥)

Vyāghrī, jīraka and dhātrī—powders of these with honey acts quickly in urdhwavāta (oppression of the chest by upward movement of gas), mahāśwāsa (severe dyspnoea) and tamaka śwāsa (asthma) (147).

अथ पञ्चनिम्बचूर्णं कुष्ठादौ—

मूलं पत्रं फलं पुष्पं त्वचं निम्बात्समाहरेत् । सूक्ष्मचूर्णमिदं कुर्यात्पलपञ्चदशोन्मितम् ॥ १४८ ॥
लोहभस्महरीतक्यौ चक्रमर्दकचित्रकौ । भल्लातकं विडङ्गानि शर्करामलकं निशा ॥ १४९ ॥

पिप्पली मरिचं शुण्ठी बाकुची कृतमालकः । गोक्षुरश्च पलोन्मानमेकैकं कारयेद्बुधः ॥ १५० ॥
सर्वमेकीकृतं चूर्णं भृङ्गराजेन भावयेत् । अष्टभागावशिष्टेन खदिरासनवारिणा ॥ १५१ ॥
भावयित्वा च संशोष्य कर्षमात्रं ततः पिबेत् । खदिरासनतोयेन सर्पिषा पयसाथवा ॥ १५२ ॥
मासेन सर्वकुष्ठानि विनिहन्ति रसायनम् । पञ्चनिम्बमिदं चूर्णं सर्वरोगप्रणाशनम् ॥ १५३ ॥

Root, leaves, fruits, flowers and bark of nimba are dried and made into nice powder. Fifteen palas of this chūrṇa is added with the powder of one pala each of lohabhasma, harītakī, chakramarda, chitraka, bhallātaka, viḍaṅga, sharkarā, āmalaka, nisha, pippalī, maricha, shunṭhī, bakuchi, kṛtamālaka and gokshura. The entire bulk of the powder is given bhāvanā (macerated and dried) with juice of bhṛṅgarāja or quatha of khadira or asana. After drying it is given in doses of one karṣa along with quatha of khadira or asana, ghee or milk. This recipe known as *Pañchanimba Chūrṇa* cures all kuṣṭha (leprosy and other skin diseases) within one month and also all other diseases acting as a a rasāyana (rejuvinator) (148–153).

शतावरीचूर्णम्—

शतावरी गोक्षुरश्च बीजं च कपिकच्छुजम् । गाङ्गेरुकी चातिबला बीजमिक्षुरकोद्भवम् ॥ १५४ ॥
चूर्णितं सर्वमेकत्र गोदुग्धेन पिबेन्निशि । न तृप्तिं याति नारीभिर्नरश्चूर्णप्रभावतः ॥ १५५ ॥

Powder of shatāvarī, gokshura, kapikacchu bīja, gāṅgerukī, atibalā and ikshuraka bīja taken at bed time with cow's milk makes man unsatiable with women (gives strength and endurance in sex act) (154–155).

अश्वगन्धादिचूर्णम्—

अश्वगन्धा दशपला तन्मात्रो वृद्धदारुकः । चूर्णीकृत्योभयं विद्वान्घृतभाण्डे निधापयेत् ॥ १५६ ॥
कर्षैकं पयसा पीत्वा नारीभिर्नैव तृप्यति । अगत्वा प्रमदां भूयाद्वलीपलितवर्जितः ॥ १५७ ॥

Ten palas each of aśwagandhā and vṛddhadāru are powdered and placed inside a pot containing a little quantity of ghee for a few days. Later on, used in doses of one karsha with milk gives strength and endurance in sex act and relieves wrinkles of the skin and greying of hairs (156–157).

मुसलीचूर्णम्—

(मुसलीकन्दचूर्णं तु गुडूचीसत्त्वसंयुतम् । वानरीगोक्षुराभ्यां च शाल्मलीशर्करामलैः ॥ १५८ ॥
आलोड्य घृतदुग्धेन पाययेत्कामवर्धनम् ।)

Choorna of musalikanda, gudūchī satwa, vānarī, gokshura, shālmalī, sharkarā and āmalakī taken with milk and ghee increases sexual vigour (158–159).

नवायसचूर्णम्—

चित्रकस्त्रिफला मुस्तं विडङ्गं त्र्यूषणानि च ॥ १५९ ॥
समभागानि कार्याणि नव भागा हतायसः । एतदेकीकृतं चूर्णं मधुसर्पियुतं लिहेत् ॥ १६० ॥
गोमूत्रमथवा तक्रमनुपाने प्रशस्यते । पाण्डुरोगं जयत्युग्रं हृद्रोगं च भगन्दरम् ॥ १६१ ॥
शोथकुष्ठोदरार्शांसि मन्दाग्निमरुचिं कृमीन् ।

Chitraka, triphala, musta, vidaṅga, tryūṣaṇa—each one part are nicely powdered and mixed with nine parts of loha bhasma. This chūrṇa taken with honey or ghee, and followed by with cow's urine or butter milk as anupāna (after drink) cures severe pāṇḍu roga (anaemia), hṛdroga (heart disease), bhagandara (fistula-in-ano), kuṣṭha (leprosy and other skin diseases), udara (abdominal enlargement), arshas (piles), mandāgnī (dyspepsia), aruchi (anorexia) and kṛmi (intestinal worms) (159–162).

आकारकरभादिचूर्णं स्तम्भनादौ—

आकारकरभः शुण्ठी कङ्कोलं कुङ्कुमं कणा ॥ १६२ ॥
जातीफलं लवङ्गं च चन्दनं चेति कार्षिकान् । चूर्णानि मानतः कुर्यादहिफेनं पलोन्मितम् ॥१६३॥
सर्वमेकीकृतं चूर्णं माषैकं मधुना लिहेत् । शुक्रस्तम्भकरं चूर्णं पुंसामानन्दकारकम् ॥ १६४ ॥
नारीणां प्रीतिजननं सेवेत निशि कामुकः ॥

One karṣa each of ākārakarabha, shunṭhī, kaṅkola, kumkuma, kaṇā, jātīphala, lavaṅga, chandana and one pala of ahiphena are all powdered together nicely. One māshā of this powder taken with honey daily by either males or females desirous of coitus, gives them enduranee (by stopping premature éjaculation) (162–165).

इति श्रीदामोदरसूनुना शार्ङ्गधराचार्येण विरचितायां शार्ङ्गधरसंहितायां मध्यमखण्डे चूर्णकल्पना नाम षष्ठोऽध्यायः ।

Thus ends the sixth chapter.

सप्तमोऽध्यायः

CHAPTER 7

Guṭikā Kalpanā (Pill)

इदानीं गुटिकाः कथ्यन्ते—

वटकाश्चाथ कथ्यन्ते तन्नाम गुटिका वटी । मोदको वटिका पिण्डी गुडो वर्तिस्तथोच्यते ॥ १ ॥
लेहवत्साध्यते वह्नौ गुडो वा शर्करा तथा । गुग्गुलुर्वा क्षिपेत्तत्र चूर्णं तन्निर्मिता वटी ॥ २ ॥
कुर्यादवह्निसिद्धेन क्वचिद्गुग्गुलुना वटीम् । द्रवेण मधुना वापि गुटिकां कारयेद्बुधः ॥ ३ ॥

Guṭikā, vaṭī, modaka, vaṭikā, piṇḍī, guḍa, varti (tablets, bolus, pills, dragees) are synonyms. It is prepared either by cooking the powder of drugs with jaggery, sugar or guggul or without cooking, by macerating the powder with any liquid, honey and guggulu and rolling into pills (1–3).

सिता चतुर्गुणा देया वटीषु द्विगुणो गुडः । चूर्णाच्चूर्णसमः कार्यो गुग्गुलुर्मधु तत्समम् ॥ ४ ॥
द्रवं च द्विगुणं देयं मोदकेषु भिषग्वरैः । कर्षप्रमाणं तन्मानं बलं दृष्ट्वा प्रयुज्यते ॥ ५ ॥

Sugar, if to be added, should be taken four times the quantity of powder of other drugs (salts, kshāras etc.); guggulu, honey are added equal in quantity. All these to be macerated with twice the quantity of water, rolled into pills of one karṣa each, dried in shade and preserved. They are used in accordance with the strength of the patient (4–5).

अथ श्रीबाहुशालो गुडः अर्शादौ—

स यथा–इन्द्रवारुणिका मुस्तं शुण्ठी दन्ती हरीतकी । त्रिवृच्छठी विडङ्गानि गोक्षुरश्चित्रकस्तथा ॥ ६ ॥
तेजोह्वा च द्विकर्षाणि पृथग्द्रव्याणि कारयेत् । सूरणस्य पलान्यष्टौ वृद्धदारु चतुष्पलम् ॥ ७ ॥
चतुष्पलं स्याद्भल्लातः क्वाथयेत्सर्वमेकतः । जलद्रोणे चतुर्थांशं गृह्णीयात्क्वाथमुत्तमम् ॥ ८ ॥
क्वाथ्यद्रव्यात्त्रिगुणितं गुडं क्षिप्त्वा पुनः पचेत् । सम्यक्पक्वं च तं ज्ञात्वा चूर्णमेतत्प्रदापयेत् ॥ ९ ॥
चित्रकत्रिवृतादन्तीतेजोह्वा पलिकाः पृथक् । पृथक्त्रिपलिकाः कार्या व्योषैलामलकत्वचः ॥ १० ॥
निक्षिपेन्मधु शीते च तस्मिन्प्रस्थप्रमाणतः । एवं सिद्धो भवेच्छ्रीमान्बाहुशालगुडाऽभिधः ॥ ११ ॥
जयेदर्शांसि सर्वाणि गुल्मं वातोदरं तथा । आढ्यवातप्रतिश्यायं महान्तं क्षयपीनसम् ॥ १२ ॥
हलीमकं पाण्डुरोगं प्रमेहं च रसायनम् ।

Indravāruṇī, musta, shuṇṭhī, dantī, harītakī, trivṛt, shaṭī, viḍaṅga, gokshura, chitraka and tejohwā, each two karṣas; eight palas of sūraṇa, four palas each of vṛddhadāru and bhallātaka should be made into a decoction by boiling in one droṇa of water and reduced to one quarter. Jaggery, three times the quantity of the powder is added to the decoction and boiled again, mixing it with powder of chitraka, trivṛt, dantī, tejohwā each one pala and three palas each of vyoṣā, elā, āmalaka and twak. After it becomes slightly cool one prastha of honey is added and rolled into pills. This recipe known as *Shrī Bāhushālā Guḍa* cures all types of arsha (piles), gulma (abdominal tumor), vātodara abdominal enlargement), āḍhyavāta (gout), pratishyāya (coryza), kshaya consumption), pīnasa (rhinitis), halīmaka (chlorosis), pāṇḍuroga (anaemia) prameha (diabetes) and acts as a rasāyana (rejuvinator, tonic) (6–13).

अथ मरिचादिगुटिका कासादौ—

मरिचं कर्षमात्रं स्यात्पिप्पली कर्षसंमिता ॥ १३ ॥
अर्धकर्षो यवक्षारः कर्षयुग्मं च दाडिमम् । एतच्चूर्णीकृतं युञ्ज्यादष्टकर्षगुडेन हि ॥ १४ ॥

शाणप्रमाणां गुटिकां कृत्वा वक्त्रेण धारयेत् । अस्याः प्रभावात्सर्वेऽपि कासा यान्त्येव संक्षयम् ॥१५॥

One karṣa each of maricha and pippalī, half karṣa of yavakṣāra and two karṣa of dāḍima are powdered, cooked in eight karṣas of jaggery and rolled into pills of one shāṇa (measure). This pill kept in the mouth and allowed to dissolve relieves all varieties of kāsa (cough) (13–15).

श्वासकासादौ गुडवटिका—

गुडशुण्ठीशिवामुस्तैर्गुटिकां धारयेन्मुखे । श्वासकासेषु सर्वेषु बिभीतं वापि केवलम् ॥ १६ ॥

Guḍa, shunṭhī, shivā and musta, rolled into pills or bark of vibhītaka fruit, alone kept in the mouth relieves śwāsa (dyspnoea) and kāsa (cough) of all types (16).

आमलक्यादिगुटिका तृष्णादौ—

आमलं कमलं कुष्ठं लाजाश्च वटरोहकः । एतच्चूर्णस्य मधुना गुटिकां धारयेन्मुखे ॥ १७ ॥
तृष्णां प्रवृद्धां हन्त्येषा मुखशोषं च दारुणम् ।

Āmalaka, kāmala, kuṣṭha, lājā, vātarohaka (sprout of vāta) are powdered, rolled into pills with honey and kept in the mouth relieves severe tṛṣṇā (thirst) and mukhashoṣa (dryness of the mouth) (17–18).

अथ ज्वरे सञ्जीवनीवटी त्रिदोषे च—

विडङ्गं नागरं कृष्णा पथ्यामलबिभीतकम् ॥ १८ ॥
वचा गुडूची भल्लातं सद्विषं चात्र योजयेत् । एतानि समभागानि गोमूत्रेणैव पेषयेत् ॥ १९ ॥
गुञ्जाभा गुटिका कार्या दद्यादार्द्रकजै रसैः । एकामजीर्णगुल्मेषु द्वे विषूच्यां प्रदापयेत् ॥ २० ॥
तिस्रश्च सर्पदष्टे तु चतस्रः सान्निपातिके । वटी संजीवनी नाम्ना संजीवयति मानवम् ॥ २१ ॥

Viḍaṅga, nāgara, kṛṣṇa, pathyā, āmalaka, vibhītaka, vachā, guḍūchī, bhallātaka and viṣa (vatsanābhī), each equal parts are powdered and macerated with cow's urine and rolled into pill of the size of guñjā. Administered with juice of green ginger, one pill relieves ajīrṇa (indigestion) and gulma (abdominal tumors), two pills in cases of vishūchī (severe diarrhoea and vomitting) three pills in cases of snake bite, four in cases of sannipāta jwara (toxic fevers). This recipe known as *Sañjīvinī Vaṭī* brings a dying man back to life (18–21).

अथ व्योषादिगुटिका पीनसादौ—

व्योषाम्लवेतसं चव्यं तालीसं चित्रकं तथा । जीरकं तिन्तिडीकं च प्रत्येकं कर्षभागिकम् ॥ २२ ॥
त्रिसुगन्धं त्रिशाणं स्याद्गुडः स्यात्कर्षविंशतिः । व्योषादिगुटिका सेयं पीनसश्वासकासजित् ॥२३॥
रुचिस्वरकरी ख्याता प्रतिश्यायप्रणाशिनी ।

Vyoṣā, amlavetasa, chavya, tālisa, chitraka, jīraka, and tintidīka each one karṣa, three shāṇas of the three sugandhas (elā, twak, patra) and twenty karṣas of jaggery are made into pills. This recipe known as *Vyoṣādi Guṭikā* relieves pīnasa (rhinitis), kāsa (cough), śwāsa (dyspnoea), pratishyāya common cold); improves taste and voice (22–24).

अथ गुडचतुष्टयगुटिका आमादौ—

आमेषु सगुडां शुण्ठीमजीर्णे गुडपिप्पलीम् ॥ २४ ॥
कृच्छ्रे जीरगुडं दद्यादर्शःसु सगुडाभयाम् ।

Shuṇṭhī and jaggery in conditions of āma; jaggery and pippalī in ajīrṇa (indigestion), jīraka and jaggery in mūtra-kṛcchra (dysuria), jaggery and abhayā in arshas (piles) are highly beneficial (24–25).

अथ वृद्धदारुमोदकः—

वृद्धदारुकभल्लातशुण्ठीचूर्णेन योजितः ॥ २५ ॥
मोदकः सगुडो हन्यात्षड्विधार्शःकृतां रुजम् ।

Pill prepared out of vṛddhadāru, bhallātaka, shuṇṭhī and jaggery will relieve the pain in all the six types of arshas (haemorrhoids) (25–26).

अथ सूरणपिण्डी अर्शोरोगे—

शुष्कसूरणचूर्णस्य भागान्द्वात्रिंशदाहरेत् ॥ २६ ॥
भागान्षोडश चित्रस्य शुण्ठ्या भागचतुष्टयम् । द्वौ भागौ मरिचस्यापि सर्वाण्येकत्र चूर्णयेत् ॥ २७ ॥
गुडेन पिण्डिकां कुर्यादर्शसां नाशनीं पराम् ।

Thirty two parts of powder of dried sūraṇa, sixteen parts of chitraka, four parts of shuṇṭhī, two parts of maricha are made into pills adding jaggery. This recipe cures arṣas (piles) effectively (26–28).

सूरणवटकाः—

सूरणो वृद्धदारुश्च भागैः षोडशभिः पृथक् ॥ २८ ॥
मुशलीचित्रकौ ज्ञेयावष्टभागमितौ पृथक् । शिवा बिभीतकी धात्री विडङ्गं नागरं कणा ॥ २९ ॥
भल्लातः पिप्पलीमूलं तालीसं च पृथक्पृथक् । चतुर्भागप्रमाणानि त्वगेला मरिचं तथा ॥ ३० ॥
द्विभागमात्राणि पृथक्ततस्त्वेकत्र चूर्णयेत् । द्विगुणेन गुडेनाथ वटकान्कारयेद्बुधः ॥ ३१ ॥
प्रबलाग्निकरा एते तथार्शोनाशनाः पराः । ग्रहणीं वातकफजां श्वासं कासं क्षयामयम् ॥ ३२ ॥
प्लीहानं श्लीपदं शोथं प्रमेहं च भगन्दरम् । निहन्युः पलितं वृष्यास्तथा मेध्या रसायनाः ॥ ३३ ॥

Sixteen parts each of sūraṇa and vṛddhadāru, eight parts each of musalī and chitraka, four parts each of shivā, vibhītakī, dhātrī, viḍaṅga, nāgara, kanā, bhallātaka, pippalīmūla and tālīsa; two parts each of twak, ela and maricha are all powdered nicely, jaggery twice the total quantity is added and rolled into pills. This recipe is a powerful carminative, cures arshas (piles), vātakapha grahanī (sprue), śwāsa (dyspnoea), kāsa (cough), kshaya (consumption), plīhā (splenic enlargement), shlīpada (filariasis), shotha (oedema), prameha (diabetes), bhagandara (fistula-in-ano), relieves palita (greying of hair) and acts as vṛṣya (aphrodisiac), medhya (tonic for the mind) and rasāyani (rejuvinator) (28–33).

मण्डूरवटकाः कामलादौ—

त्रिफला त्र्यूषणं चव्यं पिप्पलीमूलचित्रकौ । दारु माक्षिकधातुश्च दार्वी मुस्तं विडङ्गकम् ॥ ३४ ॥
प्रत्येकं कर्षमात्राणि सर्वद्विगुणितं तथा । मण्डूरं चूर्णयेच्छुद्धं गोमूत्रेऽष्टगुणे क्षिपेत् ॥ ३५ ॥
पक्त्वा च वटकान्कृत्वा दद्यात्तक्रानुपानतः । कामलापाण्डुमेहार्शः शोथकुष्ठकफामयान् ॥ ३६ ॥
ऊरुस्तम्भमजीर्णं च प्लीहानं नाशयेदपि ।

One karṣa each of triphalā, tryūshaṇa, chavya, pippalīmūla, chitraka, dāru, mākshikadhātu, darvī, musta and viḍaṅga; mandoora (iron slag); double the total quantity are powdered well, boiled in eight times of cow's urine and rolled into pills. Used along with butter milk, it relieves kāmalā (jaundice), pāṇḍu (anaemia), meha (diabetes), arshas (piles), shotha (oedema), kuṣṭha (leprosy and other skin diseases), other diseases of kapha origin, urustambha (stiffness of the leg), ajīrṇa (indigestion) and plīhā (enlargement of spleen) (34–37).

धातुगतज्वरादौ पिप्पलीमोदकः—

(क्षौद्राद्द्विगुणितं सर्पिर्घृताद्द्विगुणपिप्पली ॥ ३७ ॥
सिता द्विगुणिता तस्याः क्षीरं देयं चतुर्गुणम् । चातुर्जातं क्षौद्रतुल्यं पक्त्वा कुर्याच्च मोदकान् ॥३८॥
धातुस्थांश्च ज्वरान्सर्वान् श्वासं कासं च पाण्डुताम् । धातुक्षयं वह्निमान्द्यं पिप्पलीमोदको जयेत् ॥३९॥)

One part of honey, two parts of ghee, four parts of pippali, eight parts of sugar and thirty parts of milk and one part of chaturjata are cooked together and rolled into pills. This recipe known as *Pippalī Modaka* relieves all types of dhātugata jwara (fevers residing in the tissues), śwāsa (dyspnoea), kāsa (cough), pāṇḍu (anaemia), dhātukshaya (emaciation) and agnimāndya (dyspepsia) (37–39).

अथ चन्द्रप्रभागुग्गुलुः प्रमेहादौ—

चन्द्रप्रभा वचा मुस्तं भूनिम्बामृतदारुकम् । हरिद्रातिविषा दार्वी पिप्पलीमूलचित्रकौ ॥ ४० ॥
धान्यकं त्रिफला चव्यं विडङ्गं गजपिप्पली । व्योषं माक्षिकधातुश्च द्वौ क्षारौ लवणत्रयम् ॥ ४१ ॥
एतानि शाणमात्राणि प्रत्येकं कारयेद्बुधः । त्रिवृद्दन्तीपत्रकं च त्वगेला वंशरोचना ॥ ४२ ॥
प्रत्येकं कर्षमात्राणि कुर्यादेतानि बुद्धिमान् । द्विकर्षं हतलोहं स्याच्चतुष्कर्षा सिता भवेत् ॥ ४३ ॥
शिलाजत्वष्टकर्षं स्यादष्टौ कर्षाश्च गुग्गुलोः । एभिरेकत्र संक्षुण्णैः कर्तव्या गुटिका शुभा ॥ ४४ ॥
चन्द्रप्रभादिविख्याता सर्वरोगप्रणाशिनी । प्रमेहान्विंशतिं कृच्छ्रं मूत्राघातं तथाश्मरीम् ॥ ४५ ॥
विबन्धाऽऽनाहशूलानि मेहनं ग्रन्थिमर्बुदम् । अन्त्रवृद्धिं कटीशूलं श्वासं कासं विचर्चिकाम् ॥४६॥
अण्डवृद्धिं तथा पाण्डु कामलां च हलीमकम् । कुष्ठान्यर्शांसि कण्डूं च प्लीहोदरभगन्दरम् ॥४७॥

दन्तरोगं नेत्ररोगं स्त्रीणामार्तवजां रुजम् । पुंसां शुक्रगतान्दोषान्मन्दाग्निमरुचिं तथा ॥ ४८ ॥
वायुं पित्तं कफं हन्याद्बल्या वृष्या रसायनी । चन्द्रप्रभायां कर्षस्तु चतुःशाणो विधीयते ॥४९॥

Chandraprabha, vachā, musta, bhūnimba, amṛta, dāru, haridrā, ativiṣā, dārvī, pippalīmūla, chitraka, dhānyakā, triphalā, chavya, viḍaṅga, gajapippalī, vyoṣā, makshikādhātu, the two kshāras, the three lavaṇas—each one shāṇa; trivṛt, dantī, patraka, twak, elā, vamshalochana, each one karṣa; lohabhasma two karṣas, four karṣas of sugar, eight karṣas each of shilājātu and guggulu—all to be nicely powdered, cooked slightly and made into pills. This recipe known as "*Chardraprabhā Vaṭī*" cures all diseases, specially the twenty kinds of prameha (diabetes), mūtrakṛcchra (dysuria), mūtraghāta (retention of urine), ashmarī (renal caliculis), vibandha (constipation), ānāha (enlargement of abdomen), shūla (colic), mehana granthi and arbuda (tumors and cancers of penis), antra vṛddhi (hernia), kaṭishūla (pain in the waist), śwāsa-kāsa (dyspnoea, cough), vicharchikā (psoriasis), aṇḍavṛddhi (scrotal enlargement), pāṇḍu (anaemia), kāmalā (jaundice), halīmaka (chlorosis), kuṣṭha (leprosy and other skin diseases), arshas (piles), kaṇḍū (itching), plīhodara (splenomegaly), bhagandara (fistula in ano), dantaroga (disease of teeth), netraroga (disease of eye), ārtavaruja (menstrual pain), shukra doṣa (disorders of semen), mandāgni (dyspepsia), aruchi (anorexia), other diseases of vāta, pitta and kapha, and acts as balya (tonic), vṛṣya (aphrodisiac), rasāyanī (rejuvinator). In this recipe one karṣa (of chandraprabhā) is equal to four shāṇas (40–49).

अथ काङ्कायनगुटिका गुल्मादौ—

यमानी जीरकं धान्यं मरिचं गिरिकर्णिका । अजमोदोपकुञ्ची च चतुःशाणा पृथक्पृथक् ॥ ५० ॥
हिङ्गु षट्शाणिकं कार्यं क्षारौ लवणपञ्चकम् । त्रिवृच्चाष्टमितैः शाणैः प्रत्येकं कल्पयेत्सुधीः ॥५१॥
दन्ती शठी पौष्करं च विडङ्गं दाडिमं शिवा । चित्रोऽम्लवेतसः शुण्ठी शाणैः षोडशभिः पृथक् ॥५२॥
बीजपूररसेनैषां गुटिकां कारयेद्बुधः । घृतेन पयसा मद्यैरम्लैरुष्णोदकेन वा ॥ ५३ ॥
पिबेत्काङ्कायनप्रोक्तां गुटिकां गुल्मनाशिनीम् । मद्येन वातिकं गुल्मं गोक्षीरेण च पैत्तिकम् ॥५४॥
मूत्रेण कफगुल्मं च दशमूलैस्त्रिदोषजम् । उष्ट्रीदुग्धेन नारीणां रक्तगुल्मं विनाशयेत् ॥ ५५ ॥
हृद्रोगं ग्रहणीं शूलं क्रिमीनर्शांसि नाशयेत् ।

Four shāṇas each of yavānī, jīraka, dhānya, maricha, girikarṇikā, ajamodā and upakunchi; six shāṇas each of hiṅgu; eight shāṇas each of the two kshāras, the five lavaṇas and trivṛt; sixteen shāṇas each of dantī, shaṭhī; puṣkara, viḍaṅga dāḍima, shivā, chitraka, amlavetsa and shuṇṭhī—all are nicely powdered, macerated with juice of bījapūra and rolled into pills and taken with ghee, milk, wines, sour drinks or water. This recipe formulated by Kaṅkāyana relieves all gulmas (abdominal tumors), vātgulma if taken with wines, pitta gulma with cow's milk, kapha gulma with cow's urine, tridoṣaja gulma with dashamūla quātha, rakta gulma of women with camel's milk and also hṛdroga (heart disease), grahaṇī (sprue), shūla (colic), kṛmi (intestinal worms) and arṣas (piles) (50–56).

अथ योगराजगुग्गुलुर्वातरोगे आमवाते वा—

नागरं पिप्पली चव्यं पिप्पलीमूलचित्रकौ ॥ ५६ ॥
भृष्टं हिङ्ग्वजमोदा च सर्षपो जीरकद्वयम् । रेणुकेन्द्रयवाः पाठा विडङ्गं गजपिप्पली ॥ ५७ ॥
कटुकातिविषा भार्ङ्गी वचामूर्वे त्रिभागतः । प्रत्येकं शाणकानि स्युर्द्रव्याणीमानि विंशतिः ॥ ५८ ॥
द्रव्येभ्यः सकलेभ्यश्च त्रिफला द्विगुणा भवेत् । एभिश्चूर्णीकृतैः सर्वैः समो देयश्च गुग्गुलुः ॥५९॥
(वङ्गं रौप्यं च नागं च लोहसारस्तथाभ्रकम् । मण्डूरं रससिन्दूरं प्रत्येकं पलसंमितम्) ॥ ६० ॥
गुडपाकसमं कृत्वा इमं दद्याद्यथोचितम् । एकपिण्डं ततः कृत्वा धारयेद्घृतभाजने ॥ ६१ ॥
गुटिकाः शाणमात्रास्तु कृत्वा ग्राह्या यथोचिताः । गुग्गुलुर्योगराजोऽयं त्रिदोषघ्नो रसायनः ॥६२॥
मैथुनाहारपानानां त्यागो नैवात्र विद्यते । सर्वान्वातामयान्कुष्ठानर्शांसि ग्रहणीगदम् ॥ ६३ ॥
प्रमेहं वातरक्तं च नाभिशूलं भगन्दरम् । उदावर्तं क्षयं गुल्ममपस्मारमुरोग्रहम् ॥ ६४ ॥
मन्दाग्निं श्वासकासं च नाशयेदरुचिं तथा । रेतोदोषहरः पुंसां रजोदोषहरः स्त्रियाम् ॥ ६५ ॥
पुंसामपत्यजनको बन्ध्यानां गर्भदस्तथा । रास्नादिक्काथसंयुक्तो विविधं हन्ति मारुतम् ॥ ६६ ॥
काङ्कोल्यादिश्टतात्पित्तं कफमारग्वधादिना । दार्वीश्टतेन मेहांश्च गोमूत्रेण च पाण्डुताम् ॥ ६७ ॥
मेदोवृद्धिं च मधुना कुष्ठं निम्बश्टतेन च । छिन्नाक्काथेन वातास्रं शोथं शूलं कणाश्टतात् ॥ ६८ ॥
पाटलाक्काथसहितो विषं मूषकजं जयेत् । त्रिफलाक्काथसहितो नेत्रार्तिं हन्ति दारुणाम् ॥ ६९ ॥
पुनर्नवादिक्काथेन हन्यात्सर्वोदराण्यपि ।

Nāgara, pippalī, chavya, pippalīmūla, chitraka, fried hiṅgu, ajamoda, sarṣapa, the two jīrakas, reṇuka, indrayava, viḍaṅga, gajapippalī, kaṭuka, ativiṣā, bhārngī, vachā, mūrvā—these twenty–each one shāṇa; triphalā double the total quantity and guggulu equal to the total of all–are taken, nicely, powdered, put in a pot containing a little quantity of ghee, cooked well and rolled into pills of one shāṇa in quantity. This recipe known as *Yogarāja guggulu* alleviates all the three doṣas, acts as a rasāyana (rejuvinator); avoidance of sex, food and drinks are not necessary. It is very effective in all types of vātavyādhi (nervous disorders), kuṣṭha (leprosy and other skin diseases), arshas (piles), prameha (diabetes), vātarakta (gout), nābhishūla (pain around the umbilicus), bhagandara (fistula in ano), gulma (abdominal tumors) apasmāra (epilepsy), urograha (pain in the chest), mandāgni (dyspepsia), swāsakāsa (dyspnoea–cough), aruchi (loss of taste), seminal disorders in men and menstrual disorders in women; makes men fertile and barren women to become pregnant. Taken with rāsnādi quātha it curas all vāta (nervous) disordeɪs, with kaṅkolyādi quātha pitta disorders and kapha disorders with aragwadhādi quatha, pāṇḍu-roga (anaemia) with cow's urine, medovṛddhi

(obesity) with honey, kuṣṭha (skin diseases and leprosy) with ṇimba quath, vātarakta (gout) with chinna (amṛtavalli) quatha, shotha and shūla (colic) with kaṇā quātha, mūṣaka viṣa (poisoning by rat bite) with pātalā quatha, eyediseases with triphalā quatha and all types of udaras (abdominal enlargement) with punarnavā quatha (56–70).[1]

अथ कैशोरगुग्गुलुर्वातरक्तादौ—

त्रिफलायास्त्रयः प्रस्थाः प्रस्थैका चामृता भवेत् ॥ ७० ॥
संकुठ्य लोहपात्रेण सार्धद्रोणाम्बुना पचेत् । जलमर्धशृतं ज्ञात्वा गृह्णीयाद्वस्त्रगालितम् ॥ ७१ ॥
ततः क्वाथे क्षिपेच्छुद्धं गुग्गुलं प्रस्थसंमितम् । पुनः पचेदयःपात्रे दर्व्या संघर्षयेन्मुहुः ॥ ७२ ॥
सान्द्रीभूतं ततो ज्ञात्वा गुडपाकसमाकृतिम् । चूर्णीकृत्य ततस्तत्र द्रव्याणीमानि निक्षिपेत् ॥७३॥
त्रिफला द्विपला ज्ञेया गुडूची पलिका मता । षडक्षं त्र्यूषणं प्रोक्तं विडङ्गानां पलार्धकम् ॥ ७४ ॥
दन्ती कर्षमिता कार्या त्रिवृत्कर्षमिता स्मृता । ततः पिण्डीकृतं सर्वं घृतपात्रे विनिक्षिपेत् ॥ ७५ ॥
गुटिका शाणमात्रेण युञ्ज्याद्दोषाद्यपेक्षया । अनुपाने भिषग्दद्यात्कोष्णं नीरं पयोऽथवा ॥ ७६ ॥
मञ्जिष्ठादिशृतं वापि युक्तियुक्तमतापरम् । जयेत्सर्वाणि कुष्ठानि वातरक्तं त्रिदोषजम् ॥ ७७ ॥
सर्वव्रणानि गुल्मानि प्रमेहपिडिकास्तथा । प्रमेहोदरमन्दाग्निकासश्वयथुपाण्डुजान् ॥ ७८ ॥
हन्ति सर्वामयान्नित्यमुपयुक्तो रसायनः । कैशोरकाभिधानोऽयं गुग्गुलुः कान्तिकारकः ॥ ७९ ॥
वासादिना नेत्रगदान्गुल्मादीन्वरुणादिना । क्वाथेन खदिरस्यापि व्रणकुष्ठानि नाशयेत् ॥ ८० ॥
अम्लं तीक्ष्णमजीर्णं च व्यायामं श्रममातपम् । मद्यं रोषं त्यजेत्सम्यग्गुणार्थी पुरसेवकः ॥ ८१ ॥

Three prasthas of triphalā, one prastha of amṛta are to be boiled in an iron vessel with one and half droṇas of water, decoction reduced to half and filtered through cloth. One prastha of (purified) guggulu is added to the decoction stirring all the while with iron laddle. When the mass begins to solidify the powder of the following drugs are added–two palas of triphalā, one pala of viḍaṅga, one karṣa each of dantī and trivṛt. The mass is then transferred to a pot containing a little quantity of ghee and when slightly cool rolled into pills of one shāṇa each. Administered along with warm water, milk or mañjiṣṭhādi quatha, it cures all types of kuṣṭha (leprosy and other skin diseases) tridoṣaja vātarakta (gout), vraṇas (ulcers), gulma (abdominal tumors), prameha piḍakas (diabetic corbuncles), prameha (diabetes), udara (abdominal enlargement), mandāgni (dyspepsia), kāsa (cough), shotha of pāṇḍu roga (oedema of anaemia) and all other diseases. If used daily, acts as rasāyana (rejuvinator, tonic). This recipe known as "*Kaishora Guggulu*" imparts good lustre to the skin; with vasādi quatha it is beneficial in diseases of the eye, with varuṇādi quatha in gulma

1. **In this recipe verses No. 60. is not found in any of the manuscripts of the treatise and so not noticed by any commentators. As it a later interpotation, it has not been translated as it requires deletion.**
—Translator

(abdominal tumors), with khadirādi quatha in cases of vraṇa (ulcers) and kuṣṭha (leprosy and other diseases). During treatment the patient should avoid indigestion, foods which are sour and hot, sexual intercourse, physical exertion, exposure to sun, alconolic drinks and anger (70–81).

अथ त्रिफलागुग्गुलुर्भगन्दरादौ—

त्रिपलं त्रिफलाचूर्णं कृष्णाचूर्णं पलोन्मितम् । गुग्गुलुं पञ्चपलिकं क्षोदयेत्सर्वमेकतः ॥ ८२ ॥
ततस्तु गुटिकां कृत्वा प्रयुञ्ज्याद्वह्नयपेक्षया । भगन्दरं गुल्मशोथावर्शांसि च विनाशयेत् ॥ ८३ ॥

Three palas of triphalā powder, one pala of kṛṣṇā powder, five palas of guggulu—are all made into a paste with a little amount of ghee and rolled into pills. Used in suitable doses it relives bhagandara (fistula in ano), gulma (abdominal tumors), shotha (oedema) and arsha (piles) (80–83).

अथ गोक्षुरादिगुग्गुलुः प्रमेहादौ—

अष्टाविंशतिसंख्यानि पलान्यानीय गोक्षुरात् । विपचेत्षड्गुणे नीरे क्वाथो ग्राह्योऽर्धशेषितः ॥८४॥
ततः पुनः पचेत्तत्र पुरं सप्तपलं क्षिपेत् । गुडपाकसमाकारं ज्ञात्वा तत्र विनिक्षिपेत् ॥ ८५ ॥
त्रिकटु त्रिफला मुस्तं चूर्णितं पलसप्तकम् । ततः पिण्डीकृतस्यास्य गुटिका मुखयोजिता ॥ ८६ ॥
हन्यात्प्रमेहं कृच्छ्रं च प्रदरं मूत्रघातकम् । वातास्त्रं वातरोगांश्च शुक्रदोषं तथाश्मरीम् ॥ ८७ ॥

Twenty eight palas of gokshura is boiled in six times of water and reduced to half. Seven palas of puram (guggulu) are added and when the mass becomes solid, powder of triphalā, trikaṭu and musta—seven palas in total are added and rolled into pills. This recipe relieves prameha (diabetes), mūtra kṛcchra (dysuria), mūtraghāta (suppression of urine), pradara (menorrhagia), vātarakta (gout), vātarogas (nervous diseases), shukra doṣas (diseases of semen) and ashmarī (urinary caliculii) (84–87).

अथ त्रिफलामोदकः कुष्ठादौ—

त्रिफलाष्टपला कार्या भल्लातं च चतुष्पलम् । बाकुची पञ्चपलिका विडङ्गानां चतुष्पलम् ॥ ८८ ॥
हतलोहं त्रिवृच्चैव गुग्गुलुश्च शिलाजतु । एकैकं पलमात्रं स्यात्पलार्धं पौष्करं भवेत् ॥ ८९ ॥
चित्रकस्यं पलार्धं स्याद्द्विशाणं मरिचं भवेत् । नागरं पिप्पली मुस्ता त्वगेलापत्रकुङ्कुमम् ॥९०॥
शाणोन्मितं स्यादेकैकं चूर्णयेत्सर्वमेकतः । ततस्तत्प्रक्षिपेच्चूर्ण पक्वखण्डे च तत्समे ॥ ९१ ॥
मोदकान्पलिकान्कृत्वा प्रयुञ्जीत यथोचितान् । हन्यात् सर्वाणि कुष्ठानि त्रिदोषप्रभवामयान् ॥ ९२ ॥
भगन्दरप्लीहगुल्माजिह्वातालुगलामयान् । शिरोऽक्षिभ्रूगतान्रोगान्हन्यात्पृष्ठगतानपि ॥ ९३ ॥
प्राग्भोजनस्य देयं स्यादधःकायस्थिते गदे । भेषजं भक्तमध्ये च रोगे जठरसंस्थिते ॥ ९४ ॥
भोजनस्योपरि ग्राह्यमूर्ध्वजत्रुगदेषु च ।

Eight palas of triphalā, four palas of bhallātaka, five palas of bākuchi, four palas of viḍaṅga, one pala each of hataloha (loha bhasma), trivṛt, guggulu, shilājatu; half pala each of puṣkaramūla and chitraka; two shāṇas of maricha, one shāṇa each of nāgara, pippalī, musta, twak, elā, patra, kumkuma (kesara)—all are nicely powdered and cooked with the syrup of sugar equal in quantity of the total and rolled into pills of one pala. This recipe will cure all types of kuṣṭhas (leprosy and other skin diseases), diseases arising from tridoṣas together, bhagandhara (fistula in ano), plihā (splenic enlargement), gulma (abdominal tumor), disease of the tongue, palate, throat, head, eye, eyebrows, back and other parts of the body. It should be given before meals in diseases of lower extremities, in between meals in diseases of the abdomen and after meals in diseases of the head and neck (88-95).

अथ काञ्चनारगुग्गुलुः गण्डमालाऽपचीग्रन्थीभगन्दरादौ—

काञ्चनारत्वचो ग्राह्यं पलानां दशकं बुधैः ॥ ९५ ॥
त्रिफला षट्पला कार्या त्रिकटु स्यात्पलत्रयम् । पलैकं वरुणं कुर्यादेलात्वक्पत्रकं तथा ॥ ९६ ॥
एकैकं कर्षमात्रं स्यात्सर्वाण्येकत्र चूर्णयेत् । यावच्चूर्णमिदं सर्वं तावन्मात्रस्तु गुग्गुलुः ॥ ९७ ॥
संकुट्य सर्वमेकत्र पिण्डं कृत्वा च धारयेत् । गुटिकाः शाणमात्रेण प्रातर्ग्राह्या यथोचितम् ॥९८॥
गण्डमालां जयत्युग्रामपचीमर्बुदानि च । ग्रन्थीन्व्रणांश्च गुल्मांश्च कुष्ठानि च भगन्दरम् ॥ ९९ ॥
प्रदेयश्चानुपानार्थं क्वाथो मुण्डितकाभवः । क्वाथः खदिरसारस्य पथ्याक्वाथोऽथ कोष्णकम् ॥ १०० ॥

Ten palas of bark of kāñchanāra, six palas of triphalā, three palas of trikaṭu, one pala of bark of varunaleh, karsha each of elā, twak, patra, and guggulu equal to the total quantity of the above are rolled into pills of one shāṇa. These pills taken in the morning with decoction of muṇḍitakā, khadirasāra, pathyā, or warm water will relieve chronic gaṇḍamālā (cervical adenitis), apachī (scrofula), arbuda (cancer), granthi (tumor), vraṇas (ulcers), gulma (abdominal tumors), kuṣṭha (leprosy and other skin diseases) and bhagandara (fistula-in-ano) (95-100)

अथ माषादिमोदकः पुष्टौ—

निस्तुषं माषचूर्णं स्यात्तथा गोधूमसंभवम् । निस्तुषं यवचूर्णं च शालितण्डुलजं तथा ॥ १०१ ॥
सूक्ष्मं च पिप्पलीचूर्णं पलिकान्युपकल्पयेत् । तत एकीकृतं सर्वं भर्जयेद्गोघृतेन च ॥ १०२ ॥
अर्धमात्रेण सर्वेभ्यस्ततः खण्डं समं क्षिपेत् । जलं च द्विगुणं दत्वा पाचयेत शनैः शनैः ॥ १०३ ॥
ततः पक्वं समुद्धृत्य वृत्तान्कुर्वीत मोदकान् । भुक्त्वा सायं पलैकं च पिबेत्क्षीरं चतुर्गुणम् ॥ १०४ ॥
वर्जनीयौ विशेषेण क्षाराम्लौ द्वौ रसावपि । कृत्वैवं रमयेन्नारीर्बह्वीर्न क्षीयते नरः ॥ १०५ ॥

Powder of māṣa, godhūma, yava, shali, taṇdula (devoid of their husks) and pippalī—each one pala are fried in cow's ghee, half the total quantity of sugar candy; twice the quantity of water are cooked together on mild fire and rolled into pills of one pala each. Taken after the evening meal with four palas of cow's milk it acts as an aphrodisiac and gives strength to enjoy with many women. Kshāras and amla (foods which have alkalies and sour taste) are to be avoided specifically during treatment (101-105).

इति श्रीदामोदरसूनुना शार्ङ्गधराचार्येण विरचितायां शार्ङ्गधरसंहितायां
मध्यमखण्डे वटककल्पना नाम सप्तमोऽध्यायः ॥

Thus ends the seventh chapter.

अष्टमोऽध्यायः

CHAPTER 8

Avaleha Kalpanā (*Confections*)

अधुनावलेहानां प्रथमतस्तत्स्वरूपविषयं दर्शयन्नाह—

काथादीनां पुनः पाकाद्घनत्वं सा रसक्रिया । सोऽवलेहश्च लेहः स्यात्तन्मात्रा स्यात्पलोन्मिता ॥ १ ॥

The solid mass obtained by boiling a quatha (decoction) is called rasakriyā, avaleha or leha. Its dose is one pala (1).

इदानीमनुक्ते सितादीनां परिमाणमाह—

सिता चतुर्गुणा कार्या चूर्णाच्च द्विगुणो गुडः । द्रवं चतुर्गुणं दद्यादिति सर्वत्र निश्चयः ॥ २ ॥

If sugar is to be added, it should be four times the quantity of the powder of drugs, if jaggery, it should be double the quantity, if any liquid, it should be four times (2).

अथावलेहस्य सिद्धिलक्षणमाह—

सुपक्वे तन्तुमत्त्वं स्यादवलेहोऽप्सु मज्जति । खरत्वं पीडिते मुद्रागन्धवर्णरसोद्भवः ॥ ३ ॥

Well prepared avaleha should come up thread like (if taken out in a rod), sink in water, take finger prints or shapes if rolled between fingers, give pleasant smell, posses good colour and taste (3).

इदानीमनुक्तेष्वनुपानमाह—

दुग्धमिक्षुरसो यूषः पञ्चमूलीकषायजम् । वासाक्वाथो यथायोग्यमनुपानं प्रशस्यते ॥ ४ ॥

Milk, cane juice, decoction of grains (yūṣa), decoction of pañchamūlas, vasā, etc., are good vehicles (4).

अथ कासश्वासादौ कण्टकार्यवलेहः—

स यथा—

कण्टकारीतुलां नीरद्रोणे पक्त्वा कषायकम् । पादशेषं गृहीत्वा च तस्मिंश्चूर्णानि दापयेत् ॥ ५ ॥
पृथक्पलानि चैतानि गुडूचीचव्यचित्रकाः । मुस्तं कर्कटशृङ्गी च त्र्यूषणं धन्वयासकः ॥ ६ ॥
भार्गी रास्ना शठी चैव शर्करा पलविंशतिः । प्रत्येकं च पलान्यष्टौ प्रदद्याद्घृततैलयोः ॥ ७ ॥
पक्त्वा लेहत्वमानीय शीते मधुपलाष्टकम् । चतुष्पलं तुगाक्षीर्याः पिप्पलीनां चतुष्पलम् ॥ ८ ॥
क्षिप्त्वा निदध्यात्सुदृढे मृण्मये भाजने शुभे । लेहोऽयं हन्ति हिक्कार्तिश्वासकासानशेषतः ॥ ९ ॥

One tulā (100 palas) of kaṇṭakārī is boiled in one droṇa of water and decoction reduced to one fourth, one pala each of guḍūchī, chavya, chitraka, musta, karkaṭashṛngī, tryūṣaṇa, dhānwayasa, bhārngī, rāsnā and shaṭhī; twenty palas of sugar, eight palas each of ghee and sesame oil—are added and made into a solid mass. When cool, eight palas of honey, four palas each of tugākshīrī and pippalī are added. It is then kept in a tightly covered mud pot for a few days and later used. It cures all types of hikkā (hiccough), śwāsa (dyspnoea) and kāsa (cough) (5–9).

अथ च्यवनप्राशः क्षयक्षीणादौ—

पाटलाऽरणिकाश्मर्यबिल्वारलुकगोक्षुराः । पर्ण्यौ बृहत्यौ पिप्पल्यः शृङ्गी द्राक्षामृताभयाः ॥ १० ॥
बला भूम्यामली वासा ऋद्धिर्जीवन्तिका शठी । जीवकर्षभकौ मुस्तं पौष्करं काकनासिका ॥ ११ ॥
मुद्गपर्णी माषपर्णी विदारी च पुनर्नवा । काकोल्यौ कमलं मेदे सूक्ष्मैलागरुचन्दनम् ॥ १२ ॥
एकैकं पलसंमानं स्थूलचूर्णितमौषधम् । एकीकृत्य महत्पात्रे पञ्चामलशतानि च ॥ १३ ॥
पचेद्द्रोणजले क्षिप्त्वा ग्राह्यमष्टावशेषितम् । ततस्तु तान्यामलानि निष्कुलीकृत्य वाससा ॥ १४ ॥
दृढहस्तेन संपीड्य क्षिप्त्वा तत्र ततो घृतम् । पलसप्तमितं तानि किंचिद्भृष्ट्वाल्पवह्निना ॥ १५ ॥
ततस्तत्र क्षिपेत्क्वाथं खण्डं चार्धतुलोन्मितम् । लेहवत्साधयित्वा च चूर्णानीमानि दापयेत् ॥ १६ ॥
पिप्पली द्विपला देया तुगाक्षीरी चतुष्पला । प्रत्येकं च त्रिशाणं स्यात्त्वगेलापत्रकेशरम् ॥ १७ ॥
ततस्त्वेकीकृतं सर्वं क्षिपेत्क्षौद्रं च षट्पलम् । इत्येतच्च्यवनप्रोक्तं च्यवनप्राशसंज्ञितम् ॥ १८ ॥
लेहं वह्निबलं दृष्ट्वा खादेत्क्षीणो रसायनम् । बालवृद्धक्षतक्षीणा नारीक्षीणाश्च शोषिणः ॥ १९ ॥
हृद्रोगिणः स्वरक्षीणा ये नरास्तेषु युज्यते । कासं श्वासं पिपासां च वातास्रमुरसो ग्रहम् ॥ २० ॥
वातपित्तं शुक्रदोषं मूत्रदोषं च नाशयेत् । मेधां स्मृतिं स्त्रीषु हर्षं कान्तिं वर्णप्रसन्नताम् ॥ २१ ॥
अस्य प्रयोगादाप्नोति नरो जीर्णविवर्जितः ।

Pāṭalā, araṇi, kāshmarya, bilwa, aralu, gokshura, the two parnis, the two bṛhatis, pippalī, sringi, drākshā, amṛta, abhayā, balā, bhūmyāmalakī, vasā, ṛddhi, jīvantī, shaṭī, jīvaka, riṣabhaka, musta, puṣkaramūla, kakanasika, mudgaparṇī, māṣaparṇī, vidārī, punarnava, two kākolīs, kamala puṣpa, two medas, sūkshma elā, agaru and chandana—each one pala are boiled in one droṇa of water; well ripened āmalakas five hundred by count are tied in a cloth and the bag is hung inside the boiling water when the liquid is reduced to one eighth part, it is filtered out separately. The baked āmalakas are now made into a fine paste after removing the seeds inside them, the paste is then fried with about seven palas of ghee over mild fire. The decoction is again kept for boiling adding to it the paste of āmalaka, and half tulā (fifty palas) of sugar candy, when the decoction begins to solidify a nice powder of two palas of pippalī, four palas of tugākshīrī; three shanas each of twak, elā, patra and keśara are added and allowed to cool. Afterwards six palas of honey is mixed and stored in containers. This recipe known as *'Chyavanaprāsha'* formulated by sage Chyavana is a rasāyana (rejuvinator) for young and old, for persons suffering from shosha (consumption caused by excessive sex), hṛdroga (heart diseases), śwara kshīṇā (loss of voice), kāsa (cough), śwāsa (dyspnoea), pipāsā (thirst), vātarakta (gout), urograha

(plurecy), shukra doṣa (disorders of semen), mūtradoṣa (urinary disorders). It promotes intelligence, memory, sexual desire, complexion and colour. By its long use man can avoid old age (10–22).

अथ कूष्माण्डावलेहः—

निष्कुलीकृत्य कूष्माण्डखण्डात्पलशतं पचेत् ॥ २२ ॥
निक्षिप्य द्विगुणं नीरमर्धशिष्टं च गृह्यते । तानि कूष्माण्डखण्डानि पीडयेद्दृढवाससा ॥ २३ ॥
आतपे शोषयेत्किंचिच्छूलाग्रैर्बहुशो व्यधेत् । क्षिप्त्वा ताम्रकटाहे च दद्यादष्टपलं घृतम् ॥ २४ ॥
तेन किंचिद्भर्जयित्वा पूर्वोक्तं तज्जलं क्षिपेत् । खण्डात्पलशतं दत्त्वा सर्वमेकत्र पाचयेत् ॥ २५ ॥
सुपक्वे पिप्पली शुण्ठी जीरकं द्विपलं पृथक् । पृथक्पलार्धं धान्याकं पत्रैला मरिचं त्वचम् ॥ २६ ॥
चूर्णीकृत्य क्षिपेत्तत्र घृतार्धं क्षौद्रमावपेत् । खादेदग्निबलं दृष्ट्वा रक्तपित्ती क्षयी ज्वरी ॥ २७ ॥
शोषतृष्णावमिच्छर्दिश्वासकासक्षतातुरः । कूष्माण्डकावलेहोऽयं बालवृद्धेषु युज्यते ॥ २८ ॥
उरःसन्धानकृद्वृष्यो बृंहणो बलकृन्मतः ।

One hundred palas of kernel of kūṣmāṇḍa (devoid of outer skin and seeds) is boiled in two hundred palas of water. When well cooked the pulp is pierced with numerous thick needles (to make it a paste), then fried in a copper vessel with eight palas of ghee. The earlier decoction is kept over fire, hundred palas of sugar candy is added, when it attains semisolid consistence the paste of kūṣmāṇḍa, fine powder of two palas each of pippalī, shuṇṭhī, jīraka; half pala each of dhānyaka; patra, elā, maricha, twak are added. When cooled four palas of honey is added and stored. This recipe known as '*kūṣmāṇḍ avalehya*' is beneficial for both young and old. It is effective for persons suffering from raktapitta (purpura), kshaya (consumption), jwara (fever), shoṣa (emaciation), tṛṣṇā (thirst), bhrama (giddiness), chardi (vomiting), swāsa (dyspnoea), kāsa (cough), kshata (ulcers of the lungs) is an aphrodisiac, builds the body and strengthens it (22–29).

अथ खण्डसूरणावलेहः अर्शोरोगे—

युक्त्या कूष्माण्डखण्डस्य सूरणं विपचेत्सुधीः ॥ २९ ॥
अर्शसां मूढवातानां मन्दाग्नीनां च युज्यते ।

Sūraṇa kanda is prepared into leha in the same way as that of kūṣmāṇdavalehya. This recipe will be effective in cases of arshas (piles), mūḍhavāta (sluggishness of bowels), and mandāgni (dyspepsia) (29–30).

अथ अगस्त्यहरीतक्यवलेहः—

हरीतकीशतं भद्रं यवानामाढकं तथा ॥ ३० ॥
पलानि दशमूलस्य विंशति च नियोजयेत् । चित्रकः पिप्पलीमूलमपामार्गः शठी तथा ॥ ३१ ॥
कपिकच्छुः शङ्खपुष्पी भार्ङ्गी च गजपिप्पली । बला पुष्करमूलं च पृथग्द्विपलमात्रया ॥ ३२ ॥

पचेत्पश्चाढके नीरे यवैः स्विन्नैः शृतं नयेत् । तच्चाभयाशतं दद्यात्क्वाथे तस्मिन्विचक्षणः ॥ ३३ ॥
सर्पिस्तैलाष्टपलकं क्षिपेद्गुडतुलां तथा । पक्त्वा लेहत्वमानीय सिद्धे शीते पृथक्पृथक् ॥ ३४ ॥
क्षौद्रं च पिप्पलीचूर्णं दद्यात्कुडवमात्रया । हरीतकीद्वयं खादेत्तेन लेहेन नित्यशः ॥ ३५ ॥
क्षयं कासं ज्वरं श्वासं हिक्कार्शोऽरुचिपीनसान् । ग्रहणीं नाशयेदेष वलीपलितनाशनः ॥ ३६ ॥
बलवर्णकरः पुंसामवलेहो रसायनम् । विहितोऽगस्त्यमुनिना सर्वरोगप्रणाशनः ॥ ३७ ॥

Twenty palas of dashamūla, two palas each of chitraka, pippalīmūla, apāmārga, shaṭhī, kapikacchu, shankhapuṣpi, bhārṅgī, gajapippalī, balā and puṣkaramūla—are boiled in five aḍhakas of water reduced to quarter and filtered out. This decoction is again kept for boiling, harītakī one hundred by count and one aḍhaka of yava are tied in a cloth and hung inside the decoction. When reduced to quarter, harītakī are taken out, their seeds removed and readded along with yava paste, eight palas each of ghee and sesame oil and one tulā (100 palas) of jaggery are added and made into lehya. When cooled honey and powder of pippalimūla each one kuḍava are added and stored. This recipe revealed by sage Agastya, taken in doses of two harītakīs per time, relieves kshaya (consumption), kāsa (cough), jwara (fevers), swāsa (dyspnoea), hikkā (hiccough), arshas (piles), aruchi (loss of taste), pīnasa (coryza); grahaṇī (sprue); removes grey hairs and wrinkles, improves strength and complexion, cures all diseases and acts as a rasāyana (rejuvinator) (30–37).

अर्शादौ कुटजावलेहः—

कुटजत्वक्तुलां द्रोणे जलस्य विपचेत्सुधीः । कषायं पादशेषं च गृह्णीयाद्वस्त्रगालितम् ॥ ३८ ॥
त्रिंशत्पलं गुडस्यात्र दत्त्वा च विपचेत्पुनः । सान्द्रत्वमागतं दृष्ट्वा चूर्णानीमानि दापयेत् ॥ ३९ ॥
रसाञ्जनं मोचरसं त्रिकटु त्रिफलां तथा । लज्जालुं चित्रकं पाठां बिल्वमिन्द्रयवं त्वचाम् ॥ ४० ॥
भल्लातकं प्रतिविषां विडङ्गानि च बालकम् । प्रत्येकं पलसंमानं घृतस्य कुडवं तथा ॥ ४१ ॥
सिद्धशीते ततो दद्यान्मधुनः कुडवं तथा । जयेदेषोऽवलेहस्तु सर्वाण्यर्शांसि वेगतः ॥ ४२ ॥
दुर्नामप्रभवान्रोगानतीसारमरोचकम् । ग्रहणीं पाण्डुरोगं च रक्तपित्तं च कामलाम् ॥ ४३ ॥
अम्लपित्तं तथा शोथं कार्श्यं चैव प्रवाहिकाम् । अनुपाने प्रोक्तव्यमाजं तक्रं पयो दधि ॥ ४४ ॥
घृतं जलं वा जीर्णे च पथ्यभोजी भवेन्नरः ।

One tulā (100 palas) of bark of kuṭaja is boiled in one droṇa of water, reduced to quarter and filtered out. To this decoction, thirty palas of jaggery is added, when the liquid becomes semisolid, nice powder of one pala each of rasāñjana, mocharasa, trikaṭu, triphalā, lajjālu, chitraka, pāṭhā, bilwa, indrayava, twak, bhallātaka, prativiṣa, viḍaṅga and vālaka; one kuḍava each of ghee and honey are added and made into leha. This recipe quickly cures all types of arshas (piles) and disorders arising from it, atisāra (diarrhoea), arochaka

(loss of taste), grahaṇī (sprue), pāṇḍuroga (anaemia), raktapitta (purpura), kāmalā (jaundice), amlapitta (hyperchlorhydria), shotha (oedema), kārshya (emaciation) and pravāhikā (dysentery). During its use milk, butter milk and ghee (obtained from goats milk) or warm water are ideal for good digestion (38-45)

अतीसारादौ कुटजाष्टकावलेहमाह

कुटजत्वक्तुलामार्द्रां द्रोणनीरे विपाचयेत् ॥ ४५ ॥
पादशेषं शृतं नीत्वा चूर्णान्येतानि दापयेत् । लज्जालुर्धातकी बिल्वं पाठा मोचरसस्तथा ॥ ४६ ॥
मुस्तं प्रतिविषा चैव प्रत्येकं स्यात्पलं पलम् । ततस्तु विपचेद्भूयो यावद्दर्वीप्रलेपनम् ॥ ४७ ॥
जलेन छागदुग्धेन पीतो मण्डेन वा जयेत् । सर्वातिसारान्घोरांस्तु नानावर्णान्सवेदनान् ॥ ४८ ॥
असृग्दरं समस्तं च सर्वार्शांसि प्रवाहिकाम् ।

One tulā of green bark of kuṭaja is boiled in one droṇa of water and decoction reduced to quarter. Nice powder of one pala each of lajjālu, dhātaki, bilwa, pāṭha, mocharasa, musta, prativiṣa are added to the decoction and lehya prepared. This recipe taken along with water, goats milk, or other gruels relieves all types of severe atisāra (diarrhoea), asṛgdara (menorrhagia), arshas (piles) and pravāhikā (dysentery) (45–49).

इति श्रीदामोदरसूनुना श्रीशार्ङ्गधराचार्येण विरचितायां शार्ङ्गधरसंहितायां
मध्यमखण्डेऽवलेहकल्पना नामाष्टमोऽध्यायः ॥ ८ ॥

Thus ends the eighth chapter.

नवमोऽध्यायः

CHAPTER 9

Sneha Kalpanā (Medicated Ghee and Oils)

अथ स्नेहपरिभाषा—

कल्काच्चतुर्गुणीकृत्य घृतं वा तैलमेव वा । चतुर्गुणे द्रवे साध्यं तस्य मात्रा पलोन्मिता ॥ १ ॥
निक्षिप्य क्वाथयेत्तोयं क्वाथ्यद्रव्याच्चतुर्गुणम् । पादशिष्टं गृहीत्वा च स्नेहं तेनैव साधयेत् ॥ २ ॥

जलप्रमाणमाह—

चतुर्गुणं मृदुद्रव्ये कठिनेऽष्टगुणं जलम् । तथा च मध्यमे द्रव्ये दद्यादष्टगुणं पयः ॥ ३ ॥
अत्यन्तकठिने द्रव्ये नीरं षोडशिकं मतम् ।

Medicated sneha i. e., ghṛta or taila (ghee or oil) is prepared by mixing one part of kalka (paste of drugs), four of ghee or oil and four parts of any decoction. The dose of sneha is one pala. For preparing decoction, one part of drugs is boiled in four parts of water and reduced to a quarter. If the drugs are of soft nature water is taken four times of their quantity; if medium or moderately hard, eight times and if very hard sixteen parts of water are taken and reduced to quarter (1–4).

मतान्तरे परिमाणविशेषमाह —

कर्षादितः पलं यावत्क्षिपेत्षोडशिकं जलम् ॥ ४ ॥

तदूर्ध्वं कुडवं यावद्द्रवेदष्टगुणं पयः । प्रस्थादितः क्षिपेन्नीरं खारी यावच्चतुर्गुणम् ॥ ५ ॥

If the quantity of each drug varies from one karṣa to one pala, water should be sixteen times; if from pala to kuḍava water should be eight times, if from prastha to khārī, water is taken four times the quantity only (4–5).

अम्बुक्वाथरसैर्यत्र पृथक्स्नेहस्य साधनम् । कल्कस्यांशं तत्र दद्याच्चतुर्थं षष्ठमष्टमम् ॥ ६ ॥

दुग्धे दध्नि रसे तक्रे कल्को देयोऽष्टमांशकः । कल्कस्य सम्यक्पाकार्थं तोयमत्र चतुर्गुणम् ॥ ७ ॥

द्रवाणि यत्र स्नेहेषु पञ्चादीनि भवन्ति हि । तत्र स्नेहसमान्याहुर्यथापूर्वं चतुर्गुणम् ॥ ८ ॥

If sneha is to be prepared with only water, decoction, meat juice or fresh juice of herbs, then their quantity should be four, six and eight times of the kalka respectively. If sneha is to be prepared with milk, curd, meat juice or buttermilk, the kalka (paste of drugs) should be one eighth part and water four times of it. If in the above sneha oil or ghee is also to be added, then it should be taken in equal quantity (as a kalka) and the quantity of milk, curds, meat juice or butter milk should be four times of it (6–8)

केवलक्वाथपाके विधानमाह

द्रव्येण केवलेनैव स्नेहपाको भवेद्यदि । तत्राम्बुपिष्टः कल्कः स्याज्जलं चात्र चतुर्गुणम् ॥ ९ ॥

क्वाथेन केवलेनैव पाको यत्रेरितः क्वचित् । क्वाथ्यद्रव्यस्य कल्कोऽपि तत्र स्नेहे प्रयुज्यते ॥ १० ॥

If sneha (ghee or oil) is to be prepared with only water the quantity of water should be four times (of the paste or sneha) and the same is also the case if only decoction it to be used or any other liquid is to be used (9–10).

कल्कहीनस्तु यः स्नेहः स साध्यः केवले द्रवे । पुष्पकल्कस्तु यः स्नेहस्तत्र तोयं चतुर्गुणम् ॥११॥

स्नेहे स्नेहाष्टमांशश्च पुष्पकल्कः प्रयुज्यते ।

If in the sneha, kalka (paste) consists of flowers, then it is taken in one eighth the quantity of sneha and water is taken four times (the quantity of sneha).

वर्तिवत्स्नेहकल्कः स्याद्यदाङ्गुल्या विमर्दितः ॥ १२ ॥

शब्दहीनोऽग्निनिक्षिप्तः स्नेहः सिद्धो भवेत्तदा । यदा फेनोद्गमस्तैले फेनशान्तिश्च सर्पिषि ॥ १३ ॥

गन्धवर्णरसोत्पत्तिः स्नेहसिद्धिस्तदा भवेत् । स्नेहपाकस्त्रिधा प्रोक्तो मृदुर्मध्यः खरस्तथा ॥ १४ ॥

ईषत्सरसकल्कस्तु स्नेहपाको मृदुर्भवेत् । मध्यपाकस्य सिद्धिश्च कल्के नीरसकोमलः ॥ १५ ॥
ईषत्कठिनकल्कश्च स्नेहपाको भवेत्खरः । तदूर्ध्वं दग्धपाकः स्याद्दाहकृन्निष्प्रयोजनः ॥ १६ ॥
आमपाकश्च निर्वीर्यो वह्निमान्द्यकरो गुरुः ।

A small quantity of kalka taken out at the end of boiling and rolled in-between the fingeis, if it assumes a wick-like shape and does not produce any cracking noise if thrown on fire it is the test for properly cooked sneha; like wise, appearance and disappearance of bubbles at the terminal stage of cooking oil and ghee respectively, and emission of good smell, colour, and taste are the other tests for properly cooked sneha (ghee or oil).

Snehapāka (cooking) is of three types : mṛdu (mild), madhya (moderate) and khara (hard boiled). A small quantity of kalka taken out and pressed between finger if yields large quantity of sneha (oil or ghee) it is said to be in mṛdupāka, if it does not yield any sneha but is soft in consistence the pāka is madhyama, if the kalka does not yield any sneha and is hard it is said to be in khara. Boiling still further will result in dagdha pāka (over burnt) which not only becomes unworthy but even causes burning sensation by using it. Even so is amapāka (deficient cooking) which is not only ineffective but also causes indigestion (12-17).

नस्यार्थं स्यान्मृदुः पाको मध्यमः सर्वकर्मसु ॥ १७ ॥
अभ्यङ्गार्थं खरः प्रोक्तो युञ्ज्यादेवं यथोचितम् । घृततैलगुडादींश्च साधयेन्नैकवासरे ॥ १८ ॥
प्रकुर्वन्त्युषिता ह्येते विशेषाद्गुणसंचयम् ।

Mṛdu pāka sneha is useful for nasya karma (nasal-drops), madhyamapāka for all other purposes; kharapaka only for abhyaṅga (bath, massage etc.).

Preparation of ghṛta, taila or guḍa (pills) should not be completed within one day. Longer the duration of preparation better the aquisition of properties of drugs into them (17-19).

अथ घृतकल्पना

अथ क्षीरषट्पलघृतम्—

पिप्पलीपिप्पलीमूलचव्यचित्रकनागरैः ॥ १९ ॥
ससैन्धवैश्च पलिकैर्घृतप्रस्थं विपाचयेत् । क्षीरं चतुर्गुणं दत्त्वा तद्घृतं प्लीहनाशनम् ॥ २० ॥
विषमज्वरमन्दाग्निहरं रुचिकरं परम् ।

Pippali, pippalīmūla, chavya, chitraka, nāgara, saindhava, each one pala, ghṛta (ghee) one prastha, cow's milk four times that of ghee,—is taken and ghṛta prepared. This will cure plīhā vṛddhi (enlargement of spleen), viṣamajwara (remittant fever), mandāgni (dyspepsia) and promotes taste (19-21).

अथ चांगेरीघृतं अतीसारग्रहण्योः—

पिप्पली पिप्पलीमूलं चित्रको हस्तिपिप्पली ॥ २१ ॥
श्वदंष्ट्रा नागरं धान्यं पाठा बिल्वं यवानिका। द्रव्यैश्च पलिकैरेतैश्चतुःषष्टिपलं घृतम् ॥ २२ ॥
घृताच्चतुर्गुणं देयं चाङ्गेरीस्वरसं बुधैः। तथा चतुर्गुणं दत्त्वा दधि सर्पिर्विपाचयेत् ॥ २३ ॥
शनैः शनैर्विपक्तव्यं चाङ्गेरीघृतमुत्तमम्। तद्घृतं कफवातघ्नं ग्रहण्यर्शोविकारनुत् ॥ २४ ॥
हन्त्यानाहं गुदभ्रंशं मूत्रकृच्छ्रं प्रवाहिकाम्।

Pippalī, pippalīmūla, chitraka, hastipippalī, swadaṃṣṭra, nāgara, dhānya, pata, bilwa, yavanikā—each one pala, ghee sixty four palas, fresh juice of chāṅgerī and curd each four times the quantity of ghee,—are all cooked together and ghṛta prepared. This recipe known as *chāṅgerī ghṛta* relieves kapha and Vata. grahaṇī (sprue), arshas (piles), ānāha (tympanitis, abdominal enlargement), gudabhraṃsha (prolapse of rectum), mūtra kṛcchra (difficulty of micturition) and pravahika (dysentery) (21–25).

अथ मसूरघृतं अतीसारादौ

मसूराणां पलशतं नीरद्रोणे विपाचयेत् ॥ २५ ॥
पादशेषं शृतं नीत्वा दत्त्वा बिल्वपलाष्टकम्। घृतप्रस्थं पचेत्तेन सर्वातीसारनाशनम् ॥ २६ ॥
ग्रहणीं भिन्नविट्कं च नाशयेच्च प्रवाहिकाम्।

One hundred palas of masūra dāl is boiled in one droṇa of water and reduced to quarter. To this decoction eight palas of bilwa and one prastha of ghee are added and ghṛtapāka done. This recipe cures all kinds of atisāras (diarrhoea), grahaṇī (sprue), bhinnaviṭ (loose motions) and pravāhikā (dysentery) (25–26).

अथ कामदेवघृतं रक्तपित्तादौ—

अश्वगन्धा पलशतं तदर्धं गोक्षुरं स्मृतम्। शतावरी विदारी च शालपर्णी बलामृता ॥ २७ ॥
अश्वत्थस्य च शुङ्गानि पद्मबीजं पुनर्नवा। कश्मर्याश्च फलं चैव माषबीजं तथैव च ॥ २८ ॥
पृथग्दशपलान्भागान् चतुर्द्रोणेऽम्भसि पचेत्। द्रोणे शेषे रसे तस्मिन् पचेच्चैव घृताढकम् ॥२९॥
मृद्वीका पद्मकं कुष्ठं पिप्पली रक्तचन्दनम्। पत्रकं नागपुष्पं च आत्मगुप्ताफलं तथा ॥ ३० ॥
नीलोत्पलं सारिवे द्वे जीवनीयो गणस्तथा। पृथक्कर्षसमान्भागान् शर्करायाः पलद्वयम् ॥ ३१ ॥
रसस्य पौण्ड्रकेक्षूणामाढकैकं समाहरेत्। चतुर्गुणेन पयसा घृताढकं विपाचयेत् ॥ ३२ ॥
घृतमेतन्निहन्त्याशु रक्तपित्तमुरःक्षतम्। हलीमकं पाण्डुरोगं वर्णभेदं स्वरक्षयम् ॥ ३३ ॥
मूत्रकृच्छ्रमुरोदाहं पार्श्वशूलं च नाशयेत्। एतत्सर्पिः प्रयोक्तव्यं बह्वन्तःपुरवासिनाम् ॥ ३४ ॥
स्त्रीणां चैवाप्रजातानां दुर्बलानां च देहिनाम्। श्रेष्ठं बलकरं वर्ण्यं हृद्यं पुष्टिरसायनम् ॥ ३५ ॥
ओजस्तेजस्करं हृद्यमायुष्यं प्राणवर्धनम्। संवर्धयति शुक्रं हि पुरुषं दुर्बलेन्द्रियम् ॥ ३६ ॥
सर्वरोगविनिर्मुक्तौ पयःसिक्तो यथा द्रुमः। कामदेव इति ख्यातं सर्पिरुक्तं महागुणम् ॥ ३७ ॥

One tulā (hundred palas) of ashwagandhā and ardha tulā (fifty palas) of gokshura, ten palas each of shatāvarī, vidārī, shaliparṇī, balā, amṛtā, tender leaves of aśwatha, padmabīja, punarnavā, kāshmarī phala and māṣabīja are powdered and boiled in four droṇas of water, reduced to quarter and decoction filtered out, one āḍhaka of ghee and powder of one karṣa each of mṛdwīkā, padmaka, kuṣṭha, pippalī, raktachandana, patra, nāgapuṣpa, ātmaguptāphala, nīlotpala, two sārivās and drugs of jīvanīya gaṇa, two palas of sugar, one āḍhaka of sugarcane juice (poundraka-variety), four āḍhakas of cow's milk are added and ghṛta prepared. This known as '*Kāmadeva ghṛta*' relieves quickly raktapitta (purpura), urakshata (injury to lungs), halīmaka (severe jaundice), panduroga (anaemia), varṇabheda (discolouration), swara-kshaya (loss of voice), mūtra kṛcchra (difficulty of urination), urodāha (heart burn), pārshwa shūla, it is specially useful for women who have no issues, and are weak, it restores strength, colour, good for mind, acts as rasāyana (rejuvinator), lengthens the life span, promotes production of semen and strengthens the genital organs. Just as a tree fed with water grows well free from diseases so also does man become free from all ailments by the use of this Kamadeva Ghṛta (27–37).

अपस्मारादौ पानीयकल्याणकं घृतं—

त्रिफला द्वे निशे कौन्ती सारिवे द्वे प्रियङ्गुका । शालिपर्णी पृष्ठिपर्णी देवदार्व्यैलवालुकम् ॥ ३८ ॥
नतं विशाला दन्ती च दाडिमं नागकेशरम् । नीलोत्पलैला मञ्जिष्ठा विडङ्गं कुष्ठपद्मकम् ॥ ३९ ॥
जातिपुष्पं चन्दनं च तालीसं बृहती तथा । एतैः कर्षसमैः कल्कैर्जलं दत्वा चतुर्गुणम् ॥ ४० ॥
घृतप्रस्थं पचेद्धीमानपस्मारे ज्वरे क्षये । उन्मादे वातरक्ते च कासे मन्दानले तथा ॥ ४१ ॥
प्रतिश्याये कटीशूले तृतीयकचतुर्थके । मूत्रकृच्छ्रे विसर्पे च कण्डूपाण्ड्वामये तथा ॥ ४२ ॥
विषद्वये प्रमेहेषु सर्वथैवोपयुज्यते । वन्ध्यानां पुत्रदं भूतयक्षरक्षोहरं स्मृतम् ॥ ४३ ॥

Triphalā, the two nishās, kauntī (renuka), two sārivās, priyaṅgu, shaliparṇī, pṛṣṭhiparṇī, devadāru, elavāluka, vāta, vishālā, dantī, dāḍima, nāgakesara; nīlotpala, elā, mañjiṣṭhā, viḍaṅga, kuṣṭha, padmaka, jātīpuṣpa, chandana, tālīsa and bṛhatī—each one karṣa are made into a kalka (paste) boiled in four times their quantity of water. During boiling one prastha of ghee is added and ghṛta prepared. This recipe is beneficial in apasmāra (epilepsy), jwara (fevers), kshaya (consumption), unmāda (insanity), vātarakta (gout), kāsa (cough), mandānala (poor digestive capacity), pratishyāya (running in the nose), kaṭishūla (lumbago), tritīyaka and chaturtika jwara (tertian and quartan fevers), mūtrakṛcchra (dysurea), visarpa (erysepalas), kaṇḍū (itching), pāṇḍu (anaemia), the two kinds of viṣas (poisons), prameha (diabetes). It helps sterile women to get children, dispells bhūta, yakshas and rākshasas (evil spirits and bacteria) (38–43).

अमृताघृतं कुष्ठादौ—

अमृताक्वाथकल्काभ्यां सक्षीरं विपचेद्घृतम् । वातरक्तं जयत्याशु कुष्ठं जयति दुस्तरम् ॥ ४४ ॥

Ghṛta prepared with decoction and paste (kalka) of amṛtā with the addition of milk cures vātarakta (gout) quickly and even intractible kuṣṭha (leprosy and other skin diseases) (44).

अथ महातिक्तकघृतं वातरक्तकुष्ठादौ—

सप्तच्छदः प्रतिविषा श्यामाकः कटुरोहिणी । पाठा मुस्तमुशीरं च त्रिफला पर्पटस्तथा ॥ ४५ ॥
पटोलनिम्बमञ्जिष्ठाः पिप्पली पद्मकं शठी । चन्दनं धन्वयासश्च विशाले द्वे निशे तथा ॥ ४६ ॥
गुडूची सारिवे द्वे च मूर्वा वासा शतावरी । त्रायन्तीन्द्रयवायष्टीभूनिम्बश्चाक्षभागिका: ॥ ४७ ॥
घृतं चतुर्गुणं दद्याद्घृतादामलकीरसः । द्विगुणः सर्पिषश्चात्र जलमष्टगुणं भवेत् ॥ ४८ ॥
तत्सिद्धं पाययेत्सर्पिर्वातरक्तेषु सर्वथा । कुष्ठानि रक्तपितं च रक्तार्शांसि च पाण्डुताम् ॥ ४९ ॥
हृद्रोगगुल्मवीसर्पप्रदरं गण्डमालिकाम् । क्षुद्ररोगान् ज्वरांश्चैव महातिक्तमिदं जयेत् ॥ ५० ॥

Saptachhada, prativiṣa, shyāmāka, kaṭurohiṇī, pāṭhā, musta, usheera, triphalā, parpaṭa, paṭola, nimba, mañjiṣṭhā, pippalī, padmaka, shaṭhī, chandana, dhanwayāsa, vishālā, the two nishās, gudūchi, two sarivas, mūrvā, vāsā, shatāvarī, trāyantī, indrayava, yaṣṭi and bhūnimba—each one aksha (karṣa) in quantity are made into kalka (paste), ghee is taken four times the quantity of this kalka (paste), amalakī rasa (juice of myrobalans) double the quantity of ghee and water eight times the quantity of ghee—all these are cooked and ghṛta prepared in the usual way. This recipe known as *mahātikta ghṛta* is very useful in vātarakta (gout), kuṣṭha (leprosy and other skin diseases), rakta pitta (purpura), rakta arshas (bleeding piles), pāṇḍu (anaemia), hṛdroga (heart diseases), gulma (abdominal tumors), visarpa (erysepalas), pradara menorrhagia), gaṇḍamālā (scrofula), kshudra rogas (minor skin diseases) and jwara (fevers) (45–50).

अथ कासीसाद्यं घृतं कुष्ठे दद्रूपामाशिरःस्फोटादौ—

कासीसं द्वे निशे मुस्तं हरितालं मनःशिलाम् । कम्पिल्लकं गन्धकं च विडङ्गं गुग्गुलुं तथा ॥ ५१ ॥
सिक्थकं मरिचं कुष्ठं तुत्थकं गौरसर्षपान् । रसाञ्जनं च सिन्दूर श्रीवासं रक्तचन्दनम् ॥ ५२ ॥
इरिमेदं निम्बपत्रं करञ्जं सारिवां वचाम् । मञ्जिष्ठां मधुकं मांसीं शिरीषं लोध्रपद्मकम् ॥ ५३ ॥
हरीतकीं प्रपुन्नाटं चूर्णयेत्कार्षिकान्पृथक् । ततस्तच्चूर्णमालोड्य त्रिंशत्पलमिते घृते ॥ ५४ ॥
स्थापयेत्ताम्रपात्रे च घर्मे सप्त दिनावधि । अस्याभ्यङ्गेन कुष्ठानि दद्रूपामाविचर्चिकाः ॥ ५५ ॥
शूकदोषा विसर्पाश्च विस्फोटा वातरक्तजाः । शिरःस्फोटोपदंशाश्च नाडीदुष्टव्रणानि च ॥ ५६ ॥
शोथोभगन्दरश्चैव लूताः शाम्यन्ति देहिनाम् । शोधनं रोपणं चैव सवर्णकरणं घृतम् ॥ ५७ ॥

Kāsīsa, the two nishās, musta, haratāla, manashilā, kampillaka, gandhaka, viḍaṅga, guggulu, sikthaka, maricha, kuṣṭha, tuttha, gaurasarṣapa, rasāñjana, sindūra, srivāsa, raktachandana, irimeda, leaves of nimba, karañja, sārivā, vachā, mañjiṣṭha, madhuka, mamsi, sireesha, lodhra padmaka, harītaki and prapunnata—each one karsha are nicely powdered and mixed with thirty palas of ghee, put in a copper vessel and kept in hot sun for seven days. This ghṛta used for abhyaṅga (anointing the body) cures kuṣṭha (leprosy), dadru (ringworm), pāmā (scabies), vicharchikā (psoriasis), shūkadoṣa (venereal diseases), visarpa (erysipelas), visphoṭas of vātarakta (tophies of gout), shirasphoṭa (abscess on the head), upadaṁsha (syphilis), nāḍīvraṇa (sinus ulcer), duṣṭavraṇa (bad ulcers), shotha (oedema), bhagandara (fistula in ano), and lūtā (spider bite). It is shodhana (purifier), ropana (healer) and savarṇakara (brings back the normal colour to the skin) (51–57).

अथ व्रणे जात्यादिघृतं—

जातीनिम्बपटोलं च द्वे निशे कटुरोहिणी । मञ्जिष्ठा मधुकं सिक्थं करञ्जोशीरसारिवाः ॥ ५८ ॥
तुत्थं च विपचेत्सम्यक्कल्कैरेभिर्घृतं बुधः । अस्य लेपाद्विरोहन्ति सूक्ष्मनाडीव्रणा अपि ॥ ५९ ॥
मर्माश्रिताः क्लेदिनश्च गम्भीराः सरुजो व्रणाः ।

Leaves of jātī, nimba, paṭola, the two nishās, kaṭukarohiṇī, mañjiṣṭha, madhuka, sikthaka, karañja, ushīra, sārivā and tuttha—are to be prepared into a ghṛta in the usual way. By its application nāḍīvraṇa (ulcers with a sinus) and ulcers situated in marmas (vital points), those with exudation, those which are very deep and those painful will all heal (58–60).

अथ बिन्दुघृतं जलोदरविरेचनादौ—

चित्रकं शङ्खिनी पथ्या कम्पिल्लस्त्रिवृतायुगम् ॥ ६० ॥

वृद्धदारुश्च शम्याको दन्ती दन्तीफलं तथा । कोशातकी देवदाली नीलिनी गिरिकर्णिका ॥ ६१ ॥
सातला पिप्पलीमूलं विडङ्गं कटुकी तथा । हेमक्षीरी च विपचेत्कल्कैरेभिः पिचून्मितैः ॥ ६२ ॥
घृतप्रस्थं स्नुहीक्षीरं षट्पले तु पलद्वयम् । अर्कक्षीरस्य मतिमांस्तत्सिद्धं गुल्मकुष्ठहृत् ॥ ६३ ॥
हन्ति शूलमुदावर्तं शोथाध्मानं भगन्दरम् । शमयत्युदराण्यष्टौ निपीतं बिन्दुसंख्यया ॥ ६४ ॥
गोदुग्धेनोष्ट्रदुग्धेन कौलत्थेन शृतेन वा । उष्णोदकेन वा पीत्वा बिन्दुवेगैर्विरिच्यते ॥ ६५ ॥

एतद्बिन्दुघृतं नाम नाभिलेपाद्विरिच्यते ।

Chitraka, shaṅkhinī, pathyā, kampilla, the two trivṛts, vṛdhadāru, shamyāka dantī, dantīphala, koshātakī, devadālī, nīlinī, girikarnikā, sātalā, pippalīmūla, viḍaṅga, kaṭukī, and hemakshīrī—each one pichu in quantity are made into a kalka; one prastha of ghee, six palas of snuhikshīra (milky sap of snuhi) and two palas of arkakshīra (milky sap of arka) are taken and ghṛta prepared. This recipe known as *Bindu ghṛta* produces purgations equal in number to the number of drops of ghṛta taken with cow's milk, camel's milk, decoction of kulattha or hot water. Even its application over the umbilical region will produce purgings. It is useful in cases of shūla (colic), udāvarta (reverse peristalisis), shotha (oedema), ādhmāna (tympanitis), bhagandara (fistula in ano), the eight kinds of udara (abdominal enlargements) (60-66).

अथ त्रिफलाघृतं नेत्ररोगे तिमिरादौ—

त्रिफलाया रसप्रस्थं प्रस्थं वासारसोद्भवम् ॥ ६६ ॥
भृङ्गराजरसप्रस्थं प्रस्थमाजं पयः स्मृतम् । दत्त्वा तत्र घृतप्रस्थं कल्कैः कर्षमितैः पृथक् ॥ ६७ ॥
त्रिफला पिप्पली द्राक्षा चन्दनं सैन्धवं बला । काकोली क्षीरकाकोली मेदा मरिचनागरम् ॥ ६८ ॥
शर्करा पुण्डरीकं च कमलं च पुनर्नवा । निशायुग्मं च मधुकं सर्वैरेभिर्विपाचयेत् ॥ ६९ ॥
नक्तान्ध्यं नकुलान्ध्यं च कण्डूं पिल्लं तथैव च नेत्रस्रावं च पटलं तिमिरं काचकं जयेत् ॥ ७० ॥
अन्येऽपि प्रशमं यान्ति नेत्ररोगाः सुदारुणाः । त्रैफलं घृतमेतद्धि पाने नस्यादिषूचितम् ॥ ७१ ॥

One prastha each of decoction of triphalā, juice of vasā, bhṛṅgarāja, goats milk and ghṛta (ghee) are taken and one karṣa each of triphalā, pippalī, drākshā, chandana, saindhava, balā, kākolī, kshīra-kākolī, medā, maricha, nāgara, sharkarā (sugar), puṇḍarīka, kamala, punarnavā, the two nishās, and madhuka are made into decoction and paste and gṛhta prepared in the usual way. This recipe known as *Triphalā ghṛta*—relieves naktāndhya (night blindness), nakulāndhya (blindness during day), kaṇḍū (irritation of the eyes), pilla (growths in the eye), netrasrāva (discharges), patala (defects of vision), timira, and kācha (disorder of lens) and many other severe eye diseases. It is used internally and also as nasya (nasal drops) (66-71).

अथ गौराद्यं घृतं व्रणे—

द्वे हरिद्रे स्थिरा मूर्वा सारिवा चन्दनद्वयम् । मधुपर्णी च मधुकं पद्मकेशरपद्मकम् ॥ ७२ ॥
उत्पलोशीरमेदाभिस्त्रिफलापञ्चवल्कलैः । कल्कैः कर्षमितैरेतैर्घृतप्रस्थं विपाचयेत् ॥ ७३ ॥
विसर्पलूताविस्फोटविषकीटव्रणापहम् । गौराद्यमिति विख्यातं सर्पिर्विषहरं परम् ॥ ७४ ॥

The two haridrās, sthirā, mūrvā, sārivā, the chandanas, madhuparṇī, madhuka, padmakeśara, padmaka, utpala, ushīra, medā, triphalā, pañchavalkala each one karṣa are made into a kalka (or qwātha); prepared into ghṛta in the usual way. This recipe known as *Gouradi ghṛta* is highly beneficial in visarpa (erysipelas), lūtā (spider bite), visphoṭa (boils) and stings of poisonous insects. It is a reputed antipoisonous drug (72-74).

अथ मयूरघृतं शिरोरोगादौ—

बलामधुकरास्नाभिर्दशमूलफलत्रिकैः । पृथग्द्विपलिकैरेभिर्द्रोणनीरेण पाचयेत् ॥ ७५ ॥
मयूरं पक्षपित्तान्त्रयकृत्पादास्यवर्जितम् । पादशेषं शृतं नीत्वा क्षीरं दत्त्वा च तत्समम् ॥ ७६ ॥

घृतप्रस्थं पचेत्सम्यग्जीवनीयैः पिचून्मितैः । तत्सिद्धं शिरसः पीडां मन्यापृष्ठग्रहं तथा ॥ ७७ ॥
अर्दितं कर्णनासाक्षिजिह्वागलरुजो जयेत् । पाने नस्ये तथाभ्यङ्गे कर्णपूरेषु युज्यते ॥ ७८ ॥
हेमन्तकालशिशिरवसन्तेषु च शस्यते ।

Balā, madhuka, rāsnā, dashamūla, triphalā—each two palas are boiled in one droṇa of water. During boiling flesh of a peacock (devoid of its feathers, bile, intestines, liver, legs, and beak) cut into small bits are put into boiling decoction and reduced to quarter. Later cow's milk equal in quantity of the decoction, one prastha of ghee and kalka prepared with one pichu each of the drugs of jīvanīya gaṇa (mudgaparni, mashaparṇī, kākolī, kshīrakākolī, medā, mahāmeda, jivaka, riṣabhaka, madhuka, jīvanti) are cooked and ghṛta prepared. This recipe known as *Mayoora ghrita* used in the form of internal potion, nasal drops, external anointing and ear drops cures aches in the head, neck, back, ardita (facial paralysis), pain of the ear, nose, eye, tongue and throat. It is ideally suited for use in Hemanta, Shishira and Vasanta kālas (winter, autumn and spring seasons) (75–79).

अथ फलघृतं वन्ध्यादोषे—

त्रिफला मधुकं कुष्ठं द्वे निशे कटुरोहिणी ॥ ७९ ॥
विडङ्गं पिप्पली मुस्तं विशाला कट्फलं वचा । द्वे मेदे द्वे च काकोल्यौ सारिवे द्वे प्रियङ्गुका ॥ ८० ॥
शतपुष्पा हिङ्गु रास्ना चन्दनं रक्तचन्दनम् जातीपुष्पं तुगाक्षीरी कमलं शर्करा तथा ॥ ८१ ॥
अजमोदा च दन्ती च कल्कैरेतैश्च कार्षिकैः । जीवद्वत्सैकवर्णाया घृतप्रस्थं च गोः क्षिपेत् ॥ ८२ ॥
चतुर्गुणेन पयसा पचेदारण्यगोमयैः । सुतिथौ पुष्यनक्षत्रे मृद्भाण्डे ताम्रजे तथा ॥ ८३ ॥
ततः पिबेच्छुभदिने नारी वा पुरुषोऽथवा । एतत्सर्पिर्नरः पीत्वा स्त्रीषु नित्यं वृषायते ॥ ८४ ॥
पुत्रानुत्पादयेद्धीमान्वन्ध्यापि लभते सुतम् । अनायुषं या जनयेद्या च सूता पुनः स्थिता ॥ ८५ ॥
पुत्रं प्राप्नोति सा नारी बुद्धिमन्तं शतायुषम् । एतत्फलघृतं नाम भारद्वाजेन भाषितम् ॥ ८६ ॥
अनुक्तं लक्ष्मणामूलं क्षिपेत्तत्र चिकित्सकः ।

Triphalā, madhuka, kuṣṭha, the two nishās, kaṭukarohiṇi, viḍaṅga, pippalī, musta, vishālā, kaṭphala, vachā, the two medas, two kākolis, the two sārivās, priyaṅguka, shatapuṣpa, hiṅgu, rāsnā, chandana, raktachandana, jātipuṣpa, tugākshīrī, kamala, sharkarā, ajamodā and dantī,—each one karṣa is made into a kalka; one prastha of ghee and four prasthas of milk of the cow (which has only one colour all over the body and whose calf is alive) are cooked with the fire of forest cow-dung on an auspicious day during Pushyanakṣatra and preserved in a mud pot or a copper vessel. This recipe known as *Phalaghrita*, propounded by sage Bharadwaja, consumed by a man or woman starting on an auspicious day. By it man becomes capable of enjoying with many women, and procreate intelligent and longlived children. Women who are childless or who give birth to short lived children procreate intelligent children, who live for hundred years. The juice of roots of Lakshmana is to be added to the recipe even though not told here (79–87).

अथ लघुफलघृतं योनिरोगे—

त्रिफलां द्वे सहचरे गुडूचीं सपुनर्नवाम् । शुकनासां हरिद्रे द्वे रास्नां मेदां शतावरीम् ॥ ८७ ॥
कल्कीकृत्य घृतप्रस्थं पचेत्क्षीरे चतुर्गुणे । तत्सिद्धं पाययेन्नारीं योनिशूलनिपीडिताम् ॥ ८८ ॥
पीडिता चलिता या च निःसृता विवृता च या । पित्तयोनिश्च विभ्रान्ता षण्ढयोनिश्च या स्मृता ॥ ८९ ॥
प्रपद्यन्ते हि ताः स्थानं गर्भं गृह्णन्ति चासकृत् । एतत्फलघृतं नाम योनिदोषहरं परम् ॥ ९० ॥

Equal quantities of triphalā, the two sahacharas, guḍuchi, punarnavā, shatāvarī—one fourth of the quantity of ghee are made into kalka, one prastha of ghrita and four times its quantity of milk are cooked in the usual way. This recipe is known as *Phalaghrita* taken by women, relieves pain of vagina, displacements, distortions and discharges of the uterus, burning in the vagina, and brings back the normal condition of the uterus, helps to conceive again. Hence this recipe is an excellent remedy for all yoni doṣas (disorders of uterus and vagina) (87–90).

अथ पञ्चतिक्तकं घृतं विषमज्वरादौ—

वृषनिम्बामृताव्याघ्रीपटोलानां शृतेन च ॥ ९१ ॥
कल्केन पक्वं सर्पिस्तु निहन्याद्विषमज्वरान् । पाण्डुं कुष्ठं विसर्पं च कृमीनर्शांसि नाशयेत् ॥ ९२ ॥

Equal quantities of vṛsa, nimba, amrthā, vyāghrī and paṭola made into kalka and ghṛta prepared in the usual way. It cures viṣamajwaras (intermittent fevers), pāṇḍu (anaemia), kuṣṭha (leprosy and other skin diseases), visarpa (erysipelas), krimi (bacteria) and arshas (piles) (91–92).

Taila Kalpana

लाक्षाढकं क्वथयित्वा जलस्य चतुराढकैः । चतुर्थांशं शृतं नीत्वा तैलप्रस्थे विनिक्षिपेत् ॥ ९३ ॥
मस्त्वाढकं च गोदध्नस्तत्रैव विनियोजयेत् । शतपुष्पामश्वगन्धां हरिद्रां देवदारु च ॥ ९४ ॥
कटुकीं रेणुकां मूर्वां कुष्ठं च मधुयष्टिकाम् । चन्दनं मुस्तकं रास्नां पृथक्कर्षप्रमाणतः ॥ ९५ ॥
चूर्णयेतत्र निक्षिप्य साधयेन्मृदुवह्निना । अस्याभ्यङ्गात्प्रशाम्यन्ति सर्वेऽपि विषमज्वराः ॥ ९६ ॥
कासश्वासप्रतिश्यायत्रिकपृष्ठग्रहास्तथा । वातं पित्तमपस्मारमुन्मादं यक्षराक्षसान् ॥ ९७ ॥
कण्डूं शूलं च दौर्गन्ध्यं गात्राणां स्फुरणं जयेत् । पुष्टगर्भा भवेदस्य गर्भिण्यभ्यङ्गतो भृशम् ॥ ९८ ॥

One adhaka of lākshā is boiled in four āḍhakas of water and reduced to quarter and filtered. To it are added one prastha of tila taila (sessame oil) one āḍhaka of mastu (whey water of curds prepared with cow's milk) and a kalka prepared with one karsa each of shatapuṣpā, ạshwagandhā, haridrā, devadāru; kaṭukī, reṇukā, mūrvā, kuṣṭha, madhuyaṣṭi, chandana, musta and rāsnā—are all cooked on mild fire and taila prepared. This oil used as for abhyaṅga (oil massage) dispells all types of viṣama jwaras (intermittent fevers), kāsa (cough) śwāsa (dyspnoea), pratishyāya (running in the nose), trikaprushta graha (stiffness and pain of the back and waist), vāta and pitta, apasmara (epilepsy), unmāda due to yakshas and rakshas (insanity caused by evil spirits), kaṇḍū (itching), shūla (pain), durgandha (bad smell), sphurana (throbbings) of the body parts; pregnant women will have a good growth of their foetus by applying this oil often over the body and taking bath later (93-98).

(अङ्गारतैलम्)—

मूर्वा लाक्षा हरिद्रे द्वे मञ्जिष्ठा सेन्द्रवारुणी । बृहती सैन्धवं कुष्ठं रास्ना मांसी शतावरी ॥ ९९ ॥
आरनालाढके तत्र तैलप्रस्थं विपाचयेत् । तैलमङ्गारकं नाम सर्वज्वरविमोक्षणम् ॥ १०० ॥

Mūrvā, lākshā, the two haridras, mañjiṣṭhk, indravāruṇı, bṛhatī, saindhava, kushta, rāsna, māmsi and śatāvari are made into kalka; one adhaka of aranala (rice wasḥ) and one prastha of taila (sessame oil) are added and taila prepared. This recipe known as *Aṅgāraka taila* cures all types of jwaras (fevers) (99–100).

अथ वातरोगादौ नारायणतैलम्—

अश्वगन्धां बलां बिल्वं पाटलां बृहतीद्वयम् । श्वदंष्ट्रातिबला निम्बं स्योनाकं च पुनर्नवा ॥ १०१ ॥
प्रसारिणीमग्निमन्थं कुर्याद्दशपलं भिषक् । चतुर्द्रोणे जले पक्त्वा पादशेषं श्तं नयेत् ॥ १०२ ॥
तैलाढकेन संयोज्य शतावर्या रसाढकम् । क्षिपेत्तत्र च गोक्षीरं तैलात्तस्माच्चतुर्गुणम् ॥ १०३ ॥
शनैर्विपाचयेदेभिः कल्कैर्द्विपलिकैः पृथक् । कुष्ठैलाचन्दनबलामांसीशैलेयसैन्धवैः ॥ १०४ ॥
अश्वगन्धावचारास्नाशतपुष्पेन्द्रदारुभिः । पर्णीचतुष्टयेनैव तगरेण च साधयेत् ॥ १०५ ॥
तत्तैलं नावनेऽभ्यङ्गे पाने बस्तौ च योजयेत् । पक्षाघातं हनुस्तम्भं मन्यास्तम्भं गलग्रहम् ॥ १०६ ॥
खल्लत्वं बधिरत्वं च गतिभङ्गं कटिग्रहम् । गात्रशोषेन्द्रियध्वंसावसृक्शुक्रज्वरक्षयान् ॥ १०७ ॥
अन्त्रवृद्धिं कुरण्डं च दन्तरोगं शिरोग्रहम् । पार्श्वशूलं च पाङ्गुल्यं बुद्धिहानिं च गृध्रसीम् ॥१०८॥
अन्यांश्च विषमान्वाताञ्जयेत्सर्वाङ्गसंश्रयान् । अस्य प्रभावाद्वन्ध्यापि नारी पुत्रं प्रसूयते ॥ १०९ ॥
मर्त्यो गजो वा तुरगस्तैलादस्मात्सुखी भवेत् । यथा नारायणो देवो दुष्टदैत्यविनाशनः ॥ ११० ॥

तथैव वातरोगाणां नाशनं तैलमुत्तमम् ।

Ten palas, each of aśwagandha, balā, bilwa, pāṭalā, the two bṛhatīs, swadaṃṣṭra, atibalā, nimba, syonaka, punarnavā, prasarine and agnimantha-are boiled in four droṇas of water and decoction reduced to quarter. To it are added one ādhaka of taila (sessame oil), one ādhaka of juice of shatavari; cow's milk four times the quantity of oil, and kalka prepared with two palas each of kuṣṭha, elā, chandana, balā, māṃsī, shaileya, saindhava, ashwagandhā, vachā, rāsnā, shatapuṣpā, indradāru, the four parṇīs (shaliparni, pṛsniparṇī, mudgaparṇi masha parni) and tagara-are all cooked on mild fire and oil prepared. This oil used as nāvana

(nasal drops), abhyaṅga (oil bath), pāna (internal potion) and basti (enema) cures pakshāghāta (hemiplegia), hanustambha (lock-jaw), manyāstambha (wry neck), gala graha (wry neck), khalli (stiffness and contractures of fingers), badhiratwa (deafness), gatibhanga (distorted gait), kaṭigraha (lumbago), gātraṣosha (wasting of body parts), indriyadhwāmsa (loss of sense faculties), jwaras (fevers), rakta and shukra kshaya (loss of blood and kshaya), antravṛddhi (inguinal hernia), kuraṇḍa (scrotal hernia), danta rogas (dental disorders), shirograha headache pārshwashūla (pain in the flanks), pāṅgulya (lameness), buddhihāni (loss of intellect), gṛdhrasī (sciatica) and other vāta (nervous) disorders else where in the body. By its use barren women will get children; not only humans but even animals like elephants or horses also become cured. Just as Lord Nārāyaṇa destroys evil demons so also this taila destroys all kinds of vāta rogas (nervous disorders) (101–111).

(वारुणीतैलं कम्परागे)

वारुण्या औत्तरं मूलं कुट्टितं तु पलत्रयम् । पलद्वादशकं तैलं क्षीणे वह्नौ विपाचितम् ॥ १११ ॥
निष्कत्रय भक्तयुक्तं सेवेतास्माद्विनश्यति । हस्तकम्पः शिरःकम्पःकम्पो मन्याशिराभवः ॥ ११२ ॥

Three palas of indravāruṇī root which has spread to northern direction is made inte a paste is taken in vessel; twelve palas of taila (sessame oil) is added and cooked on mild fire. This medicated oil in doses of three nishkas taken internally mixed with small quantity of cooked rice–relieves shaking of the hands, head and neck (111–112).

अथ बलाद्यं तैलं वातव्याधौ—

बलामूलकषायेण दशमूलश्टतेन च ॥ ११३ ॥
कुलत्थयवकोलानां क्वाथेन पयसा तथा । अष्टाष्टभागयुक्तेन भागमेकं च तैलतः ॥ ११४ ॥
गणेन जीवनीयेन शतावर्येन्द्रवारुणी । मञ्जिष्ठाकुष्ठशैलेयतगरागरुसैन्धवैः ॥ ११५ ॥
वचापुनर्नवामांसीसारिवाद्वयपत्रकैः । शतपुष्पाश्वगन्धाभ्यामेलया च विपाचयेत् ॥ ११६ ॥
गर्भार्थिनीनां नारीणां नराणां क्षीणरेतसाम् । व्यायामक्षीणगात्राणां सूतिकानां च युज्यते ॥ ११७ ॥
राजयोग्यमिदं तैलं सुखिनां च विशेषतः । बलातैलमिति ख्यातं सर्ववातामयापहम् ॥ ११८ ॥

Decoction of roots of balā, dashamūlas, kulattha, yava, kola–each eight parts, one part of taila (sessame oil) and kalka prepared with drugs of jīvanīya gaṇa, shatavari, indrādaru, mañjīṣṭhā kuṣṭha, shaileya, tagara, agaru, saindhava, vachā, punarnavā, māṃsī, the two sārivās, patra, shatapuṣpa, aśwagandhā and elā–are all cooked together and taila prepared. It is beneficial for women desiring pregency, men who are sexually feeble, exhausted by physical strain, and women after delivery. This recipe known as *Blā taila* is best suited for kings, persons of tender constitution and cures all kinds of Vata-rogas (nervous disorders) (113-118).

वातकफामयादौ प्रसारिणीतैलमाह—

प्रसारिणीपलशतं जलद्रोणेन पाचयेत् । पादशिष्टः श्रृतो ग्राह्यस्तैलं दधि च तत्समम् ॥ ११९ ॥
काञ्जिकं च समं तैलात्क्षीरं तैलाच्चतुर्गुणम् । तैलात्तथाष्टमांशेन सर्वकल्कानि योजयेत् ॥ १२० ॥
मधुकं पिप्पलीमूलं चित्रकः सैन्धवं वचा । प्रसारिणी देवदारु रास्ना च गजपिप्पली ॥ १२१ ॥
भल्लातः शतपुष्पा च मांसीचैभिर्विपाचयेत् । एतत्तैलवरं पक्वं वातश्लेष्मामयाञ्जयेत् ॥ १२२ ॥
कौब्जं पङ्गुत्वखञ्जत्वे गृध्रसीमर्दितं तथा । हनुपृष्ठशिरोग्रीवाकटीस्तम्भं च नाशयेत् ॥ १२३ ॥
अन्यांश्च विषमान्वातान्सर्वानाशु व्यपोहति ।

One hundred palas of prasāriṇī is boiled in one droṇa of water and decoction reduced to quarter. To this are added equal quantities of taila (oil), dadhi (curds or water of curds), kañjikā (sour gruel), cow's milk four times the measure and one eighth part of kalka (paste) of madhuka, pippalīmūla, chitraka, saindhava, vachā, prasāriṇī, devadāru, rāsnā, gajapippalī, bhallātaka, shatapuṣpā and jaṭāmāṃsī—are mixed together and taila prepared. This recipe is beneficial in all diseases arising from vāta and kapha, kubja (kyphosis), paṅgutwa and khañjatwa (lameness), gṛdhrasī (sciatica), ardita (facial palsy), stambha of hanu, priṣṭa, shirogrīvā and kaṭi (stiffness of jaw, back, head, neck and waist) and such other diseases of vāta are cured quickly (119-124).

अथ माषादितैलं वातविकारादौ—

माषो यवातसी क्षुद्रा मर्कटी च कुरण्टकः ॥ १२४ ॥
गोकण्टघुण्टुकश्चैषां कुर्यात्सप्तपलं पृथक् । चतुर्गुणाम्बुना पक्त्वा पादशेषं श्रृतं नयेत् ॥ १२५ ॥
कार्पासास्थीनि बदरं शणबीजं कुलत्थकम् । पृथक्चतुर्दशपलं चतुर्गुणजले पचेत् ॥ १२६ ॥
चतुर्थांशावशिष्टं च गृह्णीयात्क्वाथमुत्तमम् । प्रस्थैकं छागमांसस्य चतुःषष्टिपले जले ॥ १२७ ॥
निक्षिप्य पाचयेद्धीमान्पादशेषं श्रृतं नयेत् । तैलप्रस्थे ततः सर्वान्क्वाथानेतान्विनिक्षिपेत् ॥ १२८ ॥
कल्कैरेभिश्च विपचेदमृताकुष्ठनागरैः । रास्नापुनर्नवैरण्डैः पिप्पल्या शतपुष्पया ॥ १२९ ॥
बलाप्रसारिणीभ्यां च मांस्या कुटुकया तथा । पृथगर्धपलैरेतैः साधयेन्मृदुवह्निना ॥ १३० ॥
हन्यात्तैलमिदं शीघ्रं ग्रीवास्तम्भापबाहुकौ । अर्धाङ्गशोषमाक्षेपमूरुस्तम्भापतानकौ ॥ १३१ ॥
शाखाकम्पं शिरःकम्पं विश्वाचीमर्दितं तथा । माषादिकमिदं तैलं सर्ववातविकारनुत् ॥ १३२ ॥

Seven palas each of māṣā, yava, atasī, kshudrā, markaṭī, kuranṭaka, gokanṭa and tunṭuka-are all boiled in four times their total quantity of water and decoction reduced to quarter. Fourteen palas each of seeds of kārpāsāsthi, badara, shaṇa bīja and kulattha are boiled in four times of their total quantity of water and reduced to a quarter. One prastha of goat's flesh is boiled in sixtyfour palas of water and reduced to one fourth it's measure and juice filtered out. The two decoctions, the mutton broth and one prastha of taila (sesame oil) are all added and boiled again. Kalka (paste) prepared with half pala each of amṛtā, kuṣṭha, rāsnā. punarnavā, eraṇḍa, pippalī, shatapuṣpā, balā, prasāriṇī, and kaṭuka–is added and taila prepared over mild fire. This recipe known as *Māṣādi taila* quickly relieves grīvāstambha (stiffness of the neck), apabāhuka (stiff arm), ardhāṅga śoṣa (emaciation of hālf of the body), akshepa (convulsions), urustambha (stiff leg), apatānaka (tetanus), shākhākampa (tremors of extremities), shirakampa (shaking of the head), vishwāchī (pain of the arms), ardita (facial palsy) and all other vāta rogas (nervous diseases) (124–132).

अथ शतावरीतैलं वातादौ—

शतावरी बलायुग्मं पर्ण्यौ गन्धर्वहस्तकः । अश्वगन्धा श्वदंष्ट्रश्च बिल्वः काशः कुरण्टकः ॥ १३३ ॥
एतान् सार्धपलान्भागान्कल्कयेच्च विपाचयेत् । चतुर्गुणेन नीरेण पादशेषं शृतं नयेत् ॥ १३४ ॥
नियोज्य तैलप्रस्थे च क्षीरप्रस्थं विनिक्षिपेत् । शतावरीरसप्रस्थं जलप्रस्थं च योजयेत् ॥ १३५ ॥
शतावरीदेवदारुमांसीतगरचन्दनम् । शतपुष्पा बला कुष्ठमेला शैलेयमुत्पलम् ॥ १३६ ॥
ऋद्धिर्मेदा च मधुकं काकोली जीवकस्तथा । एषां कर्षसमैः कल्कैस्तैलं गोमयवह्निना ॥ १३७ ॥
पचेत्तन्मूर्धतैलेन नरः स्त्रीषु वृषायते । नारी च लभते पुत्रं योनिशूलं च नश्यति ॥ १३८ ॥
अङ्गशूलं शिरःशूलं कामलां पाण्डुतां गरम् । गृध्रसीप्लीहशोषांश्च मेहान्दण्डापतानकम् ॥ १३९ ॥
सदाहं वातरक्तं च वातपित्तगदार्दितम् । असृग्दरं तथाध्मानं रक्तपित्तं च नश्यति ॥ १४० ॥

शतावरीतैलमिदं कृष्णात्रेयेण भाषितम् ।

ॐ नारायण्यै स्वाहा ॥

उत्तराभिमुखो भूत्वा खनेत्खदिरशङ्कुना ॥ १४१ ॥

ॐ सर्वव्याधिनाशिन्यै स्वाहा ।

इत्युत्पाटनमन्त्रः ।

ॐ कुमारीजीवन्यै स्वाहा । इति पानमन्त्रः ।

One and a half palas each of shatāvarī, the two balās, the two parṇīs gandharvahasta, aśwagandhā, shwadaṃṣṭra, bilwa, kāsha, kuranṭaka–are all boiled in four times their total quantity of water and decoction reduced to quarter. To it are added one prastha each of taila (sesame oil) and cow's milk and juice of shatāvarī. Next, kalka (paste) prepared with one karṣa each of shatāvarī, devadāru, māṃsī, tagara, chandana, shatapuṣpā, balā, kuṣṭha, elā, shaileya, uatpala, ruddhi, meda, madhuka, kākolī and jīvaka–is added and taila (oil) prepared over mild fire of cowdung cakes. This recipe known as *Shātāvarī taila* propounded by sage Kṛṣna Ātreya, acts as an aphrodisiac to men; helps barren women to get children, cures yonishūla (pain of the vagina), aṅgashūla (body pains), shirashūla (headache), kāmala (jaundice), pānḍutā (anaemia), gara (homicidal poisoning), gṛdhrasī (sciatica), plīhā (splenic enlargement), shoṣa (consumption), daṇḍapatanaka (tetanus), vātarakta with daha (gout with sensation of burning), disorders of vāta and pitta, asṛgdara (menorrhagia), adhamāna (tympanitis) and raktapitta (purpura). At the time of collecting the roots of shatāvarī, the person should be facing north, be in a worshipful mood, should repeat 'Om' nārāyaṇa swāhā, Om sarva vyādhi vināshinyāya swāhā (let Nārāyana be pleased, let the dispeller of all diseases be pleased) and dig the ground with a pointed rod of khadira wood, collect the roots which have spread to the northern direction. At the time of consuming the medicine he should repeat "Om Kumārā jivanyaii swāhā" (let mother goddess Kumarī Jīvaṇī be pleased) continuously (133–141).

इदानीं अपराणि क्षुद्रतैलान्याह—तत्रादौ अर्शादौ कासीसाद्यं तैलं दर्शयन्नाह—

कासीसं लाङ्गली कुष्ठं शुण्ठी कृष्णा च सैन्धवम् । मनःशीलाश्वमारश्च विडङ्गं चित्रका द्रुमः ॥१४२॥
दन्ती कोशातकीबीजं हेमाह्वा हरितालकम् । कल्कैः कर्षमितैरेतैस्तैलप्रस्थं विपाचयेत् ॥ १४३ ॥
स्नुह्यर्कपयसी दद्यात्पृथग्द्विपलसंमिते । चतुर्गुणं गवां मूत्रं दत्वा सम्यक्प्रसाधयेत् ॥ १४४ ॥
कथितं खरनादेन तैलमर्शोविनाशनम् । क्षारवत्पातयत्येतदर्शांस्यभ्यङ्गतो भृशम् ॥ १४५ ॥
वलीर्न दूषयत्येतत्क्षारकर्मकरं स्मृतम् ।

One karṣa each of kāsīsa, lāṅgalī, kuṣṭha, shuṇṭhī, kṛṣṇā, saindhava, manashilā, aswamāra, viḍaṅga, chitraka, druma, dantī, koshātakībīja, hemāhwā and haritāla are made into a kalka (paste), added to one prastha of taila (sesame oil) and kept for boiling. Two palas each of milky sap of snuhi and arka, and cow's urine four times the quantity (of taila) are added during boiling and taila (oil) prepared in the usual way. The oil formulated by sage Kharanāda is a cure for arshas (piles). By applying it often to the piles it acts like kshāra (caustic) and casts off the pile masses. Without damaging the folds of the rectum it does the actions of a kshāra (142–146).

अथ पिण्डतैलं वातरक्ते—

मञ्जिष्ठासारिवासर्जयष्टीसिक्थैः पलोन्मितैः ॥ १४६ ॥
पिण्डाख्यं साधयेत्तैलमभ्यङ्गाद्वातरक्तनुत् ।

Taila prepared with one pala each of mañjīṣṭhā, sārivā, sarja, yaṣṭī and siktaka known as *Piṇḍa taila* it cures vatarakta (gout), if anointed over the body often (147).

कुष्ठरोगादौ अर्कतैलम्—

अर्कपत्ररसे पक्वं हरिद्राकल्कसंयुतम् ॥ १४७ ॥
नाशयेत्सार्षपे तैलं पामां कच्छूं विचर्चिकाम् ।

Sarshapa taila (mustard oil) mixed with juice of leaves of arka and paste of tender haridra and cooked as usual is an effective cure for pama (scabies), kachu (itching skin) and vicharchika (psoriasis) (147–148).

अथ मरिचादितैलं कुष्ठव्रणादौ—

मरिचं हरितालं च त्रिवृतं रक्तचन्दनम् ॥ १४८ ॥
मुस्तं मनःशिला मांसी द्वे निशे देवदारु च । विशाला करवीरं च कुष्ठमर्कपयस्तथा ॥ १४९ ॥
तथैव गोमयरसं कुर्यात्कर्षमितान्पृथक् । विषं चार्धपलं देयं प्रस्थं च कटुतैलकम् ॥ १५० ॥
गोमूत्रं द्विगुणं दद्याज्जलं च द्विगुणं भवेत् । मरिचाद्यमिदं तैलं सिद्धं कुष्ठव्रणापहम् ॥ १५१ ॥
जयेत्कुष्ठानि सर्वाणि पुण्डरीकं विचर्चिकाम् । पामां श्वित्राणि रक्तं च कण्डूं कच्छूं प्रणाशयेत् ॥१५२॥

One karsha each of maricha, haritala, trivrit, raktachandana, musta, mansshila, mamsi, two nishas, devadaru, vishala, karaveera, kushta, sap of arka and juice of cow dung; half pala of visha (vatsanabhi), one prastha of katutaila (mustard oil); gomootra (cow s urine) and water twice the total quantity-are all cooked together and thaila prepared as usual. The recipe known as *Marichadi Thaila,* cues kushta (leprosy), effectively. Similarly other kinds of kushta such as pundareeka; vicharchika (psoriasis), pama (scabies), switra (leucoderma), rakta mandala (red patches), kachu (dermatitis), etc (148–152)

अरूंषिकायां त्रिफलादितैलम्—

त्रिफलारिष्टभूनिम्बं द्वे निशे रक्तचन्दनम् । एतैः सिद्धमरूंषीणां तैलमभ्यञ्जने हितम् ॥ १५३ ॥

Taila prepared with triphala, arishta, bhoonimba, the tow nishas and raktachandana, cures aroomshi (ulcers of the scalp) if anointed with it often (153).

अथ निम्बबीजतैलं पलिते—

भावयेन्निम्बबीजानि भृङ्गराजरसेन हि । तथासनस्य तोयेन तत्तैलं हन्ति नस्यतः ॥ १५४ ॥
अकालपलितं सद्यः पुंसां दुग्धान्नभोजिनाम् ।

Nimba beeja are macerated with juice of bhringraja and decoction of wood of asana tree and this paste is put into thaila (sesame oil) and cooked well. This oil used as nasal drops is effective in premature greying of hairs of men who adhere to rice and milk only as diet (154–155).

अथ यष्टीमधुकतैलं पलिते—

यष्टीमधुकक्षीराभ्यां नवधात्रीफलैः शृतम् ॥ १५५ ॥
तैलं नस्यकृतं कुर्यात्केशाञ्श्मश्रूणि सङ्घशः ।

Yashti madhuka, kshara (yavakshara), juice of fresh amalaka and thaila are cooked together. This taila used as nasal drops brings up thick and bulky mustaches and beards (155–156).

अथ करञ्जतैलं इन्द्रलुप्ते—

करञ्जश्चित्रको जाती करवीरश्च पाचितम् ॥ १५६ ॥
तैलमेभिर्द्रुतं हन्यादभ्यङ्गादिन्द्रलुप्तकम् ।

Indralupta (alopacea) will be cured by anointing the head with oil prepared with karanja, chitraka, jati, and keraveera (156–157).

अथ नीलिकाद्यं तैलं केशकल्पादौ—

नीलिका केतकीकन्दं भृङ्गराजः कुरण्टकः ॥ १५७ ॥
तथार्जुनस्य पुष्पाणि बीजकात्कुसुमान्यपि । कृष्णास्तिलाश्च तगरं समूलं कमलं तथा ॥ १५८ ॥
अयोरजः प्रियङ्गुश्च दाडिमत्वग्गुडूचिका । त्रिफला पद्मपङ्कश्च कल्कैरेभिः पृथक् पृथक् ॥ १५९ ॥
कर्षमात्रैः पचेत्तैलं त्रिफलाक्काथसंयुतम् । भृङ्गराजरसेनैव सिद्धं केशस्थिरीकृतम् ॥ १६० ॥
अकालपलितं हन्ति दारुणं चोपजिह्विकाम् ।

Neelika, ketakikanda, bhringaraja, kurantaka, flowers of arjuna, flowers of beejaka, krishnatila, tagara. full plant of kamala, ayoraja (iron fillings). priyangu, dadima bark, gudoochi, triphala, padma panka (silt of lotus tank), each one karsha is made into (paste); triphala decoction and juice of bhringaraja both equal and four times the quantity of oil are added and cooked in the usualway. It makes the hairs firm, prevents premature greying and relieves darunaka (dand·ruf) and upajihwaka (adenoids) (157–161).

अकालपलितादौ भृङ्गराजतैलम्—

भृङ्गराजरसेनैव लोहकिट्टं फलत्रिकम् ॥ १६१ ॥
सारिवां च पचेत्कल्कैस्तैलं दारुणनाशनम् । अकालपलितं कण्डूमिन्द्रलुप्तं च नाशयेत् ॥ १६२ ॥

Taila prepared with juice of bhringaraja, lohakitta, and kalka of triphala and sariva will cure daruna (dandruf), akala palita (premature grey hair), Kandoo (itching) and Indralupta (alopecia) (161–162).

इरिमेदाद्यं तैलं मुखदन्तरोगादौ—

इरिमेदत्वचं क्षुण्णां पचेच्छतपलोन्मिताम् । जलद्रोणे ततः क्काथं गृह्णीयात्पादशेषितम् ॥ १६३ ॥
तैलस्यार्धाढकं दत्त्वा कल्कैः कर्षमितैः पचेत् । इरिमेदलवङ्गाभ्यां गैरिकागरुपद्मकैः ॥ १६४ ॥
मञ्जिष्ठालोध्रमधुकैर्लाक्षान्यग्रोधमुस्तकैः । त्वग्जातीफलकर्पूरकङ्कोलखदिरैस्तथा ॥ १६५ ॥
पतङ्गधातकीपुष्पसूक्ष्मैलानागकेशरम् । कट्फलेन च संसिद्धं तैलं मुखरुजं जयेत् ॥ १६६ ॥
प्रदुष्टमांसं पलितं शीर्णदन्तं च शौषिरम् । श्यावदन्तं प्रहर्षं च विद्रधिं कृमिदन्तकम् ॥ १६७ ॥
दन्तस्फुरणदौर्गन्ध्यं जिह्वाताल्वोष्ठजां रुजम् ।

One hundred palas of bark of irimeda is boiled in one drona of water and decoction reduced to quarter. Half Udaka of thaila is added to it, Paste prepared with one karsha each of irimeda, avanga, gairika, agaru, padmaka, manjishta, lodhra, madhuka, laksha, nyagrodha, musta, twak, jatiphala, karpoora, kankola, khadira, pattanga, dhatakipushpua, sookshmaila, nagakesara and katphala is added and thaila cooked. This oil relieves the diseases of the mouth such as dushtamamsa of dantas (bad gums), palita danta (worn out gums), sheernadanta (shaky teeth), soushira (cavity in teeth), shyavadant (black discolouration of teeth), Praharsha (tingling of gums), vidradhi (gum abscess), krimi dants (caries teeth), Danta sphutana (cracks of teeth), dourgandhya (bad smell of the mouth) and diseases of tongue, palate and lips (163–168).

जात्यादितैलम्—

(जातीनिम्बपटोलानां नक्तमालस्य पल्लवाः ॥ १६८ ॥
सिक्थं समधुकं कुष्ठं द्वे निशे कटुरोहिणी । मञ्जिष्ठा पद्मकं लोध्रमभया नीलमुत्पलम् ॥ १६९ ॥
तुत्थकं सारिवा बीजं नक्तमालस्य दापयेत् । एतानि समभागानि पिष्ट्वा तैलं विपाचयेत् ॥ १७० ॥
नाडीव्रणे समुत्पन्ने स्फोटके कच्छुरोगिषु । सद्यः शस्त्रप्रहारेषु दग्धविद्धेषु चैव हि ॥ १७१ ॥
नखदन्तक्षते देहे व्रणे दुष्टे प्रशस्यते ।)

Equal quantities of jātī nimba, paṭola, tender lives of naktamālā, siktaka, madhuka, kuṣhṭa, the two niśas, kaṭukarohiṇī, mañjiṣṭha, padmaka, lodhra, abhaya, nīlotpala, tutha, sārivā and seeds of naktamālā are made into kalka and oil prepared in the usual way. This oil is beneficial as a dressing in cases of nāḍīvraṇa (sinus ulcers), sphoṭaka (papules), kachchu (itching, scabies) incised wounds, burns, scalds, abrasions by nail, teeth and other types of dusṭa vraṇa (bad ulcers) (168–172).

अथ हिंग्वाद्यं तैलं कर्णशूले—

हिङ्गुतुम्बुरुशुण्ठीभिः कटुतैलं विपाचयेत् ॥ १७२ ॥
तस्य पूरणमात्रेण कर्णशूलं प्रणश्यति ।

Mustard oil cooked with hiṅgu, tumburu, śunṭhī and instilled into the ears relieves ear aches (172–173).

अथ बिल्वाद्यं तैलं बाधिर्ये—

बालबिल्वानि गोमूत्रे पिष्ट्वा तैलं विपाचयेत् ॥ १७३ ॥
साजक्षीरं च नीरं च बाधिर्यं हन्ति पूरणात् ।

Unripe fruits af bilwa are made into a paste with cow's urine and oil prepared by adding ajākṣira (goat's milk) and water in the usual way. This cures bādhirya (deafness) (173–174).

अथ क्षारतैलं कर्णरोगेषु—

बालमूलकशुण्ठानां क्षारः क्षारयुगं तथा ॥ १७४ ॥
लवणानि च पञ्चैव हिङ्गु शिग्रु महौषधम् । देवदारु वचा कुष्ठं शतपुष्पा रसाञ्जनम् ॥ १७५ ॥
ग्रन्थिकं भद्रमुस्तं च कल्कैः कर्षमितैः पृथक् । तैलप्रस्थं च विपचेत्कदलीबीजपूरयोः ॥ १७६ ॥

रसाभ्यां मधुशुक्तेन चातुर्गुण्यमितेन च। पूयस्रावं कर्णनादं शूलं बधिरतां कृमीन् ॥ १७७ ॥
अन्यांश्च कर्णजान्रोगान्मुखरोगांश्च नाशयेत्।

One karṣa each of kṣāras of tender mūlaka, the two kṣāras (yavakṣāra and sarjakṣāra), the five salts, hiṅgu, śigru, mahousadha, devadaru, vacha, kuṣṭha, satapuṣpa, rasāñjana, granthika and bhadramusta–are made into kalka. One prastha of sesame oil, and juice of kadalī, bījapūra and madhuśukta (described in the next verses) each four times that of oil—are all added and oil prepared. This oil instilled into the ears cures pūyasrāva (discharge of pus), karṇa nada (sound in ears), śūla (ear ache), baadhiratā (deafness), kṛmi (insects, bacteria) and other diseases of ears and mouth also (174–178).

मधुशुक्तम्—

जम्बीराणां फलरसः प्रस्थैकः कुडवोन्मितम् ॥ १७८ ॥
माक्षिकं तत्र दातव्यं पलैका पिप्पली स्मृता। एतदेकीकृतं सर्वं मृद्भाण्डे च निधापयेत् ॥ १७९ ॥
वचाम्भो मधुसंयुक्तं शृङ्गवेरगुडान्वितम्। धान्यराशौ त्रिरात्रिस्थं मधुशुक्तमुदाहृतम् ॥ १८० ॥

Juice of jambīra fruits one prastha, one kuḍava of makṣikā (honey) one pala of pippali are macerated well and put in a mud pot and kept buried underground for one month. This preparation is known as madhuśukta. Water of yava (barley), honey, śṛṅgavera and guḍa (jaggery) put in a mud pot and buried in husk for three nights also becomes madhuśukta (178–180).

अथ पाठाद्यं तैलं पीनसे—

पाठा द्वे च निशे मूर्वा पिप्पली जातिपल्लवैः ॥ १८१ ॥
दन्त्या च तैलं संसिद्धं नस्यं स्याद्दुष्टपीनसे।

Pāṭhā, the two niśhas, mūrvā, pippali tender leaves of jati and dantī are cooked with oil and taila prepared as usual. This, used as nasal drops relieves duṣṭa pīnasa (rhinitis) (181–182).

अथ व्याघ्रीतैलं पीनसे—

व्याघ्रीदन्तीवचाशिग्रुतुलसीव्योषसैन्धवैः ॥ १८२ ॥
कफस्य पाचनं तैलं पूतिनासोदकापहम्।

Vyāghrī, danti, vacha, sigru, tulasī, vyosha and saindhava are made into kalka (paste) and oil prepared. This liquifies the kapha and cures pūtināśya (bad small of the nose) and nāsodaka (running in the nose) (182–183).

अथ कुष्ठाद्यं तैलं छिकायां—

कुष्ठं बिल्वकणाशुण्ठीद्राक्षाकल्ककषायवत् ॥ १८३ ॥
साधितं तैलमाज्यं वा नस्यात्क्षवथुनाशनम्।

Kuṣṭa, bilwa, kana, śuṇthi and drākṣā made into decoction or paste and cooked with either oil or ghee and instilled into nostrills relieves kṣavathu (sneezing) (183–184).

गृहधूमतैलं नासार्शसि—

गृहभूमकणादारुक्षारनक्ताह्वसैन्धवैः ॥ १८४ ॥
सिद्धं शिखरिबीजैश्च तैलं नासार्शसां हितम् ।

Ghṛha dhūma (chimney soot), kana, dāru, kṣāra (yavaksāra), naktahwa (niśa), saindhava and śhikhri bēja prepared into an oil and put into the nose is useful in nāsārsas (nasal polyp) (184–185).

अथ वज्रीतैलं कुष्ठादौ—

वज्रीक्षीरं रविक्षीरं द्रवं धत्तूरचित्रजम् ॥ १८५ ॥
महिषीविड्भवं द्रावं सर्वांशं तिलतैलकम् । पचेत्तैलावशेषं च गोमूत्रेऽथ चतुर्गुणे ॥ १८६ ॥
तैलावशेषं पक्त्वा च तत्तैलं प्रस्थमात्रकम् । गन्धकाग्निशिलातालं विडङ्गातिविषाविषम् ॥ १८७ ॥
तिक्तकोशातकीकुष्ठवचामांसीकटुत्रयम् । पीतदारु च यष्ट्याह्वं स्वर्जिकाक्षारजीरकम् ॥ १८८ ॥
देवदारु च कर्षांशं चूर्णं तैले विनिक्षिपेत् । वज्रतैलमिदं ख्यातमभ्यङ्गात्सर्वकुष्ठनुत् ॥ १८९ ॥

Milky sap of vajri, ravi (arka), dhatūrā and chitraka, juice of buffalo's dung (filtered) all equal quantity, tila taila (sesame oil) and cows urine fourtimes its quantity are allowed to boil. One karṣa each of gandhaka, agni, śila, talaka, viḍanga, ativiṣa, viṣa, tiktakośātakī, kuṣhṭha, vacha, māṃsī, trikaṭu, pītadāru, yaṣṭi, swarjikā kṣāra, jīraka, and devadaru—are powdered nicely and added to the oil and taila prepared in the usual way. This known as *Vajrataila* cures all kinds of kuṣtha (leprosy and other skin diseases) by anointing the body with it (185–189).

करवीरादितैलम्—

करवीरशिखादन्तीत्रिवृत्कोशातकीफलम् । रम्भाक्षारोदके तैलं प्रशस्तं लोमशातनम् ॥ १९० ॥

Roots of karavīra, dantī, trivṛt, kośatakīphala and kṣāra of rambhā are dissolved in water and oil prepared as usual. This is a good lomaśātana (hair remover, depilatory) (190).

चन्दनादितैलम्—

(चन्दनाम्बुनखैर्याम्यं यष्टीशैलेयपद्मकम् । मञ्जिष्ठा सरलं दारु सेव्यैलं पूतिकेसरम् ॥ १९१ ॥
पत्रकैलं मुरा मांसी कङ्कोलं वनिताम्बुदम् । हरिद्रा सारिवा तिक्ता लवङ्गागरुकुङ्कुमम् ॥ १९२ ॥
त्वग्रेणुनलिका चेति तैलं मस्तु चतुर्गुणम् । लाक्षारससमं सिद्धं ग्रहघ्नं बलवर्धनम् ॥ १९३ ॥
अपस्मारज्वरोन्मादकृत्यालक्ष्मीविनाशनम् । आयुःपुष्टिकरं चैव वशीकरणमुत्तमम् ॥ १९४ ॥
विशेषात्क्षयरोगघ्नं रक्तपित्तहरं परम् ।)

Chandana, ambu, nakha, yamya (raktachandana), yaṣṭi; shiaileya, padmaka, mañjiṭṭā, sāralā, dāru, sevya (ushera) elā, pūtikesara, patraka, ela, mura, māṃsī, kānkola, vanitā (priyaṅgu), ambuda, haridrā sārivā, tikta, lavaṅga, agaru, kunkuma, twak, reṇu and nīlikā—all equal parts are made into kalka (paste) and added to taila (sesame oil) and four parts each of lākṣā rasa (solution of lac) and mastu (whey of curds) are mixed togther and taila prepared as usual. This oil used both internally and externally wards off all grahas (evil spirits), promotes strength, relieves apasmāra (epilepsy) jwara (fevers), unmāda (insanity), kṛtyā (effects of sorcery or witch-craft), alakṣmī (had omens), helps prolong life, attract women and specially beneficial to persons suffering from rājayakṣmā (tuberculosis) and rakta pitta (purpura) (191–195).

वचातैलम्—

(वचां शठीं हरिद्रे द्वे देवदारुमहौषधी ॥ १९५ ॥
हरीतकीमतिविषामुस्तमैन्द्रयवान्समान् । एतान्दशपलान्भागांश्चतुर्द्रोणेऽम्भसः पचेत् ॥ १९६ ॥
चक्रमर्दरसैस्तैलं कटुकं मृदुनाऽग्निना । पादशेषे विनिक्षिप्य सिन्दूरमवतारयेत् ॥ १९७ ॥
एतत्तैलं निहन्त्याशु गण्डमालां सुदारुणाम् ।)

Ten palas each of vacha, shati, the two haridrās, devadāru, mahousadhi, harītakī, ativiṣā, musta and indrayava—are boiled in four droṇas of water and reduced to quarter. To it is added kaṭu taila (mustard oil) and juice of chakramarda and cooked on mild fire as usual. After cooling, sindūra, one fourth the quantity of oil is sdded to it. This oil applied externally cures intractable gaṇḍamālā (scrofula) (195–197).

लाङ्गलीतैलम्—

(निर्गुण्डीस्वरसे तैलं लाङ्गलीमूलकल्कितम् ॥ १९८ ॥
तैलं नस्यान्निहन्त्याशु गण्डमालां सुदारुणाम् ।)

Taila prepared with juice of nirguṇḍi and paste of laṅgalī mūla and used as nasal drops cures chronic gaṇḍamālā (scrofula) (198).

धत्तूरतैलम्—

'धत्तूररसमादाय हयमारान्तिकारसम् । भृङ्गराजरसश्चैव सारिणी निम्बपत्रकम् ॥ १९९ ॥
शोभाञ्जनश्चित्रकश्च अश्वगन्धाप्रसारिणी । शिरीषः कुटजोऽनन्ता शाल्मली नक्तपत्रकम् ॥ २०० ॥
रविप्रियो महानिम्बो डिण्डिघोषा महेरणा । बला ज्योतिष्मती चैव श्यामाकश्चक्रमर्दकः ॥ २०१ ॥
एतैस्तु रसमादाय तैलतुल्यं च दीयते । देवदारु हरिद्रे द्वे मांसी कुष्ठं सचन्दनम् ॥ २०२ ॥
मरिचं त्रिवृता दन्ती हरितालं मनःशिला । कम्पिल्लको गन्धकश्च खदिरः पिप्पली वचा ॥ २०३ ॥
रसाञ्जनं च सिन्दूरं श्रीवासो रक्तचन्दनम् । इरिमेदस्तथा तुम्बी मञ्जिष्ठा सिन्दुवारकः ॥ २०४ ॥
करवीरजटा रास्ना विश्वा श्रेष्ठा च पौष्करम् । शठी तालीसपत्रं च प्रियङ्गू रेणुका तथा ॥ २०५ ॥
चातुर्जातकमञ्जीरं कङ्कोलं जातिपत्रिका । ज्योतिष्मती च पलिका विषस्य द्विपलं भवेत् ॥ २०६ ॥
आढकं कटुतैलस्य गोमूत्रं च चतुर्गुणम् । मृत्पात्रे लोहपात्रे च शनैर्मृद्वग्निना पचेत् ॥ २०७ ॥

मज्जाश्रितं त्वग्गतं च वातं चास्थिगतं तथा । ऊरुग्रहं चाढ्यवातं कुब्जं दण्डापतानकम् ॥ २०८ ॥
कुब्जत्वं चाथ शोथं च पक्षाघातं तथार्दितम् । हनुस्तम्भं शिरःकम्पं मूर्च्छितं दृष्टिविभ्रमम् ॥ २०९ ॥
अपस्मारं तथोन्मादं तथाचैवाऽपतंत्रकम् । आक्षेपकं चास्थिभग्नं सन्धिभग्नं च नाशयेत् ॥ २१० ॥

Fresh juices of dhatura, roots of hayamārā, bhṛṅgarāja, sarini nimba patra, shobāñjana, chitraka, aśwagandhā, prasāriṇī, śirīṣa, kuṭaja, ananta śālmalī, nakta-patra, ravipriyā, mahānimba, diṇdighoṣa, maherana, bala, jyotiṣmatī, shyāmaka and chakramarda—each equal in quantity; one pala each of devadāru, the two haridrās māṃsī, kuṣṭha, chandana, maricha, trivṛt, dantī, haritāla, manaśilā, kampillaka, gandhaka, khadira, pippali, vacha, rasāñjana, sindūra, śrīvasa, raktachandana, irimeda, thumbī, mañjiṣṭha, sindhuvāra, roots of karavīra, rasnā, vishwa, sreṣtha, pouṣkara, śati, tālīsapatra, priyaṅgu, reṇuka, chaturjataka, añjīra, kaṅkola, jātīpa-traka and jyotiṣmatī; and two palas of viṣa (vastannbha) one āḍhaka of kaṭu taila (mustard oil) and gomūtra (cows urine) four times the quantity of oil are cooked over mild fire in a mud pot or an iron vessel. This oil by external application cures vāta which is located in majja (bone marrow) twak (skin) asthi (bone) urugraha (stiffness of thigh), adhyavāta (gout) dandapatanaka (tetanus) kubja-twa (kyphosis), śotha (oedema), pakṣāghāta (hemiplegia), ardita (facial palsy) hanustambha (lock—jaw), śirakampa (shaking of head), mūrchā (unconciousness, convulsions) drṣtivibhrama (disorders of vision), apasmāra (epilepsy) unmāda (insanity) apatantraka (fits), ākṣepaka (convulsions) and asthi and sandhi bhagna (feactures & dislocations) (199–210).

इति श्रीदामोदरसूनुना शार्ङ्गधराचार्येण विरचितायां शार्ङ्गधरसंहितायां घृततैलकल्पना नाम नवमोऽध्यायः ।

Thus ends the ninth chapter.

दशमोऽध्यायः

CHAPTER X

Sandhana Kalpana (Galenicals, Fermented liquids)

इदानीं संधानकल्पनां दर्शयन्नाह—

द्रवेषु चिरकालस्थं द्रव्यं यत्संधितं भवेत् । आसवारिष्टभेदैस्तु प्रोच्यते भेषजोचितम् ॥ १ ॥

Water in which, drugs kept for long periods, getting fermented are known as āsavas and āristhas. Such of them useful in medical treatment are described in this chapter (1).

तत्रापि आसवारिष्टयोर्भेदमाह—

यदपक्वौषधाम्बुभ्यां सिद्धं मद्यं स आसवः । अरिष्टः क्वाथसिद्धः स्यात्तयोर्मानं जलोन्मितम् ॥ २ ॥

Āsava is prepared in cold water without boiling the drugs whereas ariṣtha is prepared by boiling. The medicinal dose of both is the same as that of water taken for early morning drink[1] (i.e., about two palas) (2).

अनुक्तमानारिष्टेषु जलादिप्रमाणमाह—

अनुक्तमानारिष्टेषु द्रवद्रोणे तुलां गुडम् । क्षौद्रं क्षिपेद्गुडादर्धं प्रक्षेपं दशमांशिकम् ॥ ३ ॥

Where not specified, the quantity of water to be taken for the preparation of ariṣta is one droṇa, that of jaggery (guda) is one tulā (hundred palas), honey half the measure of jaggery and powder of drugs one tenth (3).

अथ क्वाथभेदेन सीधुलक्षणमाह—

ज्ञेयः शीतरसः सीधुरपक्वमधुरद्रवैः ।
सिद्धः पक्वरसः सीधुः संपक्वमधुरद्रवैः ॥ ४ ॥

Juice of sweet substances (like sugarcane juice etc) fermented without boiling them is known as śitarasa sīdhu and if prepared by boiling them, it will be ealled pakwarasa sīdhu (4).

अथ सुराप्रसन्नादीनां मद्यभेदानां लक्षणमाह—

परिपक्वान्नसंधानसमुत्पन्नां सुरां जगुः । सुरामण्डः प्रसन्ना स्यात्ततः कादम्बरी घनः ॥ ५ ॥

तदधो जगलो ज्ञेयो मेदको जगलाद्घनः । वक्कसो हृतसारः स्यात्सुराबीजं च किण्वकम् ॥ ६ ॥

The fermented liquor prepared by using cooked rice, barley etc., is *sura*, The clear supernatant fluid of surā is called *prasanna*, slightly thicker than it is *kādambarī*; next thicker to it is *jagala*; still thicker is *medaka*. The residue left over after distillation is called *bakkasa, surabīja or kinwa* (5–6).

अथ वारुणीमाह—

यत्तालखर्जूररसैः संधिता सा हि वारुणी ।

अथ शुक्तमाह—

कन्दमूलफलादीनि सस्नेहलवणानि च ॥ ७ ॥

यत्र द्रवेऽभिषूयन्ते तच्छुक्तमभिधीयते । विनष्टमम्लतां यातं मद्यं वा मधुरद्रवम् ॥ ८ ॥

The liquor prepared with juice of tāla, kharjūra is called *vāruṇi*; that prepared with roots, tubers, fruits and added with sneha (oil or ghee) and salts is called as *śukta* (7).

विनष्टः संधितो यस्तु तच्चुक्रमभिधीयते ।

The liquor or syrup which gets spoiled and looses its sweetness but becomes sour is known as *chukra* (8).

1. The dose of asava and arista have not been specified here. In the present day it is usually given in doses of 1 to 2 ounces per time.

गुडाम्बुना सतैलेन कन्दमूलफलैस्तथा ॥ ९ ॥
संधितं चाम्लतां यातं गुडशुक्तं तदुच्यते ।

इक्षुशुक्तम्—

एवमेवेक्षुशुक्तं स्यान्मृद्वीकासंभवं तथा ॥ १० ॥

Water in which jaggery is dissolved, mixed with oil, bits of tubers, roots, and fruits and fermented to aquire sour taste is called *guda sukta,* that of grapes is *mrdwika śuktā* (9–10),

इदानीं तुषाम्बुकाञ्जिकमप्याह—

तुषाम्बु संधितं ज्ञेयमामैर्विदलितैर्यवैः । यवैस्तु निस्तुषैः पक्वैः सौवीरं संधितं भवेत् ॥ ११ ॥

Fermented liquor prepared by using raw husk of yava (barley) is known as *tuṣambu;* that prepared by cooking yava grain itself is called *souvīra* (11).

अथ काञ्जिकम्—

कुल्माषधान्यमण्डादि संधितं काञ्जिकं विदुः ।

अथ सण्डाकी—

सण्डाकी संधिता ज्ञेया मूलकैः सार्षपादिभिः ॥ १२ ॥

Liquor prepared with māṇda (gruel) of half boiled kulmāṣa (black gram), dhānya (rice. barley etc) is *kanjika;* that prepared with mūlaka, sarṣapa, etc., being added to it becomes *sandaki* (12).

अथ आसवाः—

रक्तपित्तादौ उशीरासवः—

उशीरं वालकं पद्मं काश्मरीं नीलमुत्पलम् । प्रियङ्गु पद्मकं लोध्रं मञ्जिष्ठां धन्वयासकम् ॥ १३ ॥
पाठां किराततिक्तं च न्यग्रोधोदुम्बरं शठीम् । पर्पटं पुण्डरीकं च पटोलं काञ्चनारकम् ॥ १४ ॥
जम्बूशाल्मलिनिर्यासं प्रत्येकं पलसंमितान् । भागान्सुचूर्णितान्कृत्वा द्राक्षायाः पलविंशतिम् ॥ १५ ॥
धातकीं षोडशपलां जलद्रोणद्वये क्षिपेत् । शर्करायास्तुलां दत्त्वा क्षौद्रस्यैकतुलां तथा ॥ १६ ॥
मासैकं स्थापयेद्भाण्डे मांसीमरिचधूपिते । उशीरासव इत्येष रक्तपित्तविनाशनः ॥ १७ ॥
पाण्डुकुष्ठप्रमेहार्शः कृमिशोथहरस्तथा ।

One pala each of uṣīra, valaka, padma, kashmarī, nīlotpala, priyaṅgu, padmaka, lodhra, mañjiṣṭha, dhānwayasa, pāṭhā, kirātatiktā, nyagrodha, udumbara, shathi, parpaṭa, puṇḍarīka, paṭola, kanchanara, jambu and shalmalīniryāsa—are nicely powdered; twenty palas of drākshā, sixteen palas of dhātakipuṣpa, one tulā each of sugar and honey—all these are put into two droṇas of water. A big mud pot, cleaned and made fragrant with fumes of māṃsī, maricha etc., is filled with the above liquid, its mouth sealed air tight and kept underground for one month. Taken out and used after that period, this preparation known as *Uṣīrāsava* cures raktapitta (purpura), pāṇḍu (anaemia), kuṣṭha (leprosy and other skin diseases), prameha (diabetes), arśa (piles), kṛmi (parasites) and śotha (oedema) (13–17).

कुमार्यासवः—

(सुपक्वरससंशुद्धं कुमार्याः पत्रमाहरेत् ॥ १८ ॥
यत्नेन रसमादाय पात्रे पाषाणमृन्मये । द्रोणे गुडतुलां दत्त्वा घृतभाण्डे निधापयेत् ॥ १९ ॥
माक्षिकं पक्वलोहं च तस्मिन्नर्धतुलां क्षिपेत् । कटुत्रिकं लवङ्गं च चातुर्जातकमेव च ॥ २० ॥
चित्रकं पिप्पलीमूलं विडङ्गं गजपिप्पली । चविकं हपुषा धान्यं क्रमुकं कटुरोहिणी ॥ २१ ॥
मुस्ता फलत्रिकं रास्ना देवदारु निशाद्वयम् । मूर्वा मधुरसा दन्ती मूलं पुष्करसंभवम् ॥ २२ ॥
बला चातिबला चैव कपिकच्छूस्त्रिकण्टकम् । शतपुष्पा हिङ्गुपत्री आकल्लकमुटिङ्गणम् ॥ २३ ॥
पुनर्नवाद्वयं लोध्रं धातुर्माक्षिकमेव च । एषां चार्धपलं दत्त्वा धातक्यास्तु पलाष्टकम् ॥ २४ ॥
पलं चार्धपलं चैव पलद्वयमुदाहृतम् । वपुर्वयःप्रमाणेन बलवर्णाग्निदीपनम् ॥ २५ ॥
बृंहणं रोचनं वृष्यं पक्तिशूलनिवारणम् । अष्टावुदरजान्रोगान्क्षयमुग्रं च नाशयेत् ॥ २६ ॥
विंशतिं मेहजान्रोगानुदावर्तमपस्मृतिम् । मूत्रकृच्छ्रमपस्मारं शुक्रदोषं तथाश्मरीम् ॥ २७ ॥
क्रिमिजं रक्तपित्तं च नाशयेत्तु न संशयः ।)

Leaves of kumārī are washed well, lightly cooked and juice extracted from it's pulp, one droṇa of this juice is poured into a stone vessel or mud pot. To it are added one tulā of guḍa (jaggery); half tulā each of honey and pakwaloha (loha bhasma); powder of half pala each of kaṭutrika, lavaṅga, chaturjataka, chitraka, pippalīmūla, viḍaṅga, gajapippalī, chavikā, hapuṣa, dhānya, kramuka, katurohini, musta, phalatrika, rāsnā, devadāru, the two nishas, mūrvā, madhurasa, dantī, puṣkaramula, bala, atibalā, kapikachu, trikaṅṭaka, śatapuṣpā, hiṅgupatrī, akallaka, mutingaṇa, the two punarnavās, lodhra and makshika dhātu and eight palas of dhātakī puspa are mixed and filled into a pot smeared in side with ghee, its mouth is sealed air tight and kept undistur bed for a month. Later on used in doses of one, one and half or two palas according to age and constitution this recipe increases strength, colour, digestive capacity, weight and taste, acts as an aphrodisic, relieves pain of indigestion, eight kinds of udara (abdominal enlargement), severe kshaya (consumption), twenty kinds of prameha (diabetes), udāvarta (reverse peristalsis), apasmāra (epilepsy), śukra doṣas (disorders of semen), ashmarī (urinary calculus) kṛmi (parasites) and raktapitta (purpura) without doubt (18–27).

पिप्पल्यासवः क्षयादौ—

पिप्पली मरिचं चव्यं हरिद्रा चित्रको घनः ॥ २८ ॥
विडङ्गं क्रमुको लोध्रः पाठा धात्र्येलवालुकम् । उशीरं चन्दनं कुष्ठं लवङ्गं तगरं तथा ॥ २९ ॥
मांसी त्वगेलापत्रं च प्रियङ्गुर्नागकेशरम् । एषामर्धपलान्भागान्सूक्ष्मचूर्णीकृतान्शुभान् ॥ ३० ॥
जलद्रोणद्वये क्षिप्त्वा दद्याद्गुडतुलात्रयम् । पलानि दश धातक्या द्राक्षा षष्टिपला भवेत् ॥ ३१ ॥

एतान्येकत्र संयोज्य मृद्भाण्डे च विनिक्षिपेत् । ज्ञात्वाऽऽगतरसं तस्य पाययेदग्न्यपेक्षया ॥ ३२ ॥
क्षयं गुल्मोदरं कार्श्यं ग्रहणीं पाण्डुतां गदम् । अर्शांसि नाशयेच्छीघ्रं पिप्पल्याद्यासवस्त्वयम् ॥३३॥

Fine powder half pala each of pippalī, maricha, chavya, haridrā, chitraka, kuṣṭha, lavaṅga, tagara, māṃsī, twak, elā, patra, priyaṅgu, nāgakeśara; three tulas of jaggery, ten palas of dhātakī, sixty palas of drākshā are all put into two dronas of water, filled in to a mud pot and allowed to ferment. Taken in suitable doses this recipe known as *Pippalyāsava* cures quickly kshaya (consumption), gulma (abdominal tumor), udara (abdominal enlargements), kārṣya (emaciation), grahaṇī (sprue), pāṇḍutā (anaemia) and arśas (haemorrhoids) (28–33).

पाण्ड्वादौ लोहासवः—

लोहच्चूर्णं त्रिकटुकं त्रिफलां च यवानिकाम् । विडङ्गं मुस्तकं चित्रं चतुःसंख्यापलं पृथक् ॥ ३४ ॥
धातकीकुसुमानां तु प्रक्षिपेत्पलविंशतिम् । चूर्णीकृत्य ततः क्षौद्रं चतुःषष्टिपलं क्षिपेत् ॥ ३५ ॥
दद्याद्गुडतुलां तत्र जलद्रोणद्वयं तथा । घृतभाण्डे विनिक्षिप्य निदध्यान्मासमात्रकम् ॥ ३६ ॥
लोहासवममुं मर्त्यः पिबेद्वह्निकरं परम् । पाण्डुश्वयथुगुल्मानि जठराण्यर्शसां रुजम् ॥ ३७ ॥
कुष्ठं प्लीहामयं कण्डूं कासं श्वासं भगन्दरम् । अरोचकं च ग्रहणीं हृद्रोगं च विनाशयेत् ॥ ३८ ॥

Four palas each of lohachurṇa (iron filings), trikaṭu, triphalā, yavānī, viḍaṅga, mustā and chitraka are nicely powdered, twenty palas of dhātakī kusuma, sixty-four palas of honey, one tulā of jaggery are all put into two droṇas of water, poured into a mud pot smeared inside with ghee, its mouth sealed airtight and kept for a month undisturbed for fermentation. This recipe known as *Lohāsava* taken in appropriate doses improves digestion and cures pāṇḍu (anemia). swayathu (oedema), gulma (abdominal tumors), jaṭhara (abdominal enlargements), pain of arśas (piles), kuṣṭha (leprosy and other skin diseases), plīhāmaya (diseases of spleen), kaṇḍū (itching), kāsa (cough), śvāsa (dyspnoes), bhagandara (fistula-in-ano), arochaka (anorexia), grahaṇī (sprue) and hṛdroga (diseases of the heart) (34–38).

मृद्वीकारिष्टः—

(मृद्वीकायाः पलशतं चतुर्द्रोणेऽम्भसः पचेत् । द्रोणशेषे सुशीते च पूते तस्मिन्प्रदापयेत् ॥ ३९ ॥
तुले द्वे क्षौद्रखण्डाभ्यां धातक्याः प्रस्थमेव च । कङ्कोलकं लवङ्गं च फलं जात्यास्तथैव च ॥ ४० ॥
पलांशकं च मरिचत्वगेलापत्रकेसरम् । पिप्पली चित्रकं चव्यं पिप्पलीमूलरेणुके ॥ ४१ ॥
घृतभाण्डे विनिक्षिप्य चन्दनागरुधूपिते । कर्पूरवासितो ह्येष ग्रहण्या दीपनः परः ॥ ४२ ॥
अर्शसां नाशने श्रेष्ठ उदावर्तस्य गुल्मनुत् । जठरक्रिमिकुष्ठानि व्रणास्तु विविधास्तथा ॥ ४३ ॥
अक्षिरोगशिरोरोगगलरोगांश्च नाशयेत् ।)

One hundred palas of mṛdwikā are boiled in four droṇas of water and decoction reduced to quarter. To it are added two tulās of sugar candy. One prasta of dhātakī and powder of one pala each of kaṅkola, lavaṅga, jātīphala, maricha, twak, elā, patra, kesara, pippalī, chitraka, chavya, pippalīmūla and reṇuka. A mud pot smeared inside with a little ghee and fumigated with chandana, agaru and karpūra is filled with the above liquid and kept undisturbed for a month. Used later this recipe acts as an excellent carminative in grahaṇī (sprue), relieves arshas (piles), udāvarta (reverse peristalisis), gulma (abdominal tumors), jaṭhara (abdominal enlargements), kṛmi (parasites), kuṣṭha (leprosy and other skin diseases) and different kinds of vraṇas (ulcers), akṣiroga (eye diseases), shiroroga (diseases of the head) and galaroga (diseases of the throat). (39–43).

अथारिष्टाः, तत्रादौ कुटजारिष्टः ज्वरादौ—

तुलां कुटजमूलस्य मृद्वीकार्धतुलां तथा ॥ ४४ ॥
मधूकपुष्पकाश्मर्यभागान्दशपलोन्मितान् । चतुर्द्रोणेऽम्भसः पक्त्वा क्वाथे द्रोणावशेषिते ॥ ४५ ॥
धातक्या विंशतिपलं गुडस्य च तुलां क्षिपेत् । मासमात्रं स्थितो भाण्डे कुटजारिष्टसंज्ञितः ॥ ४६ ॥
ज्वरान्प्रशमयेत्सर्वान्कुर्यात्तीक्ष्णं धनञ्जयम् ।

Kuṭaja bark half a tulā, mrdwika half tulā, ten palas each of madhūkapuspa and kashmarī are boiled in four droṇas of water and reduced to one droṇa. To it are added twenty palas of dhātakī, one tulā of jaggery and kept in pot for one month. This recipe known as *Kutajāriṣṭa* relieves all fevers and improves agni (digestive capacity) (44–46).

अथ विडङ्गारिष्टः विद्रध्यादौ—

विडङ्गं ग्रन्थिकं रास्ना कुटजत्वक्फलानि च ॥ ४७ ॥
पाठैलवालुकं धात्री भागान्पञ्चपलान्पृथक् । अष्टद्रोणेऽम्भसः पक्त्वा कुर्याद्द्रोणावशेषितम् ॥ ४८ ॥
पूते शीते क्षिपेत्तत्र क्षौद्रं पलशतत्रयम् । धातकीं विंशतिपलां त्रिजातं द्विपलं तथा ॥ ४९ ॥
प्रियङ्गुकाञ्चनाराणां सलोध्राणां पलं पलम् । व्योषस्य च पलान्यष्टौ चूर्णीकृत्य प्रदापयेत् ॥ ५० ॥
घृतभाण्डे विनिक्षिप्य मासमेकं निधापयेत् । ततः पिबेद्यथार्हं तु जयेद्विद्रधिमुत्थितम् ॥ ५१ ॥
ऊरुस्तम्भाश्मरीमेहान्प्रत्यष्ठीलाभगन्दरान् । गण्डमालां हनुस्तम्भं विडङ्गारिष्टसंज्ञकम् ॥ ५२ ॥

Five palas each of viḍaṅga, granthika, rāsnā, kuṭajatwak ,kuṭaja-phala, pata, elavaluka and dhātrī are boiled in eight droṇas of water and decoction reduced to one droṇa. To it are added three hundred palas of honey, twenty palas of dhātakī; powder of two palas of trijātaka, one pala each of priyaṅgu, kanchanāra and lodhra; eight palas of vyoṣa (trikaṭu) are added and kept in apot smeared with ghee for one month. This recipe known as *Vidaṅgāriṣṭa* used in proper doses to suitable persons cures urustambha (stiffness of leg), ashmari (urinary calculus), meha (diabetes), pratyaṣṭhīlā (prostate enlargement), bhagandara (fistula-in-ano), gaṇḍamālā (scrofula) and hanustambha (lock-jaw) (47-52).

अथ देवदार्व्याद्यरिष्टः प्रमेहादौ—

तुलार्धं देवदारोः स्याद्वासा च पलविंशतिः । मञ्जिष्ठेन्द्रयवा दन्ती तगरं रजनीद्वयम् ॥ ५३ ॥
रास्ना कृमिघ्नं मुस्तं च शिरीषं खदिरार्जुनौ । भागान्दशपलान्दद्याद्यवान्या वत्सकस्य च ॥ ५४ ॥
चन्दनस्य गुडूच्याश्च रोहिण्याश्चित्रकस्य च । भागानष्टपलानेतानष्टद्रोणेऽम्भसः पचेत् ॥ ५५ ॥
द्रोणशेषे कषाये च पूते शीते प्रदापयेत् । धातक्याः षोडशपलं माक्षिकस्य तुलात्रयम् ॥ ५६ ॥
व्योषस्य द्विपलं दद्यात्त्रिजातस्य चतुष्पलम् । चतुष्पलं प्रियङ्गोश्च द्विपलं नागकेशरम् ॥ ५७ ॥
सर्वाण्येतानि संचूर्ण्य घृतभाण्डे निधापयेत् । मासादूर्ध्वं पिबेदेनं प्रमेहं हन्ति दुर्जयम् ॥ ५८ ॥
वातरोगान्ग्रहण्यर्शोमूत्रकृच्छ्राणि नाशयेत् । देवदार्वादिकोऽरिष्टः कण्डूकुष्ठविनाशनः ॥ ५९ ॥

Half tulā of devadāru, twenty palas of vasā, ten palas each of mañjiṣṭhā, indrayaya, dantī, tagara, the two rajanis, rāsnā kṛmighna musta, śirīṣa, khadira, arjuna; eight palas each of yavānī, vatsaka, chandana, guḍūchi rohiṇi and chitraka—are all boiled in eight droṇas of water and decoction reduced to one droṇa. To it are added sixteen palas of dhātakī, three tulās of honey, powder of two palas of vyoṣa, four palas of trijaṭā and priyaṅgu, two palas of nāgakesara and the liquid kept in a pot smeared inside with ghee. This recipe known as *Devadārvyādi ariṣtha*, used appropriately after one month cures intractible prameha (diabetes) vātarogas (nervous diseases), grahaṇī (sprue), arshas (piles), mūtrakṛchra (dysurea), kaṇḍū (itching) and kuṣṭha (leprosy and other skin diseases) (53–59).

अथ खदिरारिष्टं कुष्ठादौ—

खदिरस्य तुलार्धं तु देवदारु च तत्समम् । बाकुची द्वादशपला दार्वी स्यात्पलविंशतिः ॥ ६० ॥
त्रिफला विंशतिपला ह्यष्टद्रोणेऽम्भसः पचेत् । कषाये द्रोणशेषे च पूते शीते विनिक्षिपेत् ॥ ६१ ॥
तुलाद्वयं माक्षिकस्य तुलैका शर्करा मता । धातक्या विंशतिपलं कङ्कोलं नागकेशरम् ॥ ६२ ॥
जातीफलं लवङ्गैलात्वक्पत्राणि पृथक्पृथक् । पलोन्मितानि कृष्णाया दद्यात्पलचतुष्टयम् ॥ ६३ ॥
घृतभाण्डे विनिक्षिप्य मासादूर्ध्वं पिबेन्नरः । महाकुष्ठानि हृद्रोगं पाण्डुरोगार्बुदे तथा ॥ ६४ ॥
गुल्मं ग्रन्थिं कृमीन्कासं श्वासं प्लीहोदरं जयेत् । एष वै खदिरारिष्टः सर्वकुष्ठनिवारणः ॥ ६५ ॥

Half tulā each of khadira and devadāru, twelve palas of bakuchī, twenty palas of each of darvī and triphalā are boiled in eight droṇas of water and decoction reduced to one droṇa. After cooling two tulās of honey, one tulā of sugar, twenty palas of dhātakī, powder of one pala each of kaṅkola, nāgakesara, jāṭīphala, lavaṅga, elā, twak and patra; four palas kṛṣṇā—are added and kept in a pot for one month. This preparation known as *Khadirāriṣṭa* cures the mahā kuṣthas (leprosy and allied skin conditions), hṛdroga (heart diseases), pāṇḍu (anaemia), arbuda (cancer), gulma (abdominal tumor), granthi (tumors), kṛmi (intestinal parasites), kāsa (cough), śwāsa (dyspnoea) and plīhodara (splenic enlargement) and especially all varieties of kuṣṭha (leprosy) (60–65).

अथ बब्बूलारिष्टः क्षयकासादौ—

तुलाद्वयं तु बब्बूल्याश्चतुर्द्रोणे जले पचेत् । द्रोणशेषे रसे शीते गुडस्य च तुलां क्षिपेत् ॥ ६६ ॥
धातकीं षोडशपलां कृष्णां च द्विपलां तथा । जातीफलानि कङ्कोलमेलात्वक्पत्रकेशरम् ॥ ६७ ॥
लवङ्गं मरिचं चैव पलिकान्युपकल्पयेत् । मासं भाण्डे स्थितस्त्वेष बब्बूलारिष्टको जयेत् ॥ ६८ ॥
क्षयं कुष्ठमतीसारं प्रमेहश्वासकासकम् ।

Two tulās of bark of babbūla is boiled in four droṇas of water and decoction reduced to one droṇa. To it are added three tulās of jaggery; sixteen palas of dhātakī and powder of two palas of kṛṣṇā; and one pala each of jātīphala, kaṅkola elā, twak, patra, kesara, lavaṅga and maricha and kept in a pot for one month. This preparation known as *Babbūlāriṣṭa* cures kṣaya (consumption), kuṣṭha (leprosy and other skin diseases), atisāra (diarrhoea), prameha (diabetes), śwāsa (dyspnoea) and kāsa (cough) (66–69).

अथ द्राक्षारिष्टः पुष्ट्यादौ—

द्राक्षातुलार्धं द्विद्रोणे जलस्य विपचेत्सुधीः ॥ ६९ ॥
पादशेषे कषाये च पूते शीते विनिक्षिपेत् । गुडस्य द्वितुलां तत्र त्वगेलापत्रकेशरम् ॥ ७० ॥
प्रियङ्गुर्मरिचं कृष्णा विडङ्गं चेति चूर्णयेत् । पृथक्पलोन्मितैर्भागैस्ततो भाण्डे निधापयेत् ॥ ७१ ॥
समन्ततो घट्टयित्वा पिबेज्जातरसं ततः । उरःक्षतं क्षयं हन्ति कासश्वासगलामयान् ॥ ७२ ॥
द्राक्षारिष्टाह्वयः प्रोक्तो बलकृन्मलशोधनः ।

Half tulā of drakṣā is boiled in two droṇas of water and decoction reduced to quarter. After cooling are added two tulās of jaggery and powder of one pala each of twak, elā, patra, kesara, priyaṅgu, maricha, kṛṣṇā and viḍaṅga. The liquid is kept in a mud pot for a month. This recipe known as *Drākṣāriṣṭa* cures urakṣata (injury inside the lungs), kṣaya (consumption), kāsa (cough), śwāsa (dyspnoea) galamaya (throat diseases), confers strength and acts as a laxative (69–73)

अथ रोहितकारिष्टः गुदजग्रहण्यादौ—

रोहितकतुलामेकां चतुर्द्रोणे जले पचेत् ॥ ७३ ॥
पादशेषे रसे शीते पूते पलशतद्वयम् । दद्याद्गुडस्य धातक्याः पलषोडशिकं मतम् ॥ ७४ ॥
पञ्चकोलं त्रिजातं च त्रिफलां च विनिक्षिपेत् । चूर्णयित्वा पलांशेन ततो भाण्डे निधापयेत् ॥ ७५ ॥
मासादूर्ध्वं च पिबतां गुदजा यान्ति संक्षयम् । ग्रहणीपाण्डुहृद्रोगप्लीहगुल्मोदराणि च ॥ ७६ ॥
कुष्ठशोफारुचिहरो रोहितारिष्टसंज्ञकः ।

One tulā of rohitaka bark is boiled in four droṇas of water and decoction reduced to one quarter. To it are added after cooling, two hundred palas of jaggery, sixteen pala of dhātakī, and powder of one pala each of pañchakola, trijaṭā and triphalā and kept in a pot undisturbed for a month. This recipe known as *Rohitāriṣṭa* used in appropriate doses cures arshas (haemorrhoids), grahaṇī (sprue), pāṇḍu (anaemia) hṛdroga (heart diseases), plīhā (splenic enlargement), gulma (abdominal tumor), udara (abdominal enlargement), kuṣṭha (leprosy and other skin diseases), śopha (oedema) and aruchi (anorexia) (73–76).

अथ दशमूलारिष्टः वातादौ—

(पर्ण्यौ बृहत्यौ गोकण्टो बिल्वोऽग्निमन्थकोऽरलुः ॥ ७७ ॥

पाटला काश्मरी चेति दशमूलमिहोच्यते ।) दशमूलानि कुर्वीत भागैः पञ्चपलैः पृथक् ॥ ७८ ॥
पञ्चविंशत्पलं कुर्याच्चित्रकं पौष्करं तथा । कुर्याद्विंशत्पलं लोध्रं गुडूची तत्समा भवेत् ॥ ७९ ॥
पलैः षोडशभिर्धात्री रविसंख्यैर्दुरालभा । खदिरो बीजसारश्च पथ्या चेति पृथक्पलैः ॥ ८० ॥
अष्टभिर्गणितैः कुष्ठं मञ्जिष्ठा देवदारु च । विडङ्गं मधुकं भार्ङ्गी कपित्थोऽक्षः पुनर्नवा ॥ ८१ ॥
चव्यं मांसी प्रियङ्गुश्च सारिवा कृष्णजीरकम् । त्रिवृता रेणुकं रास्ना पिप्पली क्रमुकः शठी ॥ ८२ ॥
हरिद्रा शतपुष्पा च पद्मकं नागकेशरम् । मुस्तमिन्द्रयवः शुण्ठी जीवकर्षभकौ तथा ॥ ८३ ॥
मेदा चान्या महामेदा काकोल्यौ ऋद्धिवृद्धिके । कुर्यात्पृथग्द्विपलिकान्पचेदष्टगुणे जले ॥ ८४ ॥
चतुर्थांशं शृतं नीत्वा मृद्भाण्डे संनिधापयेत् । ततः षष्टिपलां द्राक्षां पचेन्नीरे चतुर्गुणे ॥ ८५ ॥
त्रिपादशेषं शीतं च पूर्वक्काथे शृतं क्षिपेत् । द्वात्रिंशत्पलिकं क्षौद्रं दद्याद्गुडचतुःशतम् ॥ ८६ ॥
त्रिंशत्पलानि धातक्याः कङ्कोलं जलचन्दनम् । जातीफलं लवङ्गं च त्वगेलापत्रकेशरम् ॥ ८७ ॥
पिप्पली चेति संचूर्ण्य भागैर्द्विपलिकैः पृथक् । शाणमात्रां च कस्तूरीं सर्वमेकत्र निक्षिपेत् ॥ ८८ ॥
भूमौ निखातयेद्भाण्डं ततो जातरसं पिबेत् । कतकस्य फलं क्षिप्त्वा रसं निर्मलतां नयेत् ॥ ८९ ॥
ग्रहणीमरुचिं श्वासं कासं गुल्मं भगन्दरम् । वातव्याधिं क्षयं छर्दिं पाण्डुरोगं च कामलाम् ॥९०॥
कुष्ठान्यर्शांसि मेहांश्च मन्दाग्निमुदराणि च । शर्करामश्मरीं मूत्रकृच्छ्रं धातुक्षयं जयेत् ॥ ९१ ॥
कृशानां पुष्टिजननो वन्ध्यानां गर्भदः परः । अरिष्टो दशमूलाख्यस्तेजःशुक्रबलप्रदः ॥ ९२ ॥

The two parṇis, the two bṛhatis, gokaṇṭa, bilwa, agnimantha, aralu, pātalā, kāshmarī—are together called as dashamūlas. Five palas each of the above; twenty five palas each of chitraka and puṣkara; twenty palas each of lodhra and guḍūchī, sixteen palas of dhātrī, twelve palas of durālabhā, eight palas each of khadira, bījasāra, pathyā and two palas each of kusṭa, mañjiṣṭha, devadāru, viḍaṅga madhuka,bhārṅgī, kapittha, akṣa, punarnavā, chavya, māṃsī, priyaṅgu, sārivā, kṛṣnā-jīraka, trivṛt, reṇuka, rāsnā, pippalī, kramuka, shaṭhi, haridrā, śatapuṣpā, padmaka, nāgakesara, mustā, indrayava, śunṭhī, jīvaka, rṣabhaka, meda, mahāmeda, the two kākolīs ṛuddhi and vṛddhi—all these are boiled in eight times their total quantity water and decoction reduced to quarter. Sixty palas of drākṣā are boiled in four times their quantity of water and decoction reduced to two—thirds. Both the decoctions are mixed together. To the mixture are added thirtytwo palas of dhātakī and powder of two palas each of kaṅkola, jala, chandana, jātīphala, lavaṅga, twak, elā, patra, kesara and pippalī are added and put in a mud pot which is later buried under ground for one month. After removal kaṭaka phala is added to clear it and filtered through cloth. One śāṇa of kastūrī is added to it and used in appropriate doses. This recipe known as *daśamūlāriṣṭa* cures grahanī (sprue), aruchi (anorexia), śwāsa (dyspnoea), kāsa (cough), gulma (abdominal tumor), bhagandara (fistula-in-ano), vātavyādhi (nervous diseases), kṣaya (consumption), chardi (vomitings) pāṇḍuroga (anaemia), kāmalā (jaundice), kuṣṭha (leprosy and other skin diseases), arshas (haemorrhoids), meha (diabetes), mandāgni (dyspepsia), udara (abdominal enlargement) śarkarā (urinary gravel), ashmarī (urinary caliculii), mūtrakṛchra (dysurea), dhātukṣaya (emaciation). It makes lean persons stout, gives progeny to the childless and quickly stimulates production of semen (87–92).

इति श्रीदामोदरसूनुना शाङ्गधराचार्येण विरचितायां शाङ्गधरसंहितायां मध्यमखण्डे आसवारिष्टकल्पना नाम दशमोऽध्यायः ॥

Thus ends the tenth chapter.

एकादशोऽध्यायः

CHAPTER 11

Dhātu Shodhanamāraṇa Kalpanā

(Purification and Killing of Minerals and Metals)

अथेदानीं धातूनां समुदायेन शोधनमारणं दर्शयन्नाह—

स्वर्णताराऽऽरताम्राणि नागवङ्गौ च तीक्ष्णकम् । धातवः सप्त विज्ञेयास्ततस्तान् शोधयेद्बुधः ॥ १ ॥

Swarṇa (gold), tārā (silver), ara (brass), tāmra (copper), nāga (lead), vaṅga (tin), tīkṣṇa (magnetic iron ore) —these seven are known as dhātus. They should be purified before use (1).

इदानीं तच्छोधनमारणमाह—

स्वर्णताराऽऽरताम्रायःपत्राण्यग्नौ प्रतापयेत् । निषिञ्चेत्तत्तत्तानि तैले तक्रे च काञ्जिके ॥ २ ॥
गोमूत्रे च कुलत्थानां कषाये च त्रिधा त्रिधा । एवं स्वर्णादिलोहानां विशुद्धिः संप्रजायते ॥ ३ ॥

Thin leaves of swarṇa, tārā, arā, tāmra and ayas are heated over fire and immediately dipped into thaila (sesame oil), takra (buttermilk), kāñjika (sour gruel), gomūtra (cow's urine) and decoction of Kulatha—three times in each liquid. By this method all these metals get purified (2–3).

नागवङ्गौ प्रतप्तौ च गालितौ तौ निषिंचयेत् । त्रिधा त्रिधा विशुद्धिः स्याद्रविदुग्धेन च त्रिधा ॥ ४॥

Nāga and vaṅga are purified by melting them over fire and pouring the molten metal into the liquids stated above and also ravidugdha (milky sap of arka plant) (4).

अथ स्वर्णमारणम्—

स्वर्णांच्च द्विगुणं सूतमम्लेन सह मर्दयेत् । तद्गोलकसमं गन्धं निदध्यादधरोत्तरम् ॥ ५ ॥
गोलकं च ततो रुन्ध्याच्छरावदृढसंपुटे । त्रिंशद्वनोपलैर्दद्यात्पुटान्येवं चतुर्दश ॥ ६ ॥
निरुत्थं जायते भस्म गन्धो देयः पुनः पुनः ।

One part of swarṇa (gold) and two parts of rasa (mercury) are macerated together with any sour liquid, and made into round pill. Equal quantity of powder of gandha (ka) (sulphur) is spread in an earthen plate, the pill is kept on it and covered again with powder of sulphur. Another earthen plate is kept inverted over the first one and both plates sealed together well with mud plaster. After drying, these sealed plates are kept inside a heap of thirty cowdung masses collected from the forests, and set fire. After the dung heap burns out and gets cooled the discs are taken out and the whole process is repeated again, every time adding fresh sulphur. By fourteen such puṭas, a niruthabhasma[1] of gold will be obtained (5–7).

अथापरो विधिः—

काञ्चने गालिते नागं षोडशांशेन निक्षिपेत् ॥ ७ ॥
चूर्णयित्वा तथाम्लेन घृष्ट्वा कृत्वा च गोलकम् । गोलकेन समं गन्धं दत्त्वा चैवाधरोत्तरम् ॥ ८ ॥
शरावसंपुटे धृत्वा पुटेत् त्रिंशद्वनोपलैः । एवं सप्तपुटैर्हेम निरुत्थं भस्म जायते ॥ ९ ॥

Gold is melted and one-sixteenth of its weight of lead is added to it. After cooling it is macerated with any sour liquid and made into discs, dried, kept inside a plate covered all over with equal quantity of powdered sulphur; plates sealed with mud plaster, dried and subjected to fire in a heap of thirty cowdung heap. Seven such putas will yield niruthabhasma of gold (7–9).

अन्यच्च स्वर्णमारणमाह—

काञ्चनाररसैर्घृष्ट्वा समसूतकगन्धयोः । कज्जल्या हेमपत्राणि लेपयेत्सममात्रया ॥ १० ॥
काञ्चनारत्वचः कल्कैर्मूषायुग्मं प्रकल्पयेत् । धृत्वा तत्संपुटे गोलं मृन्मूषासंपुटे पचेत् ॥ ११ ॥
निधाय संधिरोधं च कृत्वा संशोष्य कोकिलैः । वह्निं खरतरं कुर्यादेवं दद्यात्पुटत्रयम् ॥ १२ ॥
निरुत्थं जायते भस्म सर्वकार्येषु योजयेत् । काञ्चनारप्रकारेण लाङ्गली हन्ति काञ्चनम् ॥ १३ ॥
ज्वालामुखी यथा हन्यात्तथा हन्ति मनः शिला ।

Equal parts of rasa (mercury) and gandhaka (sulphur) are macerated with the juice of kañcanāra and kajjalī prepared. This kajjalī is pasted on either sides of thin leaves of gold. Two crucibles are prepared with the paste of bark of

1. (A bhasma is said to be nirutha when the metal from which it is prepared cannot be got back from it by any means. Such a bhasma is fit to be used as medicine).

kāñcanāra. The gold leaves are kept inside one of them and covered by another. These are in turn put inside two mud crucibles, their edges sealed by mud plaster and allowed to dry. Afterwards it is kept inside a strong fire of burning coal. When the entire heap burns out and cools, the contents of the crucibles are taken out. This process repeated three times yields a niruthabhasma of gold which can be used for all purposes. Lāṅgalī, jwālāmukhī or manshila may be used instead of kāñcanāra to prepare bhasma of gold (10–14).

अथान्यदपि स्वर्णमारणप्रकारमाह—

शिलासिन्दूरयोश्चूर्णं समयोरर्कदुग्धकैः ॥ १४ ॥

सप्तैव भावना दद्याच्छोषयेच्च पुनः पुनः । ततस्तु गालिते हेम्नि कल्कोऽयं दीयते समः ॥ १५ ॥

पुनर्धमेदतितरां यथा कल्को विलीयते । एवं वेलात्रयं दद्यात्कल्कं हेममृतिर्भवेत् ॥ १६ ॥

Equal parts of shila and sindūra are macerated with milky juice of arka plant and dried. The process is repeated seven times. Gold is melted in a crucible and equal quantity of the above powder is added to it till the total mass gets well mixed and allowed to cool. This process repeated three times kills the gold (yields good gold bhasma) (14–16).

अथान्यप्रकारमाह —

पारावतमलैर्लिम्पेदथवा कुक्कुटोद्भवैः । हेमपत्राणि तेषां च प्रदद्यादन्तरान्तरम् ॥ १७ ॥

गन्धचूर्णं समं धृत्वा शरावयुग्मसंपुटे । प्रदद्यात्कुक्कुटपुटं पञ्चभिर्गोमयोपलैः ॥ १८ ॥

एवं नवपुटान्दद्याद्दशमं च महापुटम् । त्रिंशद्वनोपलैर्देयं जायते हेमभस्मकम् ॥ १९ ॥

(सुवर्णं च भवेत्स्वादु तिक्तं स्निग्धं हिमं गुरु । बुद्धिविद्यास्मृतिकरं विषहारि रसायनम्) ॥ २० ॥

Thin leaves of gold are covered on either side with the paste of excreta of pegion or cock and dried. They are then kept in a mud plate and covered with powdered gandhaka (sulphur) all over, another mud plate is kept inverted ever the first one and both sealed with mud plaster and dried. The mud plates are kept inside five cowdung heaps and set fire. This is one kukkuṭapuṭa and nine such puṭas are given. A mahāpuṭa with thirty cowdung heaps is given as the tenth. By this method also one can obtain good gold bhasma. Suvarṇa (gold) is swādu (sweet), tikta (bitter), snigdha (unctous), hima (cold), guru (hard to digest), increases buddhi (intellegence), vidyā (common sense) and smṛti (memory), is viṣaharī (anti-poisonous) and rasāyana (rejuvinator) (17–20).

इदानीं रौप्यमारणं प्रकटयन्नाह—

भागैकं तालकं मर्द्यं जम्बेनाम्लेन केनचित् । तेन भागत्रयं तारपत्राणि परिलेपयेत् ॥ २१ ॥

धृत्वा मूषापुटे रुद्ध्वा पुटेत् त्रिंशद्वनोपलैः । समुद्धृत्य पुनस्तालं दत्त्वा रुद्ध्वा पुटे पचेत् ॥२२॥

एवं चतुर्दशपुटैस्तारं भस्म प्रजायते ।

One part of tālaka is macerated with the juice of jambīra and coated over thin leaves of silver thrice the weight of tālaka; leaves are kept inside a crucible and tightly sealed and subjected to puṭa with thirty cowdung heaps. Fourteen such puṭas with fresh tālaka every time, yields a good bhasma of silver (21–22).

अपरमपि तारमारणमाह—
स्नुहीक्षीरेण संपिष्टं माक्षिकं तेन लेपयेत् ॥ २३ ॥
तालकस्य प्रकारेण तारपत्राणि बुद्धिमान् । पुटेच्चतुर्दशपुटैस्तारं भस्म प्रजायते ॥ २४ ॥

Mākṣika made into a paste with milky sap of snuhī, applied to silver leaves and subjected to puṭa as above, yields bhasma of silver with fourteen puṭas only (23–24).

पीतलोहमारणमाह—
अर्कक्षीरेण संपिष्टो गन्धकस्तेन लेपयेत् । समेनारस्य पत्राणि शुद्धान्यम्लद्रवैर्मुहुः ॥ २५ ॥
ततो मूषापुटे धृत्वा पुटेद्गजपुटेन च । एवं पुटद्वयेनैव भस्मारं भवति ध्रुवम् ॥ २६ ॥
आरवत्कांस्यमप्येवं भस्मतां याति निश्चितम् ।

Gandhaka is made into a paste with sap of arka plant and cover thin leaves of brass (both of equal weight, washed clean with any sour juice). Leaves are placed inside a crucible sealed and subjected to gajapuṭa. With only two such puṭas, bhasma of brass can be obtained. Even kāmsya (bronze) bhasma can be obtained by this process (25–26).

अपरमप्याह—
अर्कक्षीरवदाजं स्यात्क्षीरनिर्गुण्डिका तथा ॥ २७ ॥
ताम्ररीतिध्वनिवधे समगन्धकयोगतः ।

Equal quantities of gandhaka (macerated) with goats milk and used instead will also convert tāmra (copper), rīti (brass) and dhwani (bronze) into bhasma (27).

सम्प्रति ताम्रमारणं दर्शयन्नाह—
सूक्ष्माणि ताम्रपत्राणि कृत्वा संस्वेदयेद्बुधः । वासरत्रयमम्लेन ततः खल्वे विनिक्षिपेत् ॥ २८ ॥
पादांशं सूतकं दत्त्वा याममम्लेन मर्दयेत् । तत उद्धृत्य पत्राणि लेपयेद्द्विगुणेन च ॥ २९ ॥
गन्धकेनाम्लघृष्टेन तस्य कुर्याच्च गोलकम् । ततः पिष्ट्वा च मीनाक्षीं चाङ्गेरीं वा पुनर्नवाम् ॥ ३० ॥
तत्कल्केन बहिर्गोलं लेपयेदङ्गुलोन्मितम् । धृत्वा तद्गोलकं भाण्डे शरावेण च रोधयेत् ॥ ३१ ॥
वालुकाभिः प्रपूर्याथ विभूतिलवणाम्बुभिः । दत्त्वा भांडमुखे मुद्रां ततश्चुल्ल्यां विपाचयेत् ॥ ३२ ॥
क्रमवृद्धाग्निना सम्यग्यावद्यामचतुष्टयम् । स्वाङ्गशीतलमुद्धृत्य मर्दयेत्सूरणद्रवैः ॥ ३३ ॥
दिनैकं गोलकं कुर्यादर्धगन्धेन लेपयेत् । सघृतेन ततो मूषां पुटे गजपुटे पचेत् ॥ ३४ ॥
स्वाङ्गशीतं समुद्धृत्य मृतं ताम्रं शुभं भवेत् । वान्तिं भ्रान्तिं क्लमं मूर्च्छां न करोति कदाचन ॥ ३५ ॥

Thin leaves of copper are boiled for three days in a sour juice. Later on it is macerated in a morter with quarter it's weight of pārada (mercury) and a sour juice for another three days. Gandhaka (sulphur) twice the quantity of copper is made into a paste with any sour juice and covered over the copperleaves, which are then made into a ball. A paste prepared with mīnākṣī, caṅgerī or punarnavā is covered over the copper ball and slightly dried. The ball is then kept inside a crucible and sealed, which is placed inside a pot containing sand. The mouth of the pot is sealed with plaster of soft clay and salt water. The pot is then kept over on an oven and heated in increasing fire for a period of four yāmas (12 hours). After cooling, the copper is taken out and macerated with juice of sūraṇa kanda for one day and made into a ball. Half its weight of gandhaka macerated with ghee is given as a covering over the mass, which is kept inside a crucible, sealed and subjected to fire in a gajapuṭa. After it cools off it is taken out and used. This bhasma of copper will never produce vomitting, giddiness, debility or unconciousness (28–36).

अथ सीसकमारण माह—

ताम्बूलीरससंपिष्टशिलालेपात्पुनः पुनः ॥ ३६ ॥
द्वात्रिंशद्भिः पुटैर्नागो निरुत्थो याति भस्मताम् ।

Manashila macerated with juice of tāmbūlī leaves and applied over thin leaves of nāga (lead), converts it into a nirutha bhasma with thirtytwo gajapuṭas (36–37).

अथापरमपि नागमारण माह—

अश्वत्थचिञ्चात्वक्चूर्णं चतुर्थांशेन निक्षिपेत् ॥ ३७ ॥
मृत्पात्रे द्राविते नागे लोहदर्व्या प्रचालयेत् । यामैकेन भवेद्भस्म तत्तुल्यां च मनः शिलाम् ॥ ३८ ॥
काञ्जिकेन द्वयं पिष्ट्वा पचेद्दृढपुटेन च । स्वाङ्गशीतं पुनः पिष्ट्वा शिलया काञ्जिकेन च ॥ ३९ ॥
पुनः पुटेच्छरावाभ्यामेवं षष्टिपुटैर्मृतिः ।

Nāga (lead) is melted over fire in a mud plate adding powder of bark of aswatha and ciñcā one fourth the quantity of lead and fried with an iron laddle. Within one yāma lead becomes a bhasma. It is then macerated with equal quantity of manashila and sour gruel, made into cakes, kept inside mud plates, sealed with mud plaster and subjected to gajapuṭa; sixty such puṭas with fresh manashila each time will yield a good bhasma of lead (37–40).

इदानीं वङ्गमारणं दर्शयन्नाह—

मृत्पात्रे द्राविते बङ्गे चिंञ्चाश्वत्थत्वचो रजः ॥ ४० ॥
क्षिप्त्वा क्षिप्त्वा चतुर्थांशमयोदर्व्या प्रचालयेत् । ततो द्वियाममात्रेण वङ्गभस्म प्रजायते ॥ ४१ ॥
अथ भस्मसमं तालं क्षिप्त्वाम्लेन प्रमर्दयेत् । ततो गजपुटे पक्त्वा पुनरम्लेन मर्दयेत् ॥ ४२ ॥
तालेन दशमांशेन याममेकं ततः पुटेत् । एवं दशपुटैः पक्वो वङ्गस्तु म्रियते ध्रुवम् ॥ ४३ ॥

Vaṅga (tin) is melted over fire in a mud plate and quarter its weight of powder of bark of aswatha and ciñcā are added and fried with the help of an iron laddle. Within two yāmas (six hours) of such frying a bhasma of tin is obtained. It is next macerated with equal quantity of tālaka and any sour juice; rolled into a ball, kept inside two mudplates which are sealed with mud plaster, slighty dried and subjected to a gajapuṭa. After cooling it is taken out, macerated with one tenth its weight of tālaka and a sour juice and subjected to second puṭa. Ten such puṭas will certainly kill vaṅga (yields a good bhasma of tin) (40–43).

अथ लोहमारणमाह—

शुद्धं लोहभवं चूर्णं पातालगरुडीरसैः । मर्दयित्वा पुटेद्वह्नौ दद्यादेवं पुटत्रयम् ॥ ४४ ॥
पुटत्रयं कुमार्या च कुठारकुलत्थरसैः । पुटषट्कं ततो दद्यादेवं तीक्ष्णमृतिर्भवेत् ॥ ४५ ॥

Purified loha cūrṇa (iron filings) are macerated with the juice of pātālagaruḍī; made into thin discs, kept inside mud plates, sealed and subjected to gajapuṭa. Three such puṭas are given first. Next six puṭas with juice of kumārī, kuthāra (kind of kulatha) and kuṭaja two in each juice separately is given. By so doing, iron (magnetic iron also) gets killed (44–45).

अन्यच्चेत्यपरमपि मारणमाह—

क्षिपेद्वा दशमांशेन दरदं तीक्ष्णचूर्णतः । मर्दयेत्कन्यकाद्रावैर्यामयुग्मं ततः पुटेत् ॥ ४६ ॥
एवं सप्तपुटैर्मृत्युं लोहचूर्णमवाप्नुयात् । रसैः कुठारच्छिन्नायाः पातालगरुडीरसैः ॥ ४७ ॥
स्तन्येन चार्कदुग्धेन तीक्ष्णस्यैवं मृतिर्भवेत् ।

One part of purified powder of tīkṣṇa loha (magnetic iron) and one tenth of it's weight of darada (hiṅgula) are macerated with juice of kanyakā for two yāmas (six hours) made into discs, put inside mud plates and subjected to gajapuṭa. Seven such puṭas will kill the iron. Tīkṣṇa loha (magnetic iron) will get killed by the same way by the use of juice of kuthara, chinnā, patālagaruḍī, breast milk and sap of arka plant (46–48).

अन्यदपि मारणमाह—

सूतकाद्द्विगुणं गन्धं दत्त्वा कुर्याच्च कज्जलीम् ॥ ४८ ॥
द्वयोः समं लोहचूर्णं मर्दयेत्कन्यकाद्रवैः । यामयुग्मं ततः पिण्डं कृत्वा ताम्रस्य पात्रके ॥ ४९ ॥
घर्मे धृत्वा रुबूकस्य पत्रैराच्छादयेद्बुधः । यामार्धेनोष्णतां भूयाद्धान्यराशौ न्यसेत्ततः ॥ ५० ॥
दत्त्वोपरि शरावं तु त्रिदिनान्ते समुद्धरेत् । पिष्ट्वा च गालयेद्वस्त्रादेवं वारितरं भवेत् ॥ ५१ ॥
एवं सर्वाणि लोहानि स्वर्णादीन्यपि मारयेत् । शिलागन्धार्कदुग्धाक्ताः स्वर्णाद्याः सर्वधातवः ॥ ५२॥
म्रियन्ते द्वादशपुटैः सत्यं गुरुवचो यथा ।

Kajjalī is prepared with one part of sūta (mercury), and two parts of gandhaka (sulphur), Iron filings equal to the weight of kajjalī are added and all the three macerated with juice of kanyakā for two yāmas (six hours), made into a ball and covered with leaves of rubūka (castor plant) and kept in hot sun for half a yāma (½ hrs). After it becomes hot, the ball is kept inside a heap of grains. After three days it is taken out, iron filings are scraped, powdred nicely, filtered through cloth and used. By this method gold and all other metals can be converted to their bhasmas. Gold and all other metals macerated with manashila, gandhaka and sap of arka plant and subjected to twelve puṭas successively will become killed (gets into bhasma from) as doubtlessly as the words of the preceptor(48–52).

अथोपधातुशोधनमारणं, ते के उपधातवः ? इति दर्शयन्नाह—

माक्षिकं तुत्थकाभ्रे च नीलाञ्जनशिलालकाः ॥ ५३ ॥

रसकश्चेति विज्ञेया एते सप्तोपधातवः ।

Mākṣika (pyrites), tutha (copper sulphate), abhraka (mica), nilāñjana (antimony), manashila (realgar), tālaka (orpiment) and rasaka (calamite) these seven are know as *upadhātus* (53–54).

अथ माक्षिकशोधनमारणम्—

माक्षिकस्य त्रयो भागा भागैकं सैन्धवस्य च ॥ ५४ ॥

मातुलुङ्गद्रवैर्वाथ जम्बीरोत्थद्रवैः पचेत् । चालयेल्लोहजे पात्रे यावत्पात्रं तु लोहितम् ॥ ५५ ॥

भवेत्ततस्तु संशुद्धिं स्वर्णमाक्षिकमृच्छति । कुलत्थस्य कषायेण घृष्ट्वा तैलेन वा पुटेत् ॥ ५६ ॥

तक्रेणवाजमूत्रेण म्रियते स्वर्णमाक्षिकम् ।

Three parts of mākṣika and one part of saindhava are cooked with juice of mātuluṅga or jambīra in an iron vessel till the vessel become red hot. By this the mākṣikā gets purified. Purified mākṣika is macerated with the decoction of kulatha, tilataila, takra or goat's urine and subjected to gajapuṭa becomes killed (54–56).

कर्कोटीमेषशृङ्गयुत्थैर्द्रवैर्जम्बीरजैर्दिनम् ॥ ५७ ॥

भावयेदातपे तीव्रे विमला शुध्यति ध्रुवम् ।

Vimala (another variety of mākṣika) macerated with juice of karkoṭī, meṣaśṛṅgī and jambīra one day in each and kept in hot Sun becomes purified (57–58).

अथ तुत्थकशोधनमाह—

विष्ठया मर्दयेत्तुत्थं मार्जारककपोतयोः ॥ ५८ ॥

दशांशं टङ्कणं दत्वा पचेन्मृदुपुटेन तु । पुटं दध्ना पुटं क्षौद्रैर्देयं तुत्थविशुद्धये ॥ ५९ ॥

Tutha (copper sulphate) is macerated with the excreta of cat and pegion and one tenth part of taṅkaṇa is added, placed inside earthen plates sealed and subjected to a laghupuṭa. Second and third puṭas are done by using curds and honey respectively. By this tutha becomes purified and fit for use (58–59)

अथाभ्रकशोधनम्—

कृष्णाभ्रकं धमेद्वह्नौ ततः क्षीरे विनिक्षिपेत् । भिन्नपत्रं तु तत्कृत्वा तण्डुलीयाम्लयोर्द्रवैः ॥ ६० ॥
भावयेदष्टयामं तदेवं शुद्धयति चाभ्रकम् ।

Kṛṣṇābhraka (black mica ore) is heated over strong fire and immersed into milk several times. When it attains powder from it is macerated for eight yāmas (24 hours) with the juice of tāṇḍulīya and any sour juice. By this method abhraka becomes purified (60-61).

अथ मारणम्—

कृत्वा धान्याभ्रकं तत्तु शोषयित्वाथ मर्दयेत् ॥ ६१ ॥
अर्कक्षीरैर्दिनं खल्वे चक्राकारं च कारयेत् । वेष्टयेदर्कपत्रैश्च सम्यग्गजपुटे पचेत् ॥ ६२ ॥
पुनर्मर्द्यं पुनः पाच्यं सप्तवारं प्रयत्नतः । ततो वटजटाक्वाथैस्तद्वद्देयं पुटत्रयम् ॥ ६३ ॥
म्रियते नात्र संदेहः सर्वयोगेषु योजयेत् ।

Dhanyābhraka is then prepared[1] and macerated with the juice of sap of arka plant made into discs, covered with leaves of arka plant kept inside earthen plates, sealed and subjected to seven gajapuṭas. Next, three puṭas are given in decoction of vātajata (areal roots of baniyan tree). By three puṭas abhraka gets killed (becomes bhasma) without doubt, fit to be used in all recipes (61–63).

तुल्यं घृतं मृताभ्रेण लोहपात्रे विपाचयेत् ॥ ६४ ॥
घृते जीर्णे तदभ्रं तु सर्वयोगेषु योजयेत् ।

Equal quantities of abhraka bhasma and ghee are fried in an iron pan till the ghee dries up. This bhasma is used in all recipes (64).

मृतं त्वभ्रं हरेन्मृत्युं जरापलितनाशनम् ॥ ६५ ॥
अनुपानैश्च संयुक्तं तत्तद्रोगहरं परम् ।

Abhraka bhasma wards off death, oldage, grey hairs and all other diseases when used with appropriate vehicles (65–66).

अथान्यप्रकारोऽभ्रकमारणस्य तमपि व्याचष्टे—

शुद्धं धान्याभ्रकं मुस्तं शुण्ठीषड्भागयोजितम ॥ ६६ ॥
मर्दयेत्काञ्जिकेनैव दिनं चित्रकजै रसैः । ततो गजपुटं दद्यात्तस्मादुद्धृत्य मर्दयेत् ॥ ६७ ॥
त्रिफलावारिणा तद्वत्पुटेदेवं पुटैस्त्रिभिः । बलागोमूत्रमुसलीतुलसीसूरणद्रवैः ॥ ६८ ॥
मर्दितं पुटितं वह्नौ त्रिस्त्रिवेलं व्रजेन्मृतम् ।

1. (Powder of abhraka and paddy are tied in a gunny bag, immersed in a vessel containing sour gruel, rice-wash or plain-water and kept overnight. Next morning the bag is massaged inside the liquid so that fine powder of abhraka exudes out through the pores of the bag and collects in the vessel. This is later taken out, dried in sun. Fine shining powder of mica thus obtained, is called dhanyābhraka).

Purified dhanyābhraka with six parts it's weight of mustā and shunṭhī are macerated with sour gruel and juice of citraka for one day each, made into discs and subjected to gajapuṭa. The next three puṭas are to be done with decoction of triphalā and further three puṭas with juice of balā, gomūtra, musalī, tulasī and sūraṇa together. By these, abhraka becomes converted to bhasma (66–69).

अभ्रसत्वप्रकारः—

धान्याभ्रकस्य भागैकं द्वौ भागौ टङ्कणस्य च । पिष्ट्वा तदन्धमूषायां रुद्ध्वा तीव्राग्निना पचेत् ॥ ६९ ॥
स्वभावशीतलं चूर्णं सर्वयोगेषु योजयेत् ।

One part of dhanyābhraka, and two parts of ṭaṅkaṇa are kept in an andhamūṣā (crucible covered over by another and both tightly sealed and dried). Later they are kept in a coal furnace and subjected to high heat. After the fire cools of it is taken out. The powder inside the crucible–satva (the essence of abhraka) can be used in all recipes for treatment of diseases (69–70).

अथ नीलाञ्जनम्—

नीलाञ्जनं चूर्णयित्वा जम्बीरद्रवभावितम् ॥ ७० ॥
दिनैकमातपे शुद्धं भवेत्कार्येषु योजयेत् । एवं गैरिककासीसटङ्कणानि वराटिका ॥ ७१ ॥
तौरी शङ्खं च कङ्कुष्ठं शुद्धिमायाति निश्चितम् ।

Nīlāñjana (antimony sulphide) macerated for one full day with juice of jambīra and dried in sun becomes purified and fit to be used. By the same process gairika, kāsīra, ṭaṅkaṇa, varāṭikā, tuvarī, shaṅkha and kaṅkuṣṭha—all become purified (70–72).

अथ मनःशिलाशोधनम्—

पचेत्त्र्यहमजामूत्रैर्दोलायन्त्रे मनःशिलाम् ॥ ७२ ॥
भावयेत्सप्तधा पित्तैरजायाः शुद्धिमृच्छति ।

Manashila is tied in a cloth, hung inside a pot containing goat's urine and boiled for three days (dolāyantra method). Later it is macerated for seven times with the bile of goat, each time using fresh bile. By this, manashila becomes purified (72–73).

अथ तालकशुद्धिः—

तालकं कणशः कृत्वा सचूर्णं काञ्जिके क्षिपेत् ॥ ७३ ॥
दोलायन्त्रेण यामैकं ततः कूष्माण्डजैर्द्रवैः । तिलतैले पचेद्यामं यामं च त्रिफलाजलैः ॥ ७४ ॥
एवं यन्त्रे चतुर्यामं पाच्यं शुध्यति तालकम् ।

Tālaka made into powder is tied in a cloth and kept hanging inside a pot containing kāñjika (sour gruel) and boiled for one yāma (3 hours). It is later boiled in juice of kūṣmāṇḍa, taila and decoction of triphalā separately for one yāma each. By this tālaka gets purified (73–75).

अथ रसकशुद्धिः—

नरमूत्रैश्च गोमूत्रैः सप्ताहं रसकं पचेत् ॥ ७५ ॥
दोलायन्त्रेण शुद्धिः स्यात्ततः कार्येषु योजयेत् ।

Rasaka gets purified if boiled for seven times by dolāyantra method using either human urine or cow's urine (75–76).

अथेदानीं समुदायेन सत्वनिर्गमं प्रकटयन्नाह—

लाक्षा मीना पयश्छागं टङ्कणं मृगश्टङ्गकम् ॥ ७६ ॥
पिण्याकं सर्षपाः शिग्रुर्गुञ्जोर्णागुडसैन्धवाः । यवास्तिक्ता घृतं क्षौद्रं यथालाभं विचूर्णयेत् ॥ ७७ ॥
एभिर्विमिश्रिताः सर्वे धातवो गाढवह्निना । मूषाध्माताः प्रजायन्ते मुक्तसत्वा न संशयः ॥ ७८ ॥

All the dhātus (minerals or ores) leave off their satwa (essence) if they are kept in a crucible, mixed with the powder of lākṣā, fish, goats milk, ṭankaṇa, mṛga śṛṅga, piṇyāka (oil cake of sesame), sarṣap, shigru, guñjā, urṇa, guḍa, saindhava, yavatiktā, ghṛta, kṣoudra—all or which ever is available and subjected to strong heat (76-78).

अथ रत्नानां शोधनमारणम्—

कुलत्थकोद्रवक्वाथैर्दोलायन्त्रे विपाचयेत् । व्याघ्रीकन्दगतं वज्रं त्रिदिनं तद्विशुध्यति ॥ ७९ ॥
तप्तं तप्तं तु तद्वज्रं खरमूत्रैर्निषेचयेत् । पुनस्तप्यं पुनः सेच्यमेवं कुर्यात्त्रिसप्तधा ॥ ८० ॥
मत्कुणैस्तालकं पिष्ट्वा यावद्भवति गोलकम् । तद्गोले निहितं वज्रं तद्गोलं वह्निना धमेत् ॥ ८१ ॥
सिञ्चयेदश्वमूत्रेण तद्गोले च क्षिपेत्पुनः । रुद्ध्वा ध्मातं पुनः सेच्यमेवं कुर्यात्त्रिसप्तधा ॥ ८२ ॥
एवं च म्रियते वज्रं चूर्णं सर्वत्र योजयेत् ।

Vajra (diamond) is kept inside vyāghrī kanda and boiled in dolāyantra for three days using decoction of kulatha and kodrava. By this varja gets purified. Such purified vajra is heated over strong fire and immersed in donkey's urine, repeating the process of twenty-one times.

Tālaka is macerated with blood of bed bugs to a thick paste and given a coating over purified vajra, which is then kept in a crucible, heated strong and immersed in horse's urine. Repeating this process for twentyone times gives a fine bhasma of vajra which can be used in all diseases (79–83).

अथान्यदपि वज्रमारणमाह—

हिङ्गुसैन्धवसंयुक्ते क्वाथे कौलत्थजे क्षिपेत् ॥ ८३ ॥
तप्तं तप्तं पुनर्वज्रं भूयाच्चूर्णं त्रिसप्तधा ।

Heated vajra may be immersed in decoction of kulatha mixed with hiṅgu and saindhava for twenty one times, to get a fine powder of vajra.

अपरमपि वज्रमारणमाह—

मण्डूकं कांस्यजे पात्रे निगृह्य स्थापयेत्सुधीः ॥ ८४ ॥

स भीतो मूत्रयेत्तत्र तन्मूत्रे वज्रमावपेत् । तप्तं तप्तं च बहुधा वज्रस्यैवं मृतिर्भवेत् ॥ ८५ ॥

Impound a frog in a vessel of bell metal and collect it's urine. Heated vajra dipped into this urine also makes it to become nice powder (84–85).

इदानीं वैक्रान्तमारणमाह—

वैक्रान्तं वज्रवच्छोध्यं नीलं वा लोहितं तथा । हयमूत्रेण तत्सेच्यं तप्तं तप्तं द्विसप्तधा ॥ ८६ ॥

ततस्तु मेषदुग्धस्य पञ्चाङ्गे गोलकं क्षिपेत् । पुटेन्मूषापुटे रुद्ध्वा कुर्यादेवं च सप्तधा ॥ ८७ ॥

वैक्रान्तं भस्मतां याति वज्रस्थाने नियोजयेत् ।

Blue or red vaikrānta (tourmuline) is purified in the same way as of vajra. Next it is heated strongly and immersed into hore's urine for 14 times. It is then given a covering with a paste prepared with all the five parts of meṣa dugdhi plant, kept inside a crucible subjected to strong heat in a gajapuṭa repeating the process for seven times. This vaikrānta bhasma finally obtained may be used as a substitute for vajra bhasma (86–88).

इदानीं शेषरत्नशोधनमारणमप्याह—

स्वेदयेद्दोलिकायन्त्रे जयन्त्याः स्वरसेन च ॥ ८८ ॥

मणिमुक्ताप्रवालानि यामैकं शोधनं भवेत् । कुमार्यास्तण्डुलीयेन स्तन्येन च निषेचयेत् ॥ ८९ ॥

प्रत्येकं सप्तवेलं च सप्ततप्तानि कृत्स्नशः । मौक्तिकानि प्रवालानि तथा रत्नान्यशेषतः ॥ ९० ॥

क्षणाद्विविधवर्णानि म्रियन्ते नात्र संशयः । उक्तमाक्षिकवन्मुक्ताः प्रवालानि च मारयेत् ॥ ९१ ॥

वज्रवत्सर्वरत्नानि शोधयेन्मारयेत्तथा ।

Maṇis (semi precious stones; gems) muktā (pearls) and pravāla (corals), become purified by boiling them in dolayantra for one yāma using juice of jayanti.

All the ratnas (gems) become killed (gets into bhasma) if heated strongly and immersed in each of the juice of kumārī, tāṇḍlīyaka and stanya (breast milk) for seven times. Pravāla and muktā are converted into bhasma in the same way as that of mākṣika described earlier. Purification and killing of all ratnas (gems) are similar to that described for vajra (88–92).

अथेदानीं शिलाजतुशोधनप्रकारं दर्शयन्नाह—

शिलाजतु समानीय ग्रीष्मतप्तशिलाच्युतम् ॥ ९२ ॥

गोदुग्धैस्त्रिफलाक्वाथैर्भृङ्गद्रावैश्च मर्दयेत् । आतपे दिनमेकैकं तच्छुद्धं शुद्धतां व्रजेत् ॥ ९३ ॥

Shilājatu that exude out of stone by the heat of grīṣma ṛtu (summer) is collected and macerated separately with cow's milk, decoction of triphalā and juice of bhriṅgarāja and dried in the sun. By this Shilājatu becomes purified (92–93).

अथान्यकरणप्रकारमाह—

मुख्यां शिलाजतुशिलां सूक्ष्मखण्डप्रकल्पिताम् । निक्षिप्यात्युष्णपानीये यामैकं स्थापयेत्सुधीः ॥९४॥
मर्दयित्वा ततो नीरं गृह्णीयाद्वस्त्रगालितम् । स्थापयित्वा च मृत्पात्रे धारयेदातपे बुधः ॥ ९५ ॥
उपरिस्थं घनं यस्यात्तत्क्षिपेदन्यपात्रके । धारयेदातपे तस्मादुपरिस्थं घनं नयेत् ॥ ९६ ॥
एवं पुनः पुनर्नीत्वा द्विमासाभ्यां शिलाजतु । भूयात्कार्यक्षमं वह्नौ क्षिप्तं लिङ्गोपमं भवेत् ॥ ९७ ॥
निर्धूमं च ततः शुद्धं सर्वकर्मसु योजयेत् । अधः स्थितं च यच्छेषं तस्मिन्नीरं विनिक्षिपेत् ॥ ९८ ॥
विमर्द्य धारयेद्धर्मे पूर्ववच्चैव तन्नयेत् ।

Stones which exude shilājatu are powdered and kept immersed in hot water for three hours. Later they are vigourously squeezed, filtered through cloth, collecting the water in a clean mud plate and exposed to bright sun. The scum that collects at the top is separated and dried in the sun till it becomes a hard mass in about two months time. This is fit to be used as medicine.

Good Shilājatu put on fire assumes the shape of a liṅga (round mass) and does not emit smoke.

The water which remains underneath in the earthen plate might also yield some shilājatu if kept in sun-light for a number of days. (94–99),

अथ मण्डूरकरणम्—

अक्षाङ्गारैर्धमेत्किट्टं लोहजं तद्गवां जलैः ॥ ९९ ॥
सेचयेत्तप्ततप्तं च सप्तवारं पुनः पुनः । चूर्णयित्वा ततः क्वाथैर्द्विगुणैस्त्रिफलाभवैः ॥ १०० ॥
आलोड्य भर्जयेद्वह्नौ मण्डूरं जायते वरम् ।

Maṇḍūra (the molten slag of iron) is placed in between burning coals of akṣa tree (vibhītaka), cow's urine sprinkled over the hot slag, repeating the process for seven times. It is then powdered nicely and boiled in the decoction of triphalā. Later on it is fried in a mud pan over strong fire and used as medicine (99–101).

अथ क्षारकल्पनां दर्शयितुमाह—

क्षीरवृक्षस्य काष्ठानि शुष्काण्यग्नौ प्रदीपयेत् ॥ १०१ ॥
नीत्वा तद्भस्म मृत्पात्रे क्षिप्त्वा नीरे चतुर्गुणे । विमर्द्य धारयेद्रात्रौ प्रातरच्छं जलं नयेत् ॥ १०२ ॥
तन्नीरं क्वाथयेद्वह्नौ यावत्सर्वं विशुष्यति । ततः पात्रात्समुल्लिख्य क्षारो ग्राह्यः सितप्रभः ॥ १०३ ॥
चूर्णाभः प्रतिसार्यः स्यात्पेयः स्यात्क्वाथवत्स्थितः । इति क्षारद्वयं धीमान्युक्तकार्येषु योजयेत् ॥ १०४ ॥

Dried wood of trees which exude milky sap are burnt to ashes in fire. The ash thus obtained is dissolved in four times of water in a mud pot and kept over-night. Next morning the clear supernatant water is decanted out into a clean vessel and boiled till all the water evoporates, leaving of a fine white powder at the bottom. This is known as kṣāra (alkali). It is used in two ways i.e. "Pratisārya"

(external application) and "Peya" (internal potion)—along with suitable vehicles (101–104).

इति श्री दामोदरसूनुना शार्ङ्गधराचार्येण विरचितायां शार्ङ्गधरसंहितायां मध्यमखण्डे धातुशोधनमारणं नामैकादशोऽध्यायः ॥

Thus ends the eleventh chapter.

द्वादशोऽध्यायः

CHAPTER 12

Rasādi Shodhana and Māraṇa Kalpanā

(Purification and Preparation of Mercurials)

अथेदानीं रसप्रशंसापूर्वकं तच्छोधनमारणादिमाह—

पारदः सर्वरोगाणां जेता पुष्टिकरः स्मृतः । सुदिने साधितः कुर्यात्संसिद्धिं देहलोहयोः ॥ १ ॥

Pārada (mercury) conquers all diseases and confers strength. Processed by specialists it endows control our the body and metals (1).

इदानीं रसराजस्य पर्यायनामान्याह—

रसेन्द्रः पारदः सूतो हरजः सूतको रसः । बुधैस्तस्येति नामानि ज्ञेयानि रसकर्मसु ॥ २ ॥

Rasendra, pārada, sūta, haraja, sūtaka, rasa and miśraka are its synonyms used in literature (2).

पूर्वं देहलोहयोरिति यल्लोहग्रहणं, तेषां लोहानां नवग्रहनामाङ्कितत्वेन नवसंख्याकथनमाह—

ताम्रतारारनागाश्च हेमवङ्गौ च तीक्ष्णकम् । कांस्यकं कान्तलोहं च धातवो नव ये स्मृताः ॥ ३ ॥
सूर्यादीनां ग्रहाणां ते कथिता नामभिः क्रमात् ।

Tāmra (copper), tārā (silver), ara (brass), nāga (lead), hema (gold), vaṅga (tin), tīkṣna (steel), kāṁsya (bronze) and kāntaloha (magnetic iron) are the nine dhātus (used in rasāyana process). Each one is known by the names of the nine planets respectively commencing with the Sun (3–4).

इदानीं रसशोधनकर्माह—

राजीरसोनमूषायां रसं क्षिप्त्वा विबन्धयेत् ॥ ४ ॥
वस्त्रेण दोलिकायन्त्रे स्वेदयेत्काञ्जिकैस्त्र्यहम् । दिनैकं मर्दयेत्सूतं कुमारीसंभवैर्द्रवैः ॥ ५ ॥
तथा चित्रकजैः क्वाथैर्मर्दयेदेकवासरम् । काकमाचीरसैस्तद्वद्दिनमेकं च मर्दयेत् ॥ ६ ॥
त्रिफलायास्तथा क्वाथै रसो मर्द्यः प्रयत्नतः । ततस्तेभ्यः पृथक्कुर्यात्सूतं प्रक्षाल्य काञ्जिकैः ॥ ७ ॥
ततः क्षिप्त्वा रसं खल्वे रसादर्धं च सैन्धवम् । मर्दयेन्निम्बुकरसैर्दिनमेकमनारतम् ॥ ८ ॥

ततो राजी रसोनश्च मुख्यश्च नवसादरः । एतै रससमैस्तद्वत्सूतो मर्द्यस्तुषाम्बुना ॥ ९ ॥
ततः संशोष्य चक्राभं कृत्वा लिप्त्वा च हिङ्गुना । द्विस्थालीसंपुटे धृत्वा पूरयेल्लवणेन च ॥ १० ॥
अधः स्थालीं ततो मुद्रां दद्याद्दृढतरां बुधः । विशोष्याग्निं विधायाधो निषिञ्चेदम्बुनोपरि ॥ ११ ॥
ततस्तु कुर्यात्तीव्राग्निं तदधः प्रहरत्रयम् । एवं निपातयेदूर्ध्वं रसो दोषविवर्जितः ॥ १२ ॥
अथोर्ध्वपिठरीमध्ये लग्नो ग्राह्यो रसोत्तमः ।

Rājī and rasona are made into a paste and a cruicible prepared out of it. Rasa is kept inside this and covered all over with the paste. The ball is then tied in a cloth and cooked in dolāyantra method using kañjika for three days.

Next it is macerated with the juice of kumāri, decoction of citraka, juce of kākamācī and decoction of triphalā, one day in each. It is later washed well with warm water, put in a stone pestle and morter; half it's a quantity of saindhava is added and macerated with juice of nimbu (lemon) continuously for one day.

Next it is macerated with equal quantities of rājī, rasona and navasādara along with tuṣāmbu (gruel prepared with husk of paddy and other grains) made into round discs and covered over with hiṅgu.

These discs are than kept inside a pot containing lavaṇa (salt bath), another empty pot kept inverted over and the mouths of both sealed with mud plaster. The pot containing salt is kept over the oven, and mild fire is given, for three hours, all the time keeping a thick pad of wet cloth over the top of the upper pot, frequently sprinkling water over it Later on the pots are separated carefully and the mercury adhering inside the upper pot is collected; pārada is by now, purified and fit to be used for further procedures (4–13).

अथ गन्धकशोधनम्—

लोहपात्रे विनिक्षिप्य घृतमग्नौ प्रतापयेत् ॥ १३ ॥
तप्ते घृते तत्समानं क्षिपेद्गन्धकजं रजः । विद्रुतं गन्धकं ज्ञात्वा दुग्धमध्ये विनिःक्षिपेत् ॥ १४ ॥
एवं गन्धकशुद्धिः स्यात्सर्वकार्येषु योजयेत् ।

Ghee is boiled in an iron vessel and equal quantity of powdered gandhaka (sulphur) is added to it. When the sulphur melts well it is poured into a vessel containing milk. By this process sulphur gets purified and can be used in all procedures (13–15).

इदानीं दरदशोधनमप्याह—

मेषीक्षीरेण दरदमम्लवर्गैश्च भावितम् ॥ १५ ॥
सप्तवारं प्रयत्नेन शुद्धिमायाति निश्चितम् ।

Darada (cinnabar) macerated with goats (or cow's) milk and drugs of amla varga (sour group) for seven times becomes purified (15).

अथ दरदाद्रसाकृष्टिर्भवति तामपि दर्शयन्नाह—
निम्बूरसैर्निम्बपत्ररसैर्वा याममात्रकम् ॥ १६ ॥
पिष्ट्वा दरदमूर्ध्वं च पातयेत्सूतयुक्तिवत् । ततः शुद्धरसं तस्मान्नीत्वा कार्येषु योजयेत् ॥ १७ ॥

Darada is macerated for one yāma (3 hours) in the juice of nimbu (lemon) or of leaves of nimba. Next ūrdhvapātana yantra is made use of as described earlier in the purification of sūta. (Paste is applied to the interior of the lower pot and an empty pot kept inverted over it, their mouths sealed, heat applied from below, keeping a wet cloth ovcr the top of the upper pot. Mercury vapours collect in the interior of the upper pot. Later, when the process is completed the mercury is taken out and used for further processes) (16–17).

अथोद्धृतस्य मुखकरणम्—
कालकूटो वत्सनाभः शृङ्गकश्च प्रदीपकः । हालाहलो ब्रह्मपुत्रो हारिद्रः सक्तुकस्तथा ॥ १८ ॥
सौराष्ट्रिक इति प्रोक्ता विषभेदा अमी नव । अर्कसेहुण्डधत्तूरलाङ्गलीकरवीरकम् ॥ १९ ॥
गुञ्जाहिफेनावित्येताः सप्तोपविषजातयः । एतैर्विमर्दितः सूतश्छिन्नपक्षः प्रजायते ॥ २० ॥
मुखं च जायते तस्य धातूंश्च ग्रसते क्षणात् ।

Kalakūṭa, vatsanābha, śṛṅgaka, pradīpaka, halāhala, brahmaputra, haridrā, saktuka, saurāṣṭrka—these nine are *visas* (powerful poisonous plants); arka, sehuṇḍa, dhattūra, lāṅgalī, karavīra, guñjā and ahiphena—these seven are *upaviṣas* (less poisonous plants). Mercury macerated in each one of them looses its wings (chinna pakṣa) and gets the appetite (mukha) and quickly devours the dhātus (becomes amalgam with metals), (dhatugrasa). (18–21).

अन्यदपि मुखकरणमाह—
अथवा कटुकक्षारौ राजी लवणपञ्चकम् ॥ २१ ॥
रसोनो नवसारश्च शिग्रुश्चैकत्र चूर्णितः । समांशैः पारदादेतैर्जम्बीरेण द्रवेण वा ॥ २२ ॥
निम्बुतोयैः काञ्जिकैर्वा सोष्णखल्वे विमर्दयेत् । अहोरात्रत्रयेण स्याद्रसे धातुचरं मुखम् ॥ २३ ॥

Trikaṭu, the two kṣāras, rājī, the five lavaṇas, rasona, navasāra and śigru are powdered; mixed with equal quantity of rasa (mercury) and both macerated in an iron pestle and morter warmed up with mild fire, along with the juice of nimbu or kañjika. Maceration is done continuously for three days and nights will make the mercury devour all metals (21–23).

अपरमपि मुखकरं दर्शयितुमाह—
अथवा बिन्दुलीकीटै रसो मर्द्यस्त्रिवासरम् । लवणाम्लैर्मुखं तस्य जायते धातुहृत्त्वरा ॥ २४ ॥

Pārad (mercury) macerated with bindulī kīṭa (a kind of insect) along with lavaṇas and amlas, for three days becomes capable of devouring the dhātus quickly (24).

इदानीं गन्धकजारणनिमित्तं कर्म दर्शयन्नाह—

अथ कच्छपयन्त्रेण गन्धजारणमुच्यते। मृत्कुण्डे निक्षिपेत्तोयं तन्मध्ये च शरावकम् ॥ २५ ॥
महत्कुण्डपिधानाभं मध्ये मेखलया युतम्। लिप्त्वा च मेखलामध्यं चूर्णनात्र रसं क्षिपेत् ॥ २६ ॥
रसस्योपरि गन्धस्य रजो दद्यात्समांशकम्। दत्त्वोपरि शरावं च भस्ममुद्रां प्रदापयेत् ॥ २७ ॥
तस्योपरि पुटं दद्याच्चतुर्भिर्गोमयोपलैः। एवं पुनः पुनर्गन्धं षड्गुणं जारयेद्बुधः ॥ २८ ॥
गन्धे जीर्णे भवेत्सूतस्तीक्ष्णाग्निः सर्वकर्मसु।

Further on, gandhaka jāraṇa using kachapa yantra will be described.

An earthen plate which has a small depression in the centre is taken and a coating of slaked lime is made inside the depression. Purified mercury is kept in it and covered with equal quantity of powdered sulphur. The depression is sealed with a plaster of ash. This plate is placed on pot containing water in such a way that its entire lower surface is touching the water. Another plate is covered over the first plate, the mouths of all are well sealed with mud plaster. After it dries the pot is placed under the ground and fire is kindled on the top with only four cow-dung heaps. After it cools off, the mercury is taken out and process repeated for six times. The mercury which has been treated thus with six times its quantity of sulphur becomes capable of eating all metals and giving all other effects (25–29).

अथ पारदमारणम्—

धूमसारं रसं तोरीं गन्धकं नवसादरम् ॥ २९ ॥
यामैकं मर्दयेदम्लैर्भागं कृत्वा समांशकम्। काचकुप्यां विनिक्षिप्य तां च मृद्वस्त्रमुद्रया ॥ ३० ॥
विलिप्य परितो वक्त्रे मुद्रां दत्त्वा च शोषयेत्। अधःसच्छिद्रपिठरीमध्ये कूपीं निवेशयेत् ॥ ३१ ॥
पिठरीं वालुकापूरैर्भृत्वा चाकूपिकागलम्। निवेश्य चुल्ल्यां तदधः कुर्याद्वह्निं शनैः शनैः ॥ ३२ ॥
तस्मादप्यधिकं किंचित्पावकं ज्वालयेत्क्रमात्। एवं द्वादशभिर्यामैर्म्रियते सूतकोत्तमः ॥ ३३ ॥
स्फोटयेत्स्वाङ्गशीतं तमूर्ध्वगं गन्धकं त्यजेत्। अधःस्थं मृतसूतं च सर्वकर्मसु योजयेत् ॥ ३४ ॥

Dhūmasāra (chimneysoot), pārada (mercury), tuvarī, gandhaka and navasādara each equal parts are macerated for one yāma (3 hours) with any sour juice. It is then filled into a glass bottle which is covered over with thick mud plaster and dried. The bottle is then kept in a sand bath inside a pot, keeping the mouth of the bottle above the level of the sand. Pot is now kept over an oven and heat applied continuously for twelve yāmas (36 hours) increasing its intensity gradually. Afterwards, when it cools off, the bottle is taken out, broken open, the gandhaka (sulphur) adhereing at the top is discarded. The bhasma of pārada settled at the bottom is nicely powered and used for all purposes (29–34).

अन्यदपि रसमारणमाह—

अपामार्गस्य बीजानां मूषायुग्मं प्रकल्पयेत्। तत्संपुटे न्यसेत्सूतं मलयूदुग्धमिश्रितम् ॥ ३५ ॥

द्रोणपुष्पीप्रसूनानि विडङ्गमिरिमेदकः । एतच्चूर्णमधोर्ध्वं च दत्त्वा मुद्रां प्रदीयते ॥ ३६ ॥
तं गोलं सन्धयेत्सम्यग्मृन्मूषासंपुटे सुधीः । मुद्रां दत्त्वां शोषयित्वा ततो गजपुटे पचेत् ॥ ३७ ॥
एकमेवपुटेनैव जायते भस्म सूतकम् ।

Sūṭa (mercury) is macerated with the sap of malayū (Kāṣṭhaudambarikā) tree and rolled into a ball. Two crucibles are prepared with the seeds of apāmārga plant made into a paste with water. Mercury ball is kept inside these crucibles, their edges sealed and dried. Flowers of droṇa puṣpī, viḍaṅga, and irimedaka are powdered nicely, spread over an earthen plate, the crucibles kept in it, covered with some more powder. Another plate is kept inverted over the first one. Their edges sealed with mud plaster and dried. Later these plates are subjected to gajapuṭa. Mercury becomes bhasma even with only one such puṭa (35–38).

अन्यदपि रसमारणं प्रकटयन्नाह—

काष्ठोदुम्बरिकादुग्धै रसं किंचिद्विमर्दयेत् ॥ ३८ ॥
तद्दुग्धघृष्टहिङ्गोश्च षामूयुग्मं प्रकल्पयेत् । क्षिप्त्वा तत्संपुटे सूतं तत्र मुद्रां प्रदापयेत् ॥ ३९ ॥
धृत्वा तं गोलकं प्राज्ञो मृन्मूषासंपुटेऽधिके । पचेन्मृदुपुटेनैव सूतको याति भस्मताम् ॥ ४० ॥

Pārada (mercury) is macerated with the sap of kāṣthaudumbarikā tree and rolled into a ball. Hiṅgu is made into a paste with the same juice and two crucibles are made out of it. Mercury ball is enclosed within them and sealed. The crucibles are later kept in between two mud plates, which are sealed and subjected to mṛdupuṭa (small heap of cowdung). Mercury attains bhasma form by one such puṭa itself (38–40).

अपरमपि पारदमारणं दर्शयन्नाह—

नागवल्लीरसैर्घृष्टः कर्कोटीकन्दगर्भितः । मृण्मूषासंपुटे पक्त्वा सूतो यात्येव भस्मताम् ॥ ४१ ॥

Rasa (mercury) is macerated with the juice of nāgavallī (betel leaves), kept inside the stem of karkoṭī, which is, in turn kept inside two mud plates. They are then sealed and subjected to an ordinary puṭa process. By one such cooking, bhasma of mercury can be obtained (41–42).

अथ ज्वरादौ रसाः प्रोच्यन्ते ज्वराङ्कुशः—

खण्डितं मृगश्रृङ्गं च ज्वालामुख्या रसैः समम् । रुद्ध्वा भाण्डे पचेच्चुल्यां यामयुग्मं ततो नयेत् ॥४२॥
अष्टांशं त्रिकटुं दद्यान्निष्कमात्रं च भक्षयेत् । नागवल्लीरसैः सार्धं वातपित्तज्वरापहम् ॥ ४३ ॥
अयं ज्वरांकुशो नाम रसः सर्वज्वरापहः । ऐकाहिकं द्व्याहिकं च त्र्याहिकं वा न संशयः ॥ ४४ ॥

Hariṇaśṛṅga (stag's horns) is made into small pieces and macerated with the juice of jwālāmukhī (jayantī) plant, filled into an earthen pot, its mouth sealed, kept on an oven and strong heat applied underneath, for two yāmas (six hours). It is then taken out, made into nice powder, with one—eighth it's quantity of trikaṭu. Administered in doses of one or one and half niṣka with the juice of nāgavallī, it cures jwaras (fevers) due to vātapitta origin. This recipe known as *Jwaraṅkuśa rasa* cures all fevers and fevers which comes daiy, alternate day and once in three day also without doubt (42–44).

अथ ज्वरारिरसः—

पारदं रसकं तालं तुत्थं टङ्कणगन्धकै । सर्वमेतत्समं शुद्धं कारवेल्लीरसैर्दिनम् ॥ ४५ ॥
मर्दयेल्लेपयेत्तेन ताम्रपात्रोदरं भिषक् । अङ्गुल्यर्धप्रमाणेन ततो रुद्ध्वा च तन्मुखम् ॥ ४६ ॥
पचेत्तं वालुकायन्त्रे क्षिप्त्वा धान्यानि तन्मुखे ॥ ४७ ॥
यदा स्फुटन्ति धान्यानि तदा सिद्धं विनिर्दिशेत् । ततो नयेत्स्वाङ्गशीतं ताम्रपात्रोदराद्भिषक् ॥४८॥
रसं ज्वरारिनामानं विचूर्ण्य मरिचैः समम् । माषैकं पर्णखण्डेन भक्षयेन्नाशयेज्ज्वरम् ॥ ४९ ॥
त्रिदिनैर्विषमं तीव्रमेकद्वित्रिचतुर्थकम् ।

Pārada, rasaka, tālaka, tuttha, ṭaṅkaṇa and gandhaka—each equal quantity are macerated for one day with the juice of kāravellaka. The paste is then applied into the interior of a small copper vessel and its mouth sealed. A vālukāyantra (sand bath) is prepared, the copper vessel kept inside it, the mouth of the earthen pot also sealed with another plate covered over it. Heat is applied from below and continued till such time that paddy grains kept over the cover plate, swell up and fly away by heat. After the pot cools off the contents of the copper vessel is taken out, made into a nice powder with equal quantity of marica. This recipe known as *jwarāri rasa*, taken in doses of one māṣa with the parṇa (nāgavallī) leaves cures within three days; viṣama jwaras (intermittant fevers) be it of daily alternate day, every third day or of every fourth day type (45–49).

अथ शीतज्वरारिरसः—

तालकं तुत्थकं ताम्रं रसं गन्धं मनः शिलाम् ॥ ५० ॥
कर्षं कर्षं प्रयोक्तव्यं मर्दयेत्त्रिफलाम्बुभिः । गोलं न्यसेत्संपुटके पुटं दद्यात्प्रयत्नतः ॥ ५१ ॥
ततो नीत्वार्कदुग्धेन वज्रीदुग्धेन सप्तधा । क्वाथेन दन्त्याः श्यामाया भावयेत्सप्तधा पुनः ॥ ५२ ॥
माषमात्रं रसं दिव्यं पञ्चाशन्मरिचैर्युतम् । गुडं गद्याणकं चैव तुलसीदलयुग्मकम् ॥ ५३ ॥
भक्षयेत्त्रिदिनं भक्त्या शीतारिर्दुर्लभः परः । पथ्यं दुग्धौदनं देयं विषमं शीतपूर्वकम् ॥ ५४ ॥
दाहपूर्वं हरत्याशु तृतीयकचतुर्थकौ । द्व्याहिकं सततं चैव वैवर्ण्यं च नियच्छति ॥ ५५ ॥

One karṣa each of tutthaka, tāmrabhasma, rasa, gandhaka and manaśila are macerated with the decoction of triphalā, made into discs, placed in between two mud plates. Their mouths sealed with mud plaster and subjected to puṭa. After cooling, the contents are taken out, macerated for seven times in each of milky sap of arka, vajrī, decoction of dantī and Śyāma and subjected to puṭa after each maceration. This recipe known as *shītāri rasa* (*or shītajwarāri*) is administered in doses of one māṣa, mixed with fifty marica (pepper) seeds, one gadyāṇa of guḍa (jaggery) and two leaves of tulasī, for three days, keeping the patient on rice and milk diet only. By this all types of viṣama jwaras (intermittant fevers) such as shītapūrvaka (fevers preceeded by rigors), dāhapūrvaka (fevers preceded by burning sensation), tritīyaka (terttian fever), caturthaka (fever on every fourth day), dwyāhaka (fever which comes twice a day) and satata (continuous for some days), vaivarṁyakara jwara (fevers which cause discolouration of the body) are cured quickly (50–55).

ज्वरघ्नी गुटिका—

भागैकः स्याद्रसाच्छुद्धादैलेयः पिप्पली शिवा । आकारकरभो गन्धः कटुतैलेन शोधितः ॥ ५६ ॥
फलानि चेन्द्रवारुण्याश्चतुर्भागमिता अमी । एकत्र मर्दयेच्चूर्णमिन्द्रवारुणिकारसैः ॥ ५७ ॥
माषोन्मितां गुटीं कृत्वा दद्यात्सर्वज्वरे वुधः । छिन्नारसानुपानेन ज्वरघ्नी गुटिका मता ॥ ५८ ॥

One part of rasa, four parts each of ileya, pippalī, shiva, ākārakarabha, gandhaka purifled with kaṭu taila (mustard oil) and fruits of indravāruṇī are all powdered and macerated with the juice of indravāruṇī and rolled into pills of one māṣā quantity. Given along with the juice of chinna (gudūcī), this recipe known as *Jwaraghnī guṭikā* cures all fevers (56–58).

अथ लोकनाथरसः क्षयादौ—

शुद्धो बुभुक्षितः सूतो भागद्वयमितो भवेत् । तथा गन्धस्य भागौ द्वौ कुर्यात्कज्जलिकां तयोः ॥ ५९ ॥
सूताच्चतुर्गुणेष्वेव कपर्देषु विनिक्षिपेत् । भागैकं टङ्कणं दत्त्वा गोक्षीरेण विमर्दयेत् ॥ ६० ॥
तथा शङ्खस्य खण्डानां भागानष्टौ प्रकल्पयेत् । क्षिपेत्सर्वं पुटस्यान्तश्चूर्णलिप्तशरावयोः ॥ ६१ ॥
गर्ते हस्तोन्मिते धृत्वा पुटेद्गजपुटेन च । स्वाङ्गशीतं समुद्धृत्य पिष्ट्वा तत्सर्वमेकतः ॥ ६२ ॥
षड्गुञ्जासंमितं चूर्णमेकोनत्रिंशदूषणैः । घृतेन वातजे दद्यान्नवनीतेन पित्तजे ॥ ६३ ॥
क्षौद्रेण श्लेष्मजे दद्यादतीसारे क्षये तथा । अरुचौ ग्रहणीरोगे कार्श्ये मन्दानले तथा ॥ ६४ ॥
कासश्वासेषु गुल्मेषु लोकनाथरसः हितः । तस्योपरि घृतान्नं च भुञ्जीत कवलत्रयम् ॥ ६५ ॥
मञ्चे क्षणैकमुत्तानः शयीतानुपधानके । अनम्लमन्नं सघृतं भुञ्जीत मधुरं दधि ॥ ६६ ॥
प्रायेण जाङ्गलं मांसं प्रदेयं घृतपाचितम् । सुदुग्धभक्तं दद्याच्च जातेऽग्नौ सांध्यभोजने ॥ ६७ ॥
सघृतान्मुद्गवटकान्व्यञ्जनेष्ववचारयेत् । तिलामलककल्केन स्नापयेत्सर्पिषाऽथवा ॥ ६८ ॥
अभ्यञ्जयेत्सर्पिषा च स्नानं कोष्णोदकेन च । क्वचित्तैलं न गृह्णीयान्न बिल्वं कारवेल्लकम् ॥ ६९ ॥
वार्ताकं शफरीं चिञ्चां त्यजेद्व्यायाममैथुने । मद्यं संधानकं हिङ्गु शुण्ठीं माषान्मसूरकान् ॥ ७० ॥
कूष्माण्डं राजिकां कोपं काञ्जिकं चैव वर्जयेत् । त्यजेदयुक्तनिद्रां च कांस्यपात्रे च भोजनम् ॥७१॥
ककारादियुतं सर्वं त्यजेच्छाकफलादिकम् । पथ्योऽयं लोकनाथस्तु शुभनक्षत्रवासरे ॥ ७२ ॥
पूर्णातिथौ सिते पक्षे जाते चन्द्रबले तथा । पूजयित्वा लोकनाथं कुमारीं भोजयेत्ततः ॥ ७३ ॥
दानं दत्त्वा द्विघटिकामध्ये ग्राह्यो रसोत्तमः । रसाच्चेज्जायते तापस्तथा शर्करया युतम् ॥ ७४ ॥

सत्त्वं गुडूच्या गृह्णीयाद्वंशरोचनया युतम् । खर्जूरं दाडिमं द्राक्षामिक्षुखण्डानि चारयेत् ॥ ७५ ॥
अरुचौ निस्तुषं धान्यं घृतभृष्टं सशर्करम् । दद्यात्तथा ज्वरे धान्यगुडूचीक्वाथमाहरेत् ॥ ७६ ॥
उशीरवासकक्वाथं दद्यात्समधुशर्करम् । रक्तपित्ते कफे श्वासे कासे च स्वरसंक्षये ॥ ७७ ॥
अग्निभृष्टजयाचूर्णं मधुना निशि दीयते । निद्रानाशेऽतिसारे च ग्रहण्यां मन्दपावके ॥ ७८ ॥
सौवर्चलाभयाकृष्णाचूर्णमुष्णोदकैः पिबेत् । शूलेऽजीर्णे तथा कृष्णा मधुयुक्ता ज्वरे हिता ॥ ७९ ॥
प्लीहोदरे वातरक्ते छर्द्यां चैव गुदाङ्कुरे । नासिकादिषु रक्तेषु रसं दाडिमपुष्पजम् ॥ ८० ॥
दूर्वायाः स्वरसं नस्ये प्रदद्याच्छर्करायुतम् । कोलमज्जा कणा बर्हिपक्षभस्म सशर्करम् ॥ ८१ ॥
मधुना लेहयेच्छर्दिहिक्काकोपोपशान्तये । विधिरेष प्रयोज्यस्तु सर्वस्मिन्पोट्टलीरसे ॥ ८२ ॥
मृगाङ्के हेमगर्भे च मौक्तिकाख्येऽपरेषु च । इत्ययं लोकनाथाख्यो रसः सर्वरुजो जयेत् ॥ ८३ ॥

Two parts of mercury well purified and made capable of devouring metals and two parts of purified gandhaka are macerated together and made in to kajjalī (black powder) and filled into kapardikā (cowri shells), four times the weight of pārada. Ṭaṅkaṇa mixed with milk is made into a paste and applied to the mouths of the shells. Small pieces of shaṅkha (conch shell) are placed in a mud plate, the cowrishells containing the drugs are kept in the centre and covered with pieces of shaṅkha, another plate is covered over, their mouths sealed with mud plaster, dried the subjected to gaja puṭa in a pit of one hasta cube (one elbow long, wide and deep), After cooling, the plates are removed and all their contents niecly powdered. This powder, six guñjās by weight mixed with twentynine maricas (pepper) makes up one dose. This recipe is adiministered with ghee in diseases of vāta, with butter in diseases of pitta, with honey in diseases of kapha and with other suitable vehicles in atisāra (diarrhoea), kṣaya (consumption), aruci (anorexia), grahaṇī (sprue), kārshya (wasting), mandāgni (dyspepsia), kāsa-swāsa (cough-dyspnoea), and gulma (abdominal tumors). The patient should then take three morsels of rice mixed with ghee and lie down on a cot without a head rest. He should take foods devoid of sour but having sweet taste mixed with ghee, sweet curds, mutton of jāṅgala animals cooked in ghee, rice with milk and ghee, condiments of green gram powder fried in ghee etc. Paste of āmalaka and tila or ghee to be applied over the body and given bath in warm water. During the course of treatment the person should avoid the use of oil, bilva, kāravella, vārtāka, shapharī, ciñcā; physical exercise, sex acts, alcoholic drinks, fermented liquors, hiṅgu, shuṇthi, māṣa, masūraka, kūṣmāṇḍa, rājika, kopa, (anger), kañjika (sour gruel), unwanted sleep and all articles (foods, vegetable) whose names commence with sylable "KA'. A bronze plate should be used for dining. This *Lokanātha rasa* should be administered during auspicious days, constellation and bright half of the moon. The patient should worship Lokanātha (Shiva), feed kumārīs

(unmarried young women), offer donations and commence taking the medicine within the first two hours of the morning. If the patient develops burning sensation in the body during the course of the drug, he should be given guḍūchi satwa mixed with sugar and vaṁsharocana, kharjūra, drākṣā and sugar cane juice can also be given much as desired. In cases of aruci (anorexia) the medicine is to be taken with grains fried in ghee and mixed with sugar; in jwaras (fevers) with decoction of dhānya and guḍūcī; in raktapitta (purpura), kapha kāsa and swāsa (cough and dyspnoea), swara kṣaya (loss of voice) with the decoction of ushīra and vāsa mixed with honey and sugar; in nidrānāsha (loss of sleep), atisāra (diarrhoea), grahaṇī, (sprue), agnimāndya (dyspepsia) with powder of fried jaya (bhaṅg) mixed with honey at night; in shūla (colic) ajīrṇa (indigestion) mixed with powder of sauvarcala, abhaya and kṛṣna along with warm water; in jwara (fevers), plīhodara (splenomegaly), vātarakta (gout), chardi (vomitting), gudāṅkura (piles) it is given with powder of kṛṣṇa and honey; in cases of bleeding through nose and other openings, along with juice of flowers of dāḍima, or dūrva grass along with sugar; in cases of chardi (vomitting) and hikkā (hiccough) with kolamajjā (marow of kola), kaṇā, ashes of peacock feather mixed with sugar and honey; thus *Lokanātha rasa* cures all diseases.

The above procedure is to be followed during the course of treatment with all poṭalī rasas such as mṛgāṅka poṭalī, hemagarbha poṭalī, mauktika poṭalī etc. (59–83).

(वराटभस्म मण्डूरं चूर्णयित्वा घृते पचेत् । तत्समं मरिचं चूर्णं नागवल्ल्या विभावितम् ॥ ८४ ॥
तच्चूर्णं मधुना लेह्यमथवा नवनीतकैः । माषामात्रं क्षयं हन्ति यामे यामे च भक्षितम् ॥ ८५ ॥
लोकनाथरसो ह्येष मण्डलाद्राजयक्ष्मनुत् ।)

Equal part of bhasmas (ash) of varāṭika (cowri shell) and maṇḍūra (iron slag) are fried with a little ghee. Powder of marica equal to the above mixture of bhasma is added and macerated with the juice of nāgavallī (betel leaves) and stored. Used in doses of one maṣa per time along with honey or butter once in yāma (three hours). This *Lokanātha rasa* cures rājayakṣmā (tuberculosis) within one maṇḍala (40 days) (83–85).

अथ मृगाङ्कपोट्टलीरसः क्षयादौ—

भूर्जवत्तनुपत्राणि हेम्नः सूक्ष्माणि कारयेत् ॥ ८६ ॥
तुल्यानि तानि सूतेन खल्वे क्षिप्त्वा विमर्दयेत् । काञ्चनाररसेनैव ज्वालामुख्या रसेन वा ॥ ८७ ॥
लाङ्गल्या वा रसैस्तावद्यावद्भवति पिष्टिका । ततो हेम्नश्चतुर्थांशं टङ्कणं तत्र निक्षिपेत् ॥ ८८ ॥
पिष्टमौक्तिकचूर्णं च हेमद्विगुणमावपेत् । तेषु सर्वसमं गन्धं क्षिप्त्वा चैकत्र मर्दयेत् ॥ ८९ ॥
तेषां कृत्वा ततो गोलं वासोभिः परिवेष्टयेत् । पश्चान्मृदा वेष्टयित्वा शोषयित्वा च धारयेत् ॥ ९० ॥

शरावसम्पुटस्यान्तस्तत्र मुद्रां प्रदापयेत् । लवणापूरिते भाण्डे धारयेत्तं च संपुटम् ॥ ९१ ॥
मुद्रां दत्त्वा शोषयित्वा बहुभिर्गोमयैः पुटेत् । ततः शीते समाहृत्य गन्धं सूतसमं क्षिपेत् ॥ ९२ ॥
घृष्ट्वा च पूर्ववत्खल्वे पुटेद्गजपुटेन च । स्वाङ्गशीतं ततो नीत्वा गुञ्जायुग्मं प्रयोजयेत् ॥ ९३ ॥
अष्टभिर्मरिचैर्युक्तः कृष्णात्रययुतोऽथवा । विलोक्य देयो दोषादीनेकैका रसरक्तिका ॥ ९४ ॥
सर्पिषा मधुना वापि दद्याद्दोषाद्यपेक्षया । लोकनाथसमं पथ्यं कुर्यात्स्वस्थमनाः शुचिः ॥ ९५ ॥
श्लेष्माणं ग्रहणीं कासं श्वासं क्षयमरोचकम् । मृगाङ्कोऽयं रसो हन्यात्कृशत्वं बलहीनताम् ॥ ९६ ॥

Purified gold leaves beaten into thin leaves and cut to small pieces are mixed with equal quantity of purified rasa (mercury) and macerated well with the juice of kāñcanāra, jwālāmukhī or lāṅgalī till it becomes a paste. Taṅkaṇa, one-fouith the weight of gold, powder of muktā (pearls)—twice the quantity of gold, and gandhaka equal to the total of all the above are added, macerated into a pastc and rolled into a ball. It is then covered over with thick cloth, kept inside a earthen plate covered with another one, their mouths sealed with niud plaster and dried. The sealed plates are put inside a salt bath in a pot which is subjected to fire of cowdung heaps kept in all sides. After cooling the contents are removed and added with equal quantity of gandhaka (sulphur), macerated as described earlier, made into ball, kept inside earthen platcs, sealed and subjected to gaja puṭam. Afterwards it is removed and used in dose of two guñjās along either with eight maricas or three pippalīs, or in dose of one guñjā with ghee, honey or other suitable vehicle depending upon the condition of the doṣas. The dietetic and other rigimen are similar to those of lokanātha rasa. This recipe known as *Mṛgāṅka rasa* is effective in diseases of kapha, grahaṇī (sprue), kāsa (cough), swāsa (dyspnoea), kṣaya (consumption), arocaka (anorexia), kṛshatwa (emaciation) and balahīnatā (debility) (86–96).

क्षयश्वासादौ हेमगर्भपोट्टलीरसः—

सूतात्पादप्रमाणेन हेम्नः पिष्टं प्रकल्पयेत् । तयोः स्याद्द्विगुणो गन्धो मर्दयेत्काञ्चनारकैः ॥ ९७ ॥
कृत्वा गोलं क्षिपेन्मूषासम्पुटे मुद्रयेत्ततः । पचेद्भूधरयन्त्रेण वासरत्रितयं बुधः ॥ ९८ ॥
तत उद्धृत्य तत्सर्वं दद्याद्गन्धं च तत्समम् । मर्दयेदार्द्रकरसैश्चित्रकस्वरसेन च ॥ ९९ ॥
स्थूलपीतवराटांश्च पूरयेत्तेन युक्तितः । एतस्मादौषधात्कुर्यादष्टमांशेन टङ्कणम् ॥ १०० ॥
टङ्कणार्धं विषं दत्त्वा पिष्ट्वा सेहुण्डदुग्धकैः । मुद्रयेत्तेन कल्केन वराटानां मुखानि च ॥ १०१ ॥
भाण्डे चूर्णप्रलिप्ते च धृत्वा मुद्रां प्रदापयेत् । गर्ते हस्तोन्मिते धृत्वा पुटेद्गजपुटेन च ॥ १०२ ॥
स्वाङ्गशीतं रसं ज्ञात्वा प्रदद्याल्लोकनाथवत् । पथ्यं मृगाङ्कवज्ज्ञेयं त्रिदिनं लवणं त्यजेत् ॥ १०३ ॥
यदा छर्दिर्भवेत्तस्य दद्याच्छिन्नाभृतं तदा । मधुयुक्तं तथा श्लेष्मकोपे दद्याद्गुडार्द्रकम् ॥ १०४ ॥
विरेके भर्जिता भङ्गा प्रदेया दधिसंयुता । जयेत्कासं क्षयं श्वासं ग्रहणीमरुचिं तथा ॥ १०५ ॥
अग्निं च कुरुते दीप्तं कफवातं नियच्छति । हेमगर्भः परो ज्ञेयो रसः पोट्टलिकाभिधः ॥ १०६ ॥

Sūta (mercury) one part, hema (gold leaves) one foruth part and gandhaka (sulphur) double in quantity to the total of the above—are put in a morter, macerated with the juice of kañcanāra, made into a ball and kept sealed inside two earthen plates. A bhūdhara yantra (similar to that described in the previous preparation) is made, earthen plates kept inside it and cooked for three days continuously. Later, the contents are taken out, equal quantity of gandhaka (sulphur) is added again and macerated with the juice of ārdraka and citraka. The paste is then filled into big cowri shells. A paste is prepard with eight part of taṅkaṇa and half of it of viṣa (vatsanābhi) and milk of sehuṇḍa and given a thick covering over each cowri shell and dried. These shells are kept inside a pot containing powdered slaked lime, it's mouth sealed and subjected to gajapuṭa in a pit of one arm cube. After cooling the contents are taken out and used in the same way as lokanātha Rasa. The patient should avoid intake of salt for three days. If vomitting occurs, a decoction of chinna (guḍūchī) with honey be given, if kapha prakopa, he should be given ārdraka and guḍā (jaggery), if purgations occur fried bhaṅga and curds is to be given. This recipe known as *Hemagarbha poṭṭalī rasa,* cures kāsa (cough); kṣaya (consumption), swāsa (dyspnoea), grahaṇī (sprue), aruci (anorexia); improves the agni (digestion) and alleviates kapha and vāta (97-106)

अथ द्वितीयो हेमगर्भपोट्टलीरसः—

रसस्य भागाश्चत्वारस्तावन्तः कनकस्य च । तयोश्च पिष्टिकां कृत्वा गन्धो द्वादशभागिकः ॥ १०७ ॥
कुर्यात्कज्जलिकां तेषां मुक्ताभागाश्च षोडश । चतुर्विंशच्च शङ्खस्य भागैकं टङ्कणस्य च ॥ १०८ ॥
एकत्र मर्दयेत्सर्वं पक्वनिम्बूकजै रसैः । कृत्वा तेषां ततो गोलं मूषासम्पुटके न्यसेत् ॥ १०९ ॥
मुद्रां दत्त्वा ततो हस्तमात्रे गर्ते च गोमयैः । पुटेद्गजपुटेनैव स्वाङ्गशीतं समुद्धरेत् ॥ ११० ॥
पिष्ट्वा गुञ्जाचतुर्मानं दद्याद्गव्याज्यसंयुतम् । एकोनत्रिंशदुन्मानमरिचैः सह दीयते ॥ १११ ॥
रजते मृन्मये पात्रे काचजे वाऽवलेहयेत् । लोकनाथसमं पथ्यं कुर्याच्च स्वस्थमानसः ॥ ११२ ॥
कासे श्वासे क्षये वाते कफे ग्रहणिकागदे । अतिसारे प्रयोक्तव्या पोट्टली हेमगर्भिका ॥ ११३ ॥

Four parts each of rasa (mercury) and kanaka (gold) and twelve parts of gandhaka (sulphur) are made into a kajjalī (black powder prepared by constant maceration). To it are added sixteen parts of muktā (ashes of pearls), twenty-four part of shaṅkha (ash of conch shell) and one part of ṭaṅkaṇa—all these macerated with the juice of ripe lemons. Then round discs are made, kept inside earthen plates, sealed and dried. A pit one hasta (arm) cube is filled with cow-dung heaps, earthen pots kept inside and subjected to gajapuṭa. After cooling it is taken out, given in doses of four guñjās mixed with powder of twentynine maricas and cow's ghce This should be stored in a vessel of silver, mud or glass. Regimen same as of lokanātha rasa. This recipe known as *Hemagarbha poṭṭalī* is useful in kāsa (cough), swāsa (dyspnoea), kṣaya (consumption), vāta and kapha disorders, grahaṇī (sprue) and atisāra (diarrhoeas) (107–113).

अत्र महाज्वराङ्कुशः विषमज्वरादौ—

शुद्धसूतो विषं गन्धः प्रत्येकं शाणसम्मितम् । धूर्तबीजं त्रिशाणं स्यात्सर्वेभ्यो द्विगुणा भवेत् ॥११४॥
हेमाह्वा कारयेदेषां सूक्ष्मं चूर्णं प्रयत्नतः । देयं जम्बीरमज्जाभिश्चूर्णं गुञ्जाद्वयोन्मितम् ॥ ११५ ॥
आर्द्रकस्वरसैर्वापि ज्वरं हन्ति त्रिदोषजम् । ऐकाहिकं द्व्याहिकं वा त्र्याहिकं वा चतुर्थकम् ॥११६॥
विषमं च ज्वरं हन्याद्विख्यातोऽयं ज्वराङ्कुशः ।

Purified sūta (mercury), viṣa, gandhaka each one shāṇa, three shāṇas of seeds of dhūrta (dhattūra) and hemāhwā double the total quantity of all the above and macerated in a stone morter and pestle with juice of jambīra and dried in shade. Two guñjās of this recipe known as *Jwarāṅkusha rasa* given with juice of lemon or green ginger cures jwaras (fevers) such as tridoṣaja (arising for aggravation of all the three doṣas) and viṣama jwaras (remittant fevers) like ekāhika (daily), dwāhika (alternate day), trāhika (third day), carturthaka (every fourth day) (114–117).

अथानन्दभैरवः अतीसारदौ—

दरदं वत्सनाभं च मरिचं टङ्कणं कणाम् ॥ ११७ ॥
चूर्णयेत्समभागेन रसो ह्यानन्दभैरवः । गुञ्जैकं वा द्विगुञ्जं वा बलं ज्ञात्वा प्रयोजयेत् ॥ ११८ ॥
मधुना लेहयेच्चानु कुटजस्य फलं त्वचम् । चूर्णितं कर्षमात्रं तु त्रिदोषोत्थातिसारजित् ॥ ११९ ॥
दध्यन्नं दापयेत्पथ्यं गवाज्यं तक्रमेव च । पिपासायां जलं शीतं विजया च हिता निशि ॥ १२० ॥

Equal parts each of darada, vatsanābha, marica, ṭaṅkaṇa and kaṇa, are macerated well with the juice of lemons, and rolled into pills. This *Ānanda bhairava rasa* given in doses of one or two guñjās depending upon the strength of the patient mixed with honey and one karṣa of powder of bark of kuṭaja cures even tridoṣaja atisāra (diarrhoeas). The patient should be given rice with curds, ghee or butter milk. If thirst appears cold water is given as drink. A little quantity of vijaya (bhaṅg) can be given at night with great benefit (117–120).

अथ लघुसूचिकाभरणो रसस्त्रिदोषे—

विषं पलमितं सूतः शाणिकश्चूर्णयेद्द्वयम् । तच्चूर्णं सम्पुटे क्षिप्त्वा काचलिप्तशरावयोः ॥ १२१ ॥
मुद्रां दत्त्वा च संशोष्य ततश्चुल्ल्यां निवेशयेत् । वह्निं शनैः शनैः कुर्यात्प्रहरद्वयसंख्यया ॥ १२२ ॥
तत उद्घाटयेन्मुद्रामुपरिस्थां शरावकात् । संलग्नो यो भवेत्सूतस्तं गृह्णीयाच्छनैः शनैः ॥ १२३ ॥
वायुस्पर्शो यथा न स्यात्तथा कूप्यां निवेशयेत् । यावत्सूच्या मुखे लग्नं कुप्या निर्याति भेषजम् ।१२४।
तावन्मात्रो रसो देयो मूर्च्छिते सन्निपातिनि । क्षुरेण प्रच्छिते मूर्ध्नि तत्राङ्गुल्या च घर्षयेत् ॥१२५॥
रक्तभेषजसम्पर्कान्मूर्च्छितोऽपि हि जीवति । तथैव सर्पदष्टस्तु मृतावस्थोऽपि जीवति ॥ १२६ ॥
यदा तापो भवेत्तस्य मधुरं तत्र दीयते ।

One pala of viṣa and one shāṇa of sūta are well macerated together and placed inside earthen plates which are sealed with mud plaster, dried and kept inside a pot containing sand. The pot is then kept oven a over and fire applied from below for two praharas (3-4 hours) increasing it's intensity gradually. After cooling, the plates are opened, and the powder adhering to the upper plate is transferred into a glass bottle without exposing it to air. The bottle is always kept sealed and a needle introduced inside to take out the medicine. The dose will be that much only which adheres to the point of the needle. An in cised wound is made on the head, the medicine applied into it and rubbed gently. By combining with the blood it brings conciousness to a person who is under mūrchā (unconciousness, coma), sannipāta (condition of aggravation of all the three doṣas together) or sarpa dashta (bitten by a snake and lost conciousness). If the temperature of the body increases or he complains of buring sensation sweet syrups are given to him as drinks (121–126).

अथ जलबन्धुरसः सन्निपाते—

सूतभस्मसमं गन्धं धात्र्या दद्यान्मनःशिला ॥ १२७ ॥

माक्षिकं पिप्पली व्योषं प्रत्येकं शिलया समम् । चूर्णयेद्भावयेत्पित्तैर्मत्स्यमायूरसम्भवैः ॥ १२८ ॥
सप्तधा भावयेच्छुष्कं देयं गुञ्जाद्वयं हितम् । तालपर्णीरसश्चानु पञ्चकोलशृतोऽथवा ॥ १२९ ॥
जलबन्धुरसो नाम सन्निपातं नियच्छति । जलयोगश्च कर्तव्यस्तेन वीर्यं भवेद्रसे ॥ १३० ॥

Equal parts of bhasma of sūta and gandhaka, dhātri, manashila, suvarṇamākṣika, pippali and vyoṣa each equal part are macerated along with the bile of fish and peacock each for seven times and the dry powder stored. Two gunjās of the powder given with juice of tālaparṇi or decoction of pañcakola. During its usage the person should sit inside a tub of water. This recipe known as *Jalabandhu rasa* cures sannipāta (unconcious and toxic states). (127–130).

पञ्चवक्ररसः—

शुद्धं सूतं विषं गन्धं मरिचं टङ्कणं कणाम् । मर्दयेद्धूर्तजद्रावैर्दिनमेकं च शोषयेत् ॥ १३१ ॥
पञ्चवक्रो रसो नाम द्विगुञ्जः सन्निपातजित् । अर्कमूलकषायं तु सत्र्यूषमनुपाययेत् ॥ १३२ ॥
युक्तं दध्योदनं पथ्यं जलयोगं च कारयेत् । रसेनानेन शाम्यन्ति सक्षौद्रेण कफोद्भवाः ॥ १३३ ॥
मध्वार्द्रकरसं चानु पिबेदग्निविवृद्धये । यथेष्टं घृतमांसाशी शक्तो भवति पावकः ॥ १३४ ।

Purified sūta (mercury) viṣa, gandhaka, marica, ṭaṅkaṇa and kaṇa—all equal parts are macerated for one day with juice of dhūrta, dried and stored. This recipe known as *Pañcavaktra rasa,* used in doses of two guñjās followed with decoction of root of arka mixed with powder of triyūṣaṇa, cures sannipāta (toxic state), rice and curds and jalayoga (sitting in a watertub) are indicated during the course. Taken with honey it cures disorders of kapha, with honey and juice of green ginger it promotes digestion and the person becomes capable of digesting ghee and mutton even if taken every day (131–134).

अथोन्मत्तो रसः सन्निपाते—

रसं गन्धकतुल्यांशं धत्तूरफलजद्रवैः । मर्दयेद्दिनमेकं तु तत्तुल्यं त्रिकटु क्षिपेत् ॥ १३५ ॥
उन्मत्ताख्यो रसो नाम्ना नस्ये स्यात्सन्निपातजित् ।

Rasa and gandha each equal parts macerated with juice of dhattūra along with ṭrikaṭu equal in quantity to both of the above, dried and stored. This recipe known as *unmatta rasa* used as a nasya (nasal insufflation) cures sannipāta (toxic states) (135–136).

अथ सन्निपातेऽञ्जनं रसाः—

निस्त्वग्जैपालबीजं च दशनिष्कं विचूर्णयेत् ॥ १३६ ॥
मरिचं पिप्पलीं सूतं प्रतिनिष्कं विमिश्रयेत् । भाव्यो जम्बीरजैर्द्रावैः सप्ताहं सप्रयत्नतः ॥ १३७ ॥
रसोऽयमञ्जने दत्तः सन्निपातं विनाशयेत् ।

Dehusked seeds of jaipāla ten niṣka and one niṣka each of marica, pippalī and sūta are macerated with the juice of jambīra (big lime fruit) for seven days, dried and stored. This recipe applied as añjana (collyrium) to the eyes relieves sannipāta (toxic states) (136–138).

अथ महानाराचरसः शूलादौ—

सूतं टङ्कणकं तुल्यं मरिचं सूततुल्यकम् ॥ १३८ ॥
गन्धकं पिप्पलीं शुण्ठीं द्वौ द्वौ भागौ विचूर्णयेत् । सर्वतुल्यं क्षिपेद्दन्तीबीजं निस्तुषितं भिषक् ॥ १३९ ॥
द्विगुञ्जं रेचनं सिद्धं नाराचोऽयं महारसः । आध्मानं मलविष्टम्भानुदावर्तं च नाशयेत् ॥ १४० ॥

Equal parts of sūta, ṭaṅkaṇa and marica and two parts each of gandhaka pippalī and śuṇṭhi and dehusked seeds of dantī equal to the total of all the above are macerated well (with a sour juice) dried and stored. Two guñjās of this ricipe defenetely produces purgation and relives ādhmāna (tympanitis), malaviṣṭambha (constipation) and udāvarta (reverse peristalisis (138–140).

अथ इच्छाभेदी रसः शूलादौ—

दरदं टङ्कणं शुण्ठी पिप्पली चैककार्षिका । हेमाह्वा पलमात्रा स्याद्दन्तीबीजं च तत्समम् ॥ १४१ ॥
विचूर्ण्यैकत्र सर्वाणि गोदुग्धेनैव साधयेत् । त्रिगुञ्जं रेचनं दद्याद्विष्टम्भाध्मानरोगिषु ॥ १४२ ॥

Darada, ṭaṅkaṇa, śuṇṭhī and pippalī each one karṣa, one pala each of hemāhwa and dantī bīja are macerated well and stored. Administered in doses of three guñjās along with cow's milk it produces purgations and relieves viṣṭambha (indigestion) and ādhmāna (flatulence) etc. (141-142).

वसन्तकुसुमाकररसः प्रमेहादौ—

द्वौ भागौ हेमभूतेश्च गगनं चापि तत्समम् । लोहभस्म त्रयोभागाश्चत्वारो रसभस्मनः ॥ १४३ ॥
वङ्गभस्म त्रिभागं स्यात्सर्वमेकत्र मर्दयेत् । प्रवालं मौक्तिकं चैव रससाम्येन दापयेत् ॥ १४४ ॥

भावनां गव्यदुग्धेन रसैर्घृष्ट्वाटरूषकै । हरिद्रावारिणा चैव मोचकन्दरसेन च ॥ १४५ ॥
शतपत्ररसेनापि मालत्याः स्वरसेन च । पश्चान्मृगमदश्चन्द्रतुलसीरसभावितः ॥ १४६ ॥
कुसुमाकर इत्येष वसन्तपदपूर्वकः । गुञ्जाद्वयं ददीतास्य मधुना सर्वमेहनुत् ॥ १४७ ॥
सिताचन्दनसंयुक्तश्चाम्लपित्तादिरोगजित् ।

Two parts each of hemabhasma and gagana bhasma (abhraka bhasma), three parts of loha bhasma, four of rasa bhasma, two each of pravāla and mouktikā are macerated for one day in each of the following juices—cow's milk, juice of aṭarūṣa, haridrā, juice of stem of banana, śatapatra, mālatī and tulasī adding small quantities of mṛgamada (musk), and candra (camphor) during maceration. This recipe known as *Vasanta kusumākara rasa*; given in doses of two guñjās, with honey cures all types of pramehas (diabetes); with white sandal wood (decoction) syrup, it relieves amlapitta (hyperchlorhydria) and such other allied diseases (143–147).

क्षयादौ राजमृगाङ्करसः—

सूतभस्म त्रयो भागा भागैकं हेमभस्मकम् ॥ १४८ ॥
मृतताम्रस्य भागैकं शिलागन्धकतालकम् । प्रतिभागद्वयं शुद्धमेकीकृत्य विचूर्णयेत् ॥ १४९ ॥
वराटान्पूरयेत्तेनं छागीक्षीरेण टङ्कणम् । पिष्ट्वा तेन मुखं रुद्ध्वा मृद्भाण्डे तन्निरोधयेत् ॥ १५० ॥
शुष्कं गजपुटं पक्त्वा चूर्णयेत्स्वाङ्गशीतलम् । रसो राजमृगाङ्कोऽयं चतुर्गुञ्जः क्षयापहः ॥ १५१ ॥
दशपिप्पलिकाक्षौद्रैरेकोनत्रिंशदूषणैः । सघृतं दापयेत्पथ्यं स्त्रीकोपाग्निश्रमांस्त्यजेत् ॥ १५२ ॥
पथ्यं वा लघुमांसानि राजरोगप्रशान्तये ।

Three parts of sūtabhasma, one each of hemabhasma and tāmra bhasma, two parts each of purified manaśila, tālaka, gandhaka are all mixed and powdered nicely and filled into big sized cowri shells, ṭaṅkaṇa made into a paste with goats milk is pasted over them. They are then kept inside a mud pot, its mouth sealed and subjected to gajapuṭam. After cooling the cowrieshells are removed and nicely powdered. Four guñjās in weight of this recipe known as *Rāja mṛgāṅka* given along with ten pippalīs, twentynine marica, honey and ghee cures kṣaya (consumption, tuberculosis). During the course of treatement the patient should avoid sex, anger, heat of open fire and physical exertion and should take easily digestible mutton as food (148–152).

अथाग्निनामा रस क्षयश्वासादौ—

शुद्धं सूतं द्विधा गन्धं कुर्यात्खल्वेन कज्जलीम् ॥ १५३ ॥
तयोः समं तीक्ष्णचूर्णं मर्दयेत्कन्यकाद्रवैः । द्वियामान्ते कृतं गोलं ताम्रपात्रे विनिक्षिपेत् ॥ १५४ ॥
आच्छाद्यैरण्डपत्रेण यामार्धेऽत्युष्णता भवेत् । धान्यराशौ न्यसेत्पश्चादहोरात्रात्समुद्धरेत् ॥ १५५ ॥
संचूर्ण्य गालयेद्वस्त्रे सत्यं वारितरं भवेत् । भावयेत्कन्यकाद्रावैः सप्तधा भृङ्गजैस्तथा ॥ १५६ ॥
काकमाचीकुरण्टोत्थद्रवैर्मुण्ड्यापुनर्नवैः । सहदेव्यमृतानीलीनिर्गुण्डीचित्रजैस्तथा ॥ १५७ ॥
सप्तधा तु पृथग्द्रावैर्भाव्यं शोष्यं तथातपे । सिद्धयोगो ह्ययं ख्यातः सिद्धानां च मुखागतः ॥ १५८ ॥

अनुभूतो मया सत्यं सर्वरोगगणापहः । स्वर्णादीन्मारयेदेवं चूर्णीकृत्य तु लोहवत् ॥ १५९ ॥
त्रिफलामधुसंयुक्तः सर्वरोगेषु योजयेत् । त्रिकटुत्रिफलैलाभिर्जातीफललवङ्गकैः ॥ १६० ॥
नवभागोन्मितैरेतैः समः पूर्वरसो भवेत् । संचूर्ण्य लोडयेत्क्षौद्रैर्भक्ष्यं निष्कद्वयं द्वयम् ॥ १६१ ॥
स्वयमग्निरसो नाम्ना क्षयकासनिकृन्तनः ।

Purified sūta one part and twice its quantity of purified gandhaka are made into a kajjalī. To it, fine powder (or bhasma) of tīkṣṇa loha (magnetic iron), is added double in quantity of the above two and macerated with juice of kanyaka (aloes) for two yāmas (6 hours) made into a ball, kept in a copper vessel covered over with leaves of castor plant and kept in hot sun for half a yāma or till the vessel becomes hot. Next the ball is kept inside a heap of grain for a day and night. Later the ball is nicely powdered and filtered through cloth to get powder which floats on water. This powder is macerated seven times in each of the juices of kanyaka, bhṛṅgarāja, kākamācī, kuraṇṭa, muṇḍī, punarnavā, sahadevī, amṛta, nīlī, nirguṇḍī and citraka. Later it is dried in sun and stored. This recipe was revealed by siddhas (mendicant physicians) and found effective by myself in many diseases. By this even the metals like hema (gold) can be converted to bhasma. This recipe known as *Swayamagni rasas* used in doses of two niṣkas along with triphalā and honey, or powder of equal parts of trikaṭu, triphalā, elā, jatīphala and lavaṅga (total nine) and honey cures kṣaya (consumption tuberculosis) and kāsa (cough) (153–161).

अमृतार्णवरसः—

पारदं गन्धकं शुद्धं मृतलोहं च टङ्कणम् ॥ १६२ ॥
रास्नाविडङ्गत्रिफला देवदारु कटुत्रयम् । अमृता पद्मकं क्षौद्रं विश्वं तुल्यांशचूर्णितम् ॥ १६३ ॥
त्रिगुञ्जं सर्वकासार्तः सेवयेदमृतार्णवम् ।

Purified pārada and gandhaka; lohabhasma, ṭaṅkaṇa, rāsnā, viḍaṅga, triphalā, devadāru, kaṭutraya, amṛta, padmaka, kaṇṭākari and viṣa—each equal part are nicely powdered and stored. Used in doses of three guñjās, this *amṛtārṇava rasa* cures all types of kāsa (cough) (162–163).

अथ सूर्यावर्तो रसः श्वासे—

सूतार्धो गन्धको मर्द्यो यामैकं कन्यकाद्रवैः ॥ १६४ ॥
द्वयोस्तुल्यं ताम्रपत्रं पूर्वकल्केन लेपयेत् । दिनैकं स्थालिकायन्त्रे पक्वमादाय चूर्णयेत् ॥ १६५ ॥
सूर्यावर्तो रसो ह्येष द्विगुञ्जः श्वासजिद्भवेत् ।

One part of sūta and half part of gandhaka are macerated for one yāma (3 hours) with the juice of kanyaka (kumarī). This patse is applied over thin leaves of tāmra equal in weight to the total of pārada and gandhaka. Leaves are kept in a mud pot, sealed and cooked on fire for one day. Later it is removed, powdered and stored, Two guñjās of this recipe known as *Sūryāvarta rasa* cures swāsa (dyspnoeas) (164–165).

अथ स्वच्छन्दभैरवरसः वातरोगे—

शुद्धं सूतं मृतं लोहं ताप्यं गन्धकतालके ॥ १६६ ॥
पथ्याग्निमन्थं निर्गुण्डी त्र्यूषणं टङ्कणं विषम् । तुल्यांशं मर्दयेत्खल्वे दिनं निर्गुण्डिकाद्रवैः ॥ १६७ ॥
मुण्डीद्रावैर्दिनैकं तु द्विगुञ्जं वटकीकृतम । भक्षयेद्वातरोगार्तो नाम्ना स्वच्छन्दभैरवः ॥ १६८ ॥
रास्नामृतादेवदारुशुण्ठीवातारिजं श्रृतम् । सगुग्गुलुं पिबेत्कोष्णमनुपानं सुखावहम् ॥ १६९ ॥

Purified sūta, lohabhasma, tāpya, gandhaka, tālaka, pathya, agnimantha, nirguṇḍī, tryūṣaṇa, ṭaṅkaṇa and viṣam—each equal quantity is macerated with the juice of nirguṇḍī for one day, next with juice of muṇḍī, for another day, rolled into pills of two guñjās then dried and stored. This recipe known as *Swacchanda bhairava*, is useful in all types of vāta rogas (nervous disorders). A decoction of rāsnā, amṛta, devadāru, śuṇṭhī, eraṇḍamūla and guggulu, if taken warm as anupāna is beneficial (166–169).

अथ हंसपोट्टलीरसः ग्रहणीरोगे—

दग्ध्वा कपर्दकं पिष्ट्वा त्र्यूषणं टङ्कणं विषम् । गन्धकं शुद्धसूतं च तुल्यं जम्बीरजैर्द्रवैः ॥ १७० ॥
मर्दयेद्भक्षयेन्माषं मरिचाज्यं लिहेदनु । निहन्ति ग्रहणीरोगं पथ्यं तक्रौदनं हितम् ॥ १७१ ॥

Bhasma of kapardika, tryūṣaṇa, ṭaṅkaṇa, viṣa, gandhaka and purified sūta each equal parts are macerated with the juice of jambīra, dried and stored. Given in doses of one māṣā along with powder of marica and ghee it cures grahaṇī roga. The patient should take buttermilk and rice during the treatment (170–171).

अथ त्रिविक्रमरसः अश्मर्यां—

मृतं ताम्रमजाक्षीरैः पाच्यं तुल्यैर्गतद्रवम् । तत्ताम्रं शुद्धसूतं च गन्धकं च समं समम् ॥ १७२ ॥
निर्गुण्डीस्वरसैर्मर्द्यं तद्गोलं सन्धयेद्दिनम् । यामैकं वालुकायन्त्रे पाच्यं भोज्यं द्विगुञ्जकम् ॥ १७३ ॥
बीजपूरकमूलं तु सजलं चानुपाययेत् । रसस्त्रिविक्रमो नाम्ना मासैकेनाश्मरीप्रणुत् ॥ १७४ ॥

Tāmrabhasma is mixed with goat's milk and cooked till all the milk evaporates. Purified sūta and gandhaka equal in weight to tāmrabhasma are taken and all the three are macerated with the juice of nirguṇḍī, rolled into discs, kept inside mud plates which are sealed and dried. They are later kept inside a pot containing sand and subjected to increasing heat for one yāma (3 hours). After cooling it is removed and stored. This recipe known as *Trivikrama rasa* if used, in doses of two guñjās followed with juice of root of bijapūraka as anupāna, cures aśmarī (caliculii) within one month (173–174).

सर्वकुष्ठादौ महातालेश्वररसः—

तालं ताप्यं शिला सूतं शुद्धं सैन्धवटङ्कणे । समांशं चूर्णयेत्खल्वे सूताद्द्विगुणगन्धकम् ॥ १७५ ॥
गन्धतुल्यं मृतं ताम्रं जम्बीरैर्दिनपञ्चकम् । मर्द्यं षड्भिः पाच्यं भूधरे सम्पुटोदरे ॥ १७६ ॥
पुटे पुटे द्रवैर्मर्द्यं सर्वमेतत्तु षट्पलम् । द्विपलं मारितं ताम्रं लोहभस्म चतुष्पलम् ॥ १७७ ॥
जम्बीराम्लेन तत्सर्वं दिनं मर्द्यं पुटेल्लघु । त्रिंशदंशं विषं चास्य क्षिप्त्वा सर्वं विचूर्णयेत् ॥ १७८ ॥
माहिषाज्येन सम्मिश्रं निष्कार्धं भक्षयेत्सदा । मध्वाज्यैर्बाकुचीचूर्णं कर्षमात्रं लिहेदनु ॥ १७९ ॥
सर्वकुष्ठानि हन्त्याशु महातालेश्वरो रसः ।

Tālaka, tāpya, śiva, sūta (purified mercury), saindhava, ṭaṅkaṇa,-each one part, two parts each of gandhaka and tāmrabhasma are collected. Sūta and gandhaka are first made into kajjalī and all the others are added and powdered nicely. Tāmra bhasma equal in weight to gandhaka is added to the above and all are macerated with juiceof jāmbīra for five days and subjected to bhūdara puṭas for six times. Afterwards, two palas of tāmra bhasma and four palas of loha bhasma are added, macerated with juice of jambīra for one day and subjected one laghu puṭa. Later, viṣa (vatsanabhi) one thirtieth part of the whole powder is added and macerated with buffalos ghee for one day and stored. This recipe known as *Mahā tāleśwara rasa,* used in doses of half a niṣka followed with honey, ghee and half a karṣa of powder of bakucī cures all kinds of kuṣṭhas (leprosy and other skin diseases (175–179).

अथकुष्ठकुठारो रसः—

भस्मसूतसमो गन्धो मृतायस्ताम्रगुग्गुलून् ॥ १८० ॥
त्रिफला च महानिम्बश्चित्रकश्च शिलाजतु । इत्येतच्चूर्णितं कुर्यात्प्रत्येकं शाणषोडश ॥ १८१ ॥
चतुःषष्टिः करञ्जस्य बीजचूर्णं प्रकल्पयेत् । चतुःषष्टिर्मृतं चाभ्रं मध्वाजाभ्यां विलोडयेत् ॥ १८२ ॥
स्निग्धभाण्डे धृतं खादेद्द्विनिष्कं सर्वकुष्ठनुत् । रसः कुष्ठकुठारोऽयं गलत्कुष्ठनिवारणः ॥ १८३ ॥

Sixteen śāṇas each of sūtabhasma, gandhaka, lohabhasma, tāmrabhasma, guggulu, triphalā, mahānimba, citraka and śilājatu are powdered nicely and added to sixtyfour śāṇas each of powder of karañja and abhraka bhasma, All these are macerated nicely with honey and ghee and stored. Used in doses of two niṣkas, this *Kuṣṭha kuṭhāra rasa,* cures all kuṣṭhas including galat kuṣṭha (leprosy which mutilates the body parts) (180–183).

अथोदयादिरसः श्वेतकुष्ठादौ—

शुद्धं सूतं द्विधा गन्धं मर्द्यं कन्याद्रवैर्दिनम् । तद्गोलं पिठरीमध्ये ताम्रपात्रेण रोधयेत् ॥ १८४ ॥
सूतकाद्द्विगुणेनैव शुद्धेनाधोमुखेन च । पार्श्वे भस्म निधायाथ पात्रोर्ध्वं गोमयं जलम् ॥ १८५ ॥
किंचित्किंचित्प्रदातव्यं चुल्ल्यां यामद्वयं पचेत् । चण्डाग्निना तदुद्धृत्य स्वाङ्गशीतं विचूर्णयेत् ॥१८६॥
काष्ठोदुम्बरिकावह्नित्रिफलाराजवृक्षकम् । विडङ्गं बाकुचीबीजं क्वाथयेत्तेन भावयेत् ॥ १८७ ॥

दिनैकमुदयादित्यो रसो देयो द्विगुञ्जकः । विचर्चिकां दद्रुकुष्ठं वातरक्तं च नाशयेत् ॥ १८८ ॥
अनुपानं च कर्तव्यं बाकुचीफलचूर्णकम् । खदिरस्य कषायेण समेन परिपाचितम् ॥ १८९ ॥
त्रिशाणं तद्भवां क्षीरैः क्वाथैर्वा त्रैफलै पिबेत् । त्रिदिनान्ते भवेत्स्फोटः सप्ताहाद्वा किलासके ॥ १९० ॥
नीलीं गुञ्जां च कासीसं धत्तूरं हंसपादिकाम् । सूर्यभक्तां च चाङ्गेरीं पिष्ट्वा मूलात्प्रलेपयेत् ॥ १९१ ॥
स्फोटस्थानप्रशान्त्यर्थं सप्तरात्रं पुनः पुनः । श्वेतकुष्ठं निहत्याशु साध्यासाध्यं न संशयः ॥ १९२ ॥
अपरः श्वित्रलेपोऽपि कथ्यतेऽत्र भिषग्वरैः । गुञ्जाफलाग्निचूर्णं च लेपितं श्वेतकुष्ठनुत् ॥ १९३ ॥
शिलापामार्गभस्मापि लिप्तं श्वित्रं विनाशयेत् ।

One part of sūta and two parts of gandhaka are macerated with jucie of kanya for one day and made into a ball. Thin leaves of copper equal in weight as that of sūta is taken, into which the ball of kajjalī is placed. Covered all over with a paste of ash and cowdung and allowed to dry. After drying it is kept inside a pot containing a solution of cowdung and subjected to cooking over strong fire for two yāmas (six hours). Later the contents are removed and macerated for one day with the decoction prepared out of kāsṭhaudumbarikā, vahni, triphalā, rājavṛkṣa viḍaṅga and bākucī seeds. Afterwards it is dried and stored. This recipe known as *Udayāditya rasa* in doses of two guñjās cures vicarcika (psoriasis), dadru kuṣṭha (a kind of leprosy) and vātarakta (gout) if followed of bākucī seeds and decoction of khadira both equal parts. Taken in doses of three śāṇas followed with cow's milk or decoction of triphalā, it produces blebs at the end of three days or seven days in cases of kilāsa (leucoderma, vitiligo). A powder prepared with the roots of nīlī, guñjā, kāsīsa, dhattūra, haṁsapādī, sūryabhakta and cāṅgerī is dusted over the ulcers often. By so doing sweta kuṣṭha (leucoderma, vitiligo) will be cured without doubt. Another kind of paste prepared with guñjāphala and agni (citraka) or manaśila and ashes of apāmārga which also cures svitra (leucoderma) has been extolled by experts (184–193).

अथ कुष्टादौ सर्वेश्वरो रसः—

शुद्धं सूतं चतुर्गन्धं पलं यामं विचूर्णयेत् ॥ १९४ ॥
मृतताम्राभ्रलोहानां दरदस्य पलं पलम् । सुवर्णं रजतं चैव प्रत्येकं दशनिष्ककम् ॥ १९५ ॥
माषैकं मृतवज्रं च तालं शुद्धं पलद्वयम् । जम्बीरोन्मत्तवासाभिः स्नुह्यर्कविषमुष्टिभिः ॥ १९६ ॥
मर्द्यं हयारिजैर्द्रावैः प्रत्येकेन दिनंदिनम् । एवं सप्तदिनं मर्द्यं तद्गोलं वस्त्रवेष्टितम् ॥ १९७ ॥
वालुकायन्त्रगं स्वेद्यं त्रिदिनं लघुवह्निना । आदाय चूर्णयेच्छ्लक्ष्णं पलैकं योजयेद्विषम् ॥ १९८ ॥
द्विपलं पिप्पलीचूर्णं मिश्रं सर्वेश्वरो रसः । द्विगुञ्जो लिह्यते क्षौद्रैः सुप्तिमण्डलकुष्ठनुत् ॥ १९९ ॥
बाकुची देवकाष्ठं च कर्षमात्रं सुचूर्णयेत् । लिहेदैरण्डतैलाक्तमनुपानं सुखावहम् ॥ २०० ॥

One pala of purified sūta and four palas of purified gandhaka are rubbed together for one yāma (three hours) and kajjalī prepared. To this are added one pala each of bhasmas of tāmra, abhraka, loha and darada, teñ niṣkas of suvarṇa and rajata; one māṣa of vajra bhasma, to palas of purified tālaka—are all macerated for seven days, one day in each of the juices of jambīra, unmatta, vasā, snuhī, arka, viṣamuṣṭī and hayāri. The paste is made into a ball, covered over with cloth and mud plaster and dried. Later the ball is kept inside vālukāyantra (sand bath) and cooked over mild fire for three days, later taken out and mixed with powder of one pala of viṣa (vatsanābhi) and two palas of pippalī and stored. Used in doses of two guñjās each with honey this recipe known as *Sarveśwara rasa*, cures supti (aneasthetic patches on skin) and maṇḍala kuṣṭha (a veriety of leprosy). It can even be used with powder of one karṣa each of bākucī and devakāṣṭha along with eraṇḍa taila with great benefit (194–200).

अथ सुप्त्यादौ स्वर्णक्षीरीरसः—

हेमाह्वां पञ्चपलिकां क्षिप्त्वा तक्रघटे पचेत् । तक्रे जीर्णे समुद्धृत्य पुनः क्षीरघटे पचेत् ॥ २०१ ॥
क्षीरे जीर्णे समुद्धृत्य क्षालयित्वा विशोधयेत् । तच्चूर्णं पञ्चपलिकं मरिचानां पलद्वयम् ॥ २०२ ॥
पलैकं मूर्च्छितं सूतमेकीकृत्य तु भक्षयेत् । निष्कैकं सुप्तिकुष्ठार्तः स्वर्णक्षीरीरसो ह्ययम् ॥ २०३ ॥

Five palas of hemāhwa (swarṇakṣīrī plant) is cut into bits and boiled in butter milk till the fluid evaporates. Next it is boiled in cow's milk like wise. Next the bits are washed in water and dried in shade and powdered. Five palas of this powder is mixed with two palas of marica and one pala of mūrchita sūta (mercury cooked with sulphur i.e., rasa sindūra) and grinded well and stored. This recipe known as *Swarṇakṣīrī rasa* used in doses of one niṣka cures supti kuṣṭh (anaesthetic leprosy) (201–203).

अथ मेहबद्धो रसः प्रमेहे—

भस्मसूतं मृतं कान्तं मुण्डभस्म शिलाजातु । शुद्धं ताप्यं शिला व्योम त्रिफलां कोलबीजकम् ॥२०४॥
कपित्थं रजनीचूर्णं भृङ्गराजेन भावयेत् । त्रिंशद्वारं विशोष्याथ मधुयुक्तं लिहेत्सदा ॥ २०५ ॥
निष्कमात्रो हरेन्मेहान्मेहबद्धो रसो महान् । महानिम्बस्य बीजानि पिष्ट्वा षट्सम्मितानि च ॥२०६॥
पलंतण्डुलतोयेन घृतनिष्कद्वयेन च । एकीकृत्य पिबेच्चानु हन्ति मेहं चिरन्तनम् ॥ २०७ ॥

Bhasmas of sūta, kānta, muṇḍa, śilājatu, purified tāpya, manaśila; vyoma,[1] triphalā, aṅkola bīja, kapittha, rajanī—all equal parts are macerated with juices of bhṛṅgarāja for thirty times, dried and stored. This recipe known as *Mahā mehabaddha rasa*, used in doses of one niṣka each with honey cures all types of pramehas (diabetes). Six seeds of mahānimba, one pala of rice-wash and one niṣka of ghee all mixed well—should be taken as an anupāna (after drink) in cases of long standing diabetes (204–207).

1. Vyoṣa in some texts.

अथ महावह्निरसमाह—

चतुःसूतस्य गन्धाष्टौ रजनी त्रिफला शिवा । प्रत्येकं च द्विभागं स्यात्त्रिवृज्जैपालचित्रकम् ॥ २०८ ॥
प्रत्येकं च त्रिभागं स्यात्त्र्यूषं दन्ती च जीरकम् । प्रत्येकमष्टभागं स्यादेकीकृत्य विचूर्णयेत् ॥ २०९ ॥
जयन्तीस्नुकपयोभृङ्गवह्निवातारितैलकैः । प्रत्येकेन क्रमाद्भाव्यं सप्तवारं पृथक्पृथक् ॥ २१० ॥
महावह्निरसो नाम निष्कमुष्णजलैः पिबेत् । विरेचनं भवेत्तेन तक्रभक्तं ससैन्धवम् ॥ २११ ॥
दिनान्ते दापयेत्पथ्यं वर्जयेच्छीतलं जलम् । सर्वोदरहरः प्रोक्तो मूढवातहरः परः ॥ २१२ ॥

Four parts of sūta, eight of gandhaka are made into kajjalī first; to this are added two parts each of rajanī, triphalā, śiva; three parts each of trivṛt, japāla, citraka, eight parts each of tryūṣaṇa, dantī and jīraka—all are powdered and macerated with the juice of jayantī and snuhī, decoction of bhṛṅga, vahni and vātāri taila (castor oil) for seven times in each fluid, dried and stored. This recipe called *Mahāvahni rasa,* taken in doses of one niṣka followed with warm water produces purgations and there by cures all types of udaras (abdominal enlargemets) and mūḍa vāta (sluggish peristalisis). The patient is told to drink butter milk and saindhava till the evening and given rice and butter milk as diet and told to avoid drinking cold water (208–212).

अथ विद्याधरो रसः गुल्मप्लीहादौ—

गन्धकं तालकं ताप्यं मृतताम्रं मनःशिलाम् । शुद्धं सूतं च तुल्यांशं मर्दयेद्भावयेद्दिनम् ॥ २१३ ॥
पिप्पल्यास्तु कषायेण वज्रीक्षीरेण भावयेत् । निष्कार्धं भक्षयेत्क्षौद्रैर्गुल्मं प्लीहादिकं जयेत् ॥ २१४ ॥
रसो विद्याधरो नाम गोमूत्रं च पिबेदनु ।

Equal quantities of purified sūta and gandhaka are made into kajjali. Later tālaka, tāpya, tāmra bhasma, manaśila each equal in weight to that of sūta are added and macerated with the decoction of pippalī and milky juice of vajrī one day in each, dried and stored. This recipe known as *Vidyādhara rasa* taken in doses of half a niṣka along with honey cures gulma (abdominal tumor) and plīh*ā* (splenic enlargement). Taking cow's urine as an after-drink is advantageous (213–215).

अथ त्रिनेत्रो रसः पक्तिशूलादौ—

टङ्कणं हारिणं श्रृङ्गं स्वर्णं शुल्बं मृतं रसम् ॥ २१५ ॥
दिनैकमार्द्रकद्रावैर्मर्द्यं रुद्ध्वा पुटे पचेत् । त्रिनेत्राख्यरसस्यैकं माषं मध्वाज्यकैर्लिहेत् ॥ २१६ ॥
सैन्धवं जीरकं हिङ्गु मध्वाज्याभ्यां लिहेदनु । पक्तिशूलहरः ख्यातो मासमात्रान्नसंशयः ॥ २१७ ॥

Ṭaṅkaṇa, hāriṇaśṛṅgabhasma, swarṇabhasma, tāmrabhasma, mṛtarasa (bhasma of mercury)—each equal parts are macerated with juice of green ginger for one day, made into thin cakes, sealed inside earthen plates and subjected to gajapuṭa. After cooling it is used in doses of one māṣa followed by honey, ghee, saindhava, jīraka and hiṅgu. This recipe known as *Trinetra rasa* cures paktiśūla (colic due to digestive disorders) within a month without doubt (215–217).

अथ शूलगजकेसरीरसः शूले—

शुद्धं सूतं द्विधा गन्धं यामैकं मर्दयेद्दृढम् । द्वयोस्तुल्यं शुद्धताम्रं संपुटे तन्निरोधयेत् ॥ २१८ ॥
ऊर्ध्वाधो लवणं दत्त्वा मृद्भाण्डे धारयेद्भिषक् । ततो गजपुटे पक्त्वा स्वाङ्गशीतं समुद्धरेत् ॥२१९॥
संपुटं चूर्णयेत्सूक्ष्मं पर्णखण्डे द्विगुञ्जकम् । भक्षयेत्सर्वशूलार्तो हिङ्गु शुण्ठी च जीरकम् ॥ २२० ॥
वचामरिचजं चूर्णं कर्षमुष्णजलैः पिबेत् । असाध्यं नाशयेच्छूलं रसोऽयं गजकेसरी ॥ २२१ ॥

One part of purified sūta and two parts of gandhaka are macerated for one yāma, tāmrabhasma equal in weight to the above two is taken and made into two crucibles within which the mixture of rasa and gandhaka is kept. The crucible is placed in an earthen pot containing salt, the pot sealed and subjected to gajapuṭa, with cowdung heaps. After cooling the crucible is removed, powdered nicely and stored. This recipe known as *Śūla gaja kesarī* used in doses of two guñjās along with the decoction of one karṣa each of hiṅgu, śuṇṭhī, jīraka, vaca and marica and warm water cures all kinds of śūla (abdominal pain) (218–221).

अथाग्नितुण्डवटीरसः अग्निमान्द्यादौ—

शुद्धं सूतं विषं गन्धमजमोदां फलत्रयम् । स्वर्जिक्षारं यवक्षारं वह्निसैन्धवजीरकम् ॥ २२२ ॥
सौवर्चलं विडङ्गानि सामुद्रं त्र्यूषणं समम् । विषमुष्टिं सर्वतुल्यं जम्बीराम्लेन मर्दयेत् ॥ २२३ ॥
मरिचाभां वटीं खादेद्वह्निमान्द्यप्रशान्तये ।

Purified sūta, viṣa, gandhaka, ajamodā, triphalā, swarjikṣāra, yavakṣāra, vahni (citraka), saindhava, jīraka, sauvarcala, viḍaṅga, sāmudra lavaṇa and tryūṣaṇa—each equal in quantity and viṣamuṣṭi equal to the total quantity of all the above are macerated with juice of jambīra and rolled into pills of the size of black pepper. This recipe is effective in agnimāndya (dyspepsia) (222–224).

अथाजीर्णकण्टको रसः—

शुद्धं सूतं विषं गन्धं समं सर्वं विचूर्णयेत् ॥ २२४ ॥
मरिचं सर्वतुल्यांशं कण्टकार्याः फलद्रवैः । मर्दयेद्भावयेत्सर्वमेकविंशतिवारकम् ॥ २२५ ॥
वटीं गुञ्जात्रयं खादेत्सर्वाजीर्णप्रशान्तये । अजीर्णकण्टकः सोऽयं रसो हन्ति विषूचिकाम् ॥२२६॥

Purified sūta, gandhaka and viṣa all equal parts and marica equal to the total weight of all—are macerated with juice of fruits of kaṇṭakārī for twentyone times and rolled into pills of three guñjās in weight. This recipe known as *Ajīrṇakaṇṭaka rasa* relieves all types of ajīrṇa (indigestion) and cures viṣūcikā (gastro-enteritis, cholera) (224–226).

कफादौ मन्थानभैरवसः ।

मृतं सूतं मृतं ताम्रं हिङ्गु पुष्करमूलकम् । सैन्धवं गन्धकं तालं कटुकीं चूर्णयेत्समम् ॥ २२७ ॥
पुनर्नवादेवदालीनिर्गुण्डीतण्डुलीयकैः । तिक्तकोशातकीद्रावैर्दिनैकं मर्दयेद्दृढम् ॥ २२८ ॥
माषमात्रं लिहेत्क्षौद्रे रसं मन्थानभैरवम् । कफरोगप्रशान्त्यर्थं निम्बकाथं पिबेदनु ॥ २२९ ॥

Bhasmas of sūta, tāmra, hiṅgu, puṣkaramūla, saindhava, gandhaka, tālaka and kaṭuka—each equal quantity are macerated with the juices of punarnavā, devadālī, nirguṇḍī, taṇḍulīyaka, and tikta kośātakī—one day in each and dried. Used in doses of one māṣa with honey and followed with a decoction of nimba this recipe known as *Manthana bhairava* cures all kapha rogas (diseases due to increase of kapha in the body) (227–229).

अथ वातनाशनो रसः—

सूतहाटकवज्राणि ताम्रं लोहं च माक्षिकम् । तालं नीलाञ्जनं तुत्थमहिफेनं समांशकम् ॥ २३० ॥
पञ्चानां लवणानां च भागमेकं विमर्दयेत् । वज्रीक्षीरैर्दिनैकं तु रुद्ध्वाधो भूधरे पचेत् ॥ २३१ ॥
माषैकमार्द्रकद्रावैर्लेहयेद्वातनाशनम् । पिप्पलीमूलजक्वाथं सकृष्णमनुपाययेत् ॥ २३२ ॥
सर्वान्वातविकरांस्तु निहन्त्याक्षेपकादिकान् ।

Bhasmas of sūta, hāṭaka, vajra tāmra, loha, mākṣika, nīlāñjana, tuttha and ahiphena—all equal quantities and all the five lavaṇas together one part (i.e. equal in weight to any one of the above) are all macerated with the milky juice of vajrī (snuhī) and subjected to heat in bhūdhara puṭa with cowdung heaps. After cooling, it is taken out, powdered nicely and stored. Taken in doses of one māṣa mixed with juice of green ginger or decoction of pippalīmūla and kṛṣṇa—cures all vātarogas such as ākṣepaka (convulsions) etc. (230–233).

अथ कनकसुन्दरः सन्निपातादौ—

कनकस्याष्टशाणाः स्युः सूतो द्वादशभिर्मतः ॥ २३३ ॥
गन्धोऽपि द्वादश प्रोक्तस्ताम्रं शाणद्वयोन्मितम् । अभ्रकं स्याच्चतुःशाणं माक्षिकं च द्विशाणिकम् ॥२३४॥
वङ्गो द्विशाणः सौवीरं त्रिशाणं लोहमष्टकम् । विषं त्रिशाणिकं कृत्वा लाङ्गली पलसंमिता ॥२३५॥
मर्दयेद्दिनमेकं तु रसैरम्लफलोद्भवैः । दद्यान्मृदुपुटं वह्नौ ततः सूक्ष्मं विचूर्णयेत् ॥ २३६ ॥
माषमात्रो रसो देयः संनिपाते सुदारुणे । आर्द्रकस्वरसेनैव रसोनस्य रसेन वा ॥ २३७ ॥
किलासं सर्वकुष्ठानि विसर्पं च भगन्दरम् । ज्वरं गरमजीर्णं च जयेद्रोगहरो रसः ॥ २३८ ॥

Eight śāṇas of kanaka bhasma, twelve of sūta, twelve of gandhaka, two of mākṣika bhasma, four of abhraka bhasma, two of tāmra bhasma, two of vaṅga bhasma, three of sauvīrāñjana bhasma, eight of loha bhasma, three of viṣa and one pala of lāṅgalī—all are macerated with any sour liquid (lemon juice etc.) and subjected to a small puṭapāka (heat of cowdung cakes). Taken out after cooling, powdered nicely and stored. This recipe known as *Roga hara rasa* used in doses of one māṣa along with juice of green ginger of garlic cures sannipāta (toxic) states, kilāsa (white leprosy, vitiligo), all varieties of kuṣṭha (leprosy and other skin diseases), visarpa (erysepelas), bhagandara (fistula in ano) jwara (fevers), gara (homicidal poison) and ajīrṇa (indigestion) (233–238).

अथ सन्निपातभैरवो रसः—

रसो गन्धस्त्रिकर्षः स्यात् कुर्यात्कज्जलिकां तयोः । ताम्रताराभ्रवङ्गाहिसाराश्चैकैककार्षिकाः ॥ २३९ ॥
शिग्रुज्वालामुखीशुण्ठीबिल्वेभ्यस्तण्डुलीयकान् । प्रत्येकं स्वरसैः कुर्याद्यामैकैकं विमर्दनम् ॥२४०॥
कृत्वा गोलं वृतं वस्त्रे लवणापूरिते न्यसेत् । काचभाण्डे ततः स्थाल्यां काचकूपीं निवेशयेत् ॥२४१॥
वालुकाभिः प्रपूर्याथ वह्निर्यामद्वयं भवेत् । तत उद्धृत्य तं गोलं चूर्णयित्वा विमिश्रयेत् ॥ २४२ ॥
प्रवाणचूर्णकर्षेण शाणमात्रविषेण च । कृष्णसर्पस्य गरलैर्द्विवेलं भावयेत्तथा ॥ २४३ ॥
तगरं मुशली मांसी हेमाह्वा वेतसः कणा । नीलिनी पत्रकं चैला चित्रकश्च कुठेरकः ॥ २४४ ॥
शतपुष्पा देवदाली धत्तूरागस्त्यमुण्डिकाः । मधूकजातीमदनरसैरेषां विमर्दयेत् ॥ २४५ ॥
प्रत्येकमेकवेलं च ततः सशोष्य धारयेत् । बीजपूरार्द्रकद्रावैर्मरिचैः षोडशोन्मितैः ॥ २४६ ॥
रसो द्विगुञ्जामितः संनिपातेषु दीयते । प्रसिद्धोऽयं रसो नाम्ना संनिपातस्य भैरवः ॥ २४७ ॥

Three karṣas of rasa and gandhaka are first made into kajjalī and mixed with one karṣa each of bhasmas of tāra (silver), abhraka (mica), tāmra (copper), āra (brass), vaṅga (tin), ahi (lead), sāra (iron)—all are macerated with the juices of śigru, jvālāmukhī, śuṇṭhī, bilwa and taṇḍulīyaka one yāma in each, made into a ball, kept in a glass bottle putting salt above and below. The bottle is given a mud plaster sealing, kept inside a pot containing sand and subjected to strong fire for two yāmas. After cooling, the contents are powdered nicely mixing it with one karṣa of *Pravāṇa cūrṇa* (lime powder) and one śāṇa of viṣa and macerated with one śāṇa of poison of black cobra.

Later on it is macerated with the decoction of tagara, musalī, māṃsī, hemāhwa, vetasa, kaṇa, nīlinī, patraka, elā, citraka, kuṭheraka, śatapuṣpa, devadālī, dhattūra, agastya, muṇḍī, madhūka, jātī and madana—once in each, dried and stored. Used in doses of two guñjas along with marica sixteen in number and juice of bījapūra and ārdraka, it is effectively used in cases of sannipātas (toxic states). This recipe is famous as *Sannipāta bhairava* (239–247).

अतीसारादौ ग्रहणीकपाटः—

तारमौक्तिकहेमानि सारश्चैकैकभागिकाः । द्विभागो गन्धकः सूतस्त्रिभागो मर्दयेदिमान् ॥ २४८ ॥
कपित्थस्वरसैर्गाढं मृगश्रृङ्गे ततः क्षिपेत् । पुटेन्मध्यपुटेनैव तत उद्धृत्य मर्दयेत् ॥ २४९ ॥
बलारसैः सप्तवेलमपामार्गरसैस्त्रिधा । लोध्रप्रतिविषामुस्तधातकीन्द्रयवामृताः ॥ २५० ॥
प्रत्येकमेषां स्वरसैर्भावना स्यात्त्रिधा त्रिधा । माषमात्रो रसो देयो मधुना मरिचैस्तथा ॥ २५१ ॥
हन्यात्सर्वानतीसारान्ग्रहणीं सर्वजामपि । कपाटो ग्रहणीरोगे रसोऽयं वह्निदीपनः ॥ २५२ ॥

One part each of bhasmas of tāra (silver), mauktika (pearls), hema (gold) sāra (iron), two parts of gandhaka (sulphur) and three parts of (bhasma) of sūta (mercury) are macerated with the juice of kapittha and added with bhasma of mṛga śṛṅga and subjected to gajapuṭa with cowdung cakes. Next it is macerated with the juice of balā for seven times and three times in each of the juices of apāmārga, lodhra, prativiṣa, musta, dhātakī, indrayava and amṛta. This recipe used in doses of one māṣa, along with marica and honey cures all types of atisāras (diarrhoea) and grahaṇī (sprue). It acts like a kapāṭa (shutter) in grahaṇi roga and is a good dīpana (stomachic) (248-252).

अथ ग्रहणीवज्रकपाटः—

मृतसूताभ्रकं गन्धं यवक्षारं सटङ्कणम् । अग्निमन्थं वचां कुर्यात्सूततुल्यानिमान्सुधीः ॥ २५३ ॥
ततो जयन्तीजम्बीरभृङ्गद्रावैर्विमर्दयेत् । त्रिवासरं ततो गोलं कृत्वा संशोष्य धारयेत् ॥ २५४ ॥
लोहपात्रे शरावं च दत्त्वोपरि विमुद्रयेत् । अधो वह्निं शनैः कुर्याद्यामार्धं तत उद्धरेत् ॥ २५५ ॥
रसतुल्यां प्रतिविषां दद्यान्मोचरसं तथा । कपित्थविजयाद्रावैर्भावयेत्सप्तधा पृथक् ॥ २५६ ॥
धातकीन्द्रयवा मुस्ता लोध्रं बिल्वं गुडूचिका । एतद्रसैर्भावयित्वा वेलैकैकं च शोषयेत् ॥ २५७ ॥
रसं वज्रकपाटाख्यं शाणैकं मधुना लिहेत् । वह्निं शुण्ठीं बिडं बिल्वं लवणं चूर्णयेत्समम् ॥२५८॥
पिबेदुष्णाम्बुना चानु सर्वजां ग्रहणीं जयेत् ।

Bhasmas of sūta and abhraka, gandhaka, yavakṣāra, agnimantha and vaca-all equal quantities are macerated for three days with the juice of jayantī, jambīra, bhṛṅga, rolled into a ball and dried. It is then sealed in between to iron plates and cooked for about half a yāma, with mild fire underneath. After cooling it is taken out and added with prativiṣa, mocarasa each equal in quantity to that of rasa and macerated with the juice of kapittha and vijayā for seven times in each and once in each of juices of dhātakī, indrayava, musta, lodhra, bilwa and guḍūcī, dried in shade and stored. This recipe known as (Grahaṇī) *Vajrakapāṭa rasa* used in doses of one śāna along with honey or equal quantity of powder of vahni (citraka), śuṇṭhi, viḍa, bilwa lavāṇa, follwed by warm water as a drink cures all types of grahaṇī (sprue). (253-259)

अथ मदनकामदेवो वाजीकरणे—

तारं वज्रं सुवर्णं च ताम्रं सूतकगन्धकम् ॥ २५९ ॥
लोहं क्रमविवृद्धानि कुर्यादेतानि मात्रया । विमर्द्य कन्यकाद्रावैर्न्यसेत्काचमये घटे ॥ २६० ॥
विमुद्रां पिठरीमध्ये धारयेत्सैन्धवावृते । पिठरीं मुद्रयेत्सम्यक् ततश्चुल्ल्यां निवेशयेत् ॥ २६१ ॥
वह्निं शनैः शनैः कुर्याद्दिनैकं तत उद्धरेत् । स्वाङ्गशीतं च संचूर्ण्य भावयेदर्कदुग्धकैः ॥ २६२ ॥
अश्वगन्धा च काकोली वानरी मुशलीक्षुरा । त्रित्रिवेलं रसैरासां शतावर्याश्च भावयेत् ॥ २६३ ॥
पद्मकन्दकसेरूणां रसैः काशस्य भावयेत् । कस्तूरी व्योषकर्पूरकङ्कोलैलालवङ्गकम् ॥ २६४ ॥
पूर्वंचूर्णादष्टमांशमेतच्चूर्णं विमिश्रयेत् । सर्वैः समां शर्करां च दत्त्वा शाणोन्मितां पिबेत् ॥ २६५ ॥
गोदुग्धद्विपलेनैव मधुराहारसेवकः । अस्य प्रभावात्सौन्दर्यं बलं तेजोऽभिवर्धते ॥ २६६ ॥
तरुणी रमयेद्बह्वीः शुक्रहानिर्न जायते ।

Bhasma of tāra, vajra, suvarṇa, tāmra, sūta, gandhaka, lohabhasma in successively increasing proportion are maceated in the juice of kanyaka, filled into a glass bottle, its mouth sealed with saindhava. The bottle is covered with mud plaster, kept inside a lavaṇa yantra (salt bath), mounted on a oven and cooked with mild fire for one day. After cooling it is taken out and macerated for three times in each of the juices of arka dughdha (milky sap of arka), aswangandhā, kākolī, vānarī, musalī, ikṣukā (kokilākṣa), śatāvarī, padmakanda, kaseruka and kāśa. Afterwards kastūrī, vyoṣa, karpūra, kaṅkola, elā and lavaṅga each equal parts are powdered and added to the first mixture equalant to one eighth of it's total weight; sugar equal to the total weight of all is also added. Taken in doses of one śāṇa followed with two palas of warm cow's milk and indulging in sweet foods only, the person obtains by the effect of this recipe, radiance on the face, strength in the body and valour in activities, capacity to copulate with many women, without seminal loss (259-266).

वाजीकरणे कन्दर्पसुन्दररसमाह—

सूतो वज्रमहिर्मुक्ता तारं हेमासिताभ्रकम् ॥ २६७ ॥
रसैः कर्षांशकानेतान्मर्दयेदिरिमेदजैः । प्रवालचूर्णं गन्धं च द्विद्विकर्षं विमिश्रयेत् ॥ २६८ ॥
ततोऽश्वगन्धास्वरसैर्विमर्द्य मृगश्रृङ्गके । क्षिप्त्वा मृदुपुटे पक्त्वा भावयेद्धातकीरसैः ॥ २६९ ॥
काकोली मधुकं मांसी बलात्रयबिसेङ्गुदे । द्राक्षापिप्पलवन्दाकं वरी पर्णीचतुष्टयम् ॥ २७० ॥
परूषकं कसेरुश्च मधूकं वानरी तथा । भावयित्वा रसैरेषां शोषयित्वा विचूर्णयेत् ॥ २७१ ॥
एलात्वक्पत्रकं वांशी लवङ्गागरुकेशरम् । मुस्तं मृगमदः कृष्णा जलं चन्द्रश्च मिश्रयेत् ॥ २७२ ॥
एतच्चूर्णैः शाणमितैं रसं कन्दर्पसुन्दरम् । खादेच्छाणमितं रात्रौ सिता धात्री विदारिका ॥ २७३ ॥
एतासां कर्षचूर्णेन सर्पिष्कर्षेण संयुतम् । तस्यानु द्विपलं क्षीरं पिबेत्सुस्थितमानसः ॥ २७४ ॥
रमणी रमयेद्बह्वीनं हानि कापि गच्छति ।

Sūta, vajra, ahi (lead), muktā, tāra, hema, kṛṣṇa abhraka—each one karṣa is macerated with the juice of irimeda for one day. Two karṣas each of pravāla bhasma and gandhaka are added next the macerated with juice of aswagandhā, filled into a mṛga śṛṅga (stag horn) and subjected to a small puṭapāka. Afterwards it is macerated with each of the juices of dhātakī, kākolī, madhuka, māṃsī, the three balās, bisa, iṅgudī, drākṣā, pippalī, vandāka, varī, the four parṇīs, parūṣaka, kaseru, madhūka and vānarī—dried in shade. A powder of elā, twak, patra, māṃsī, lavaṅga, aguru, kesara, musta, mṛgamada, kṛṣṇa, jala (uśīra), candra (karpūra) is also made ready. One śāṇa each of the first and the second powders taken at night mixed with little quantity of powder of one karṣa of sita, dhatrī and vidārika; one karṣa of ghee followed with two palas of cow's milk, makes the user capable of copulating with many women without loss of semen (267-275).

अथ लोहरसायनम्—

शुद्धं रसेन्द्रं भागैकं द्विभागं शुद्धगन्धकम् ॥ २७५ ॥
क्षिपेत्कज्जलिकां कुर्यात्तत्र तीक्ष्णभवं रजः । क्षिप्त्वा कज्जलिकातुल्यं प्रहरैकं विमर्दयेत् ॥ २७६ ॥

ततः कन्याद्रवैर्धर्मे त्रिदिनं परिमर्दयेत् । ततः संजायते तस्य सोष्णो धूमोद्गमो महान् ॥ २७७ ॥
अत्यन्तं पिण्डितं कृत्वा ताम्रपात्रे निधापयेत् । मध्ये धान्यकुशूलस्य त्रिदिनं धारयेद्बुधः ॥ २७८ ॥
उद्धृत्य तस्मात्खल्वे च क्षिप्त्वा धर्मे निधाय च । रसैः कुठारच्छिन्नायास्त्रिवेलं परिभावयेत् ॥२७९॥
संशोष्य धर्मे काथैश्च भावयेत्त्रिकटोस्त्रिधा । वासामृताचित्रकाणारसैर्भाव्यं क्रमात्त्रिधा ॥ २८० ॥
लोहपात्रे ततः क्षिप्त्वा भावयेत्त्रिफलाजलैः । निर्गुण्डीदाडिमत्वग्भिर्बिसभृङ्गकुरण्टकैः ॥ २८१ ॥
पलाशकदलीद्रावैर्बीजकस्य श्रृतेन च । नीलिकालम्बुषाद्रावैर्बब्बूलफलिकारसैः ॥ २८२ ॥
भावयेत्त्रिस्त्रिवेलं च ततो नागबलारसैः । शतावरीगोक्षुरुभिः पातालगरुडीद्रवैः ॥ २८३ ॥
त्रिस्त्रिवेलं यथालाभं भावयेदेभिरौषधैः । ततः प्रातर्लिहेत्क्षौद्रघृताभ्यां कोलमात्रकम् ॥ २८४ ॥
पलमात्रं वराक्वाथं पिबेदस्यानुपानकम् । मासत्रयं शीलितं स्याद्वलीपलितनाशनम् ॥ २८५ ॥
मन्दाग्निं श्वासकासौ च पाण्डुतां कफमारुतौ । पिप्पलीमधुसंयुक्तं हन्यादेतन्न संशयः ॥ २८६ ॥
वातास्रं मूत्रदोषांश्च ग्रहणीं गुदजां रुजम् । अण्डवृद्धिं जयेदेतच्छिन्नासत्त्वमधुप्लुतम् ॥ २८७ ॥
बलवर्णकरं वृष्यमायुष्यं परमं स्मृतम् । जयेत्सर्वामयान्कालादिदं लोहरसायनम् ॥ २८८ ॥
कूष्माण्डं तिलतैलं च माषान्नं राजिकां तथा । मद्यमम्लरसं चैव त्यजेल्लोहस्य सेवकः ॥ २८९ ॥

One part of purified rasendra and two parts of purified gandhaka are made into kajjalī. To it is added equal quantity of fine filings of tīkṣṇa loha (magnetic iron) and macerated for three days with the juice of kanyaka, keeping the mortor and pestle in sunlight all through, till strong smoke exudes from it. It is then rolled into a mass, kept in copper vessel which is kept hidden for three days in paddy husk. Next it is macerated for three times in each of juices of kuṭhāra and chinna, next three times with decoction of trikaṭu, vāsā, amṛta, citraka and decoction of triphalā, nirguṇḍī, daḍimatwak, bisa, bhṛṅga, kuraṇṭaka, palāśa, kadalī, bījaka, nīlikā, alambuṣā, babbūla phala, nāgabalā, śatāvarī, gokṣura and pātālagaruḍī. It is then dried in shade powdered nicely and stored. It is taken in doses of one kola each, followed with varā quātha one pala and some quantity of honey and ghee. Used for a period of three months it removes loose-skin, hairs, poor appetite, swāsa (dyspnoea), kāsa (cough), pāṇḍutā (anaemia) and mitigates kapha and vāta. Used with pīppalī and honey, it cures vātasra (gout), mūtradoṣa (urinary disorders), grahaṇī (sprue), guda rujā (pain in the rectum, piles); with honey and satwa of amṛtavallī it cures andavṛddhi (scrotal enlargement). This recipe known as *Loha rasāyana*, confers complexion and strength, is an aphrodisac and bestows longevity; cures all diseases. During the course of treatment, the person should avoid kūṣmāṇḍa, tilataila, māṣa, rājika, madya (alcoholic drinks) and sour foods. (275–289)

जैपालशोधनम् —

(जैपालं रहितं त्वगङ्कुररसभिर्मले माहिषे निक्षिप्तं त्र्यहमुष्णतोयविमलं खल्वे सवासोऽर्दितम् ।
लिप्तं नूतनखर्परेषु विगतस्नेहं रजःसंनिभं । निम्बूकाम्बुविभावितं च बहुशः शुद्धं गुणाढ्यं भवेत् ॥२९०॥

The outer husk and embryo (sprout) present inside the seeds of jayapāla (croton seeds) are removed after soaking the seeds in solution of buffalo's dung. They are then boiled in the same solution of buffalo's dung for three days, later washed in warm water. It is then made into a mass in stone pestle and morter, the mass pasted over a fresh mud pot. The oil in the mass gets absorbed and a powder is then obtained. It is then macerated with lemon juice for more than once. Thus jayapāla gets purified and becomes fit for us. (290)

विषशोधनम्—

विषं तु खण्डशः कृत्वा वस्त्रखण्डेन बन्धयेत् । गोमूत्रमध्ये निक्षित्य स्थापयेदातपे त्र्यहम् ॥ २९१ ॥
गोमूत्रं च प्रदातव्यं नूतनं प्रत्यहं बुधैः । त्र्यहेऽतीते समुद्धृत्य शोषयेन्मृदु पेषयेत् ॥ २९२ ॥
शुद्ध्यत्येवं विषं तच्च योग्यं भवति चार्तजित् । खण्डीकृत्य विषं वस्त्रपरिबद्धं तु दोलया ॥ २९३ ॥
अजापयसि संस्विन्नं यामतः शुद्धिमाप्नुयात् । अजादुग्धाभावतस्तु गव्यक्षीरेण शोधयेत् ॥२९४॥)

Viśa (vastsanābha) is cut into small bits and tied in a cloth, immersed in a pot containing cow's urine and kept in strong sunlight for three days, putting fresh urine each day. After three days it is removed and made into a thin paste. By this it gets purified and fit to be used in all recipes.

Viṣa is cut into pieces tied in a cloth and boiled in goat's milk for one yāma (3 hours) or in cow's milk if goats milk is not available, by this method also it gets purified (291–294).

इति श्रीदामोदरसूनुना शार्ङ्गधराचार्येण विरचितायां शार्ङ्गधरसंहितायां मध्यमखण्डे रसकल्पना नाम द्वादशोऽध्यायः ।

Thus ends the twelvth chapter.

समाप्तोऽयं मध्यमखण्डः ।

Thus ends the Madhyama khaṇḍa of Śārṅgadhara Saṃhitā.

UTTARA KHAṆḌA

(Third Section)

प्रथमोऽध्यायः

CHAPTER 1

अथ स्नेहाध्यायः

Sneha Adhyāya (Oleation Therapy)

अथ स्नेहपानविधिः ।

स्नेहश्चतुर्विधः प्रोक्तो घृतं तैलं तथा वसा ।

मज्जा च—

'कः काल' एतस्य उत्तरमाह—

तं पिबेन्मर्त्यः किंचिदभ्युदिते रवौ ॥ १ ॥

Ghṛta (ghee), taila (oil), vasā (fat) and majā (marrow) are the four snehadravyas (oleating materials). They should be given to drink just after sunrise (1).

'कियोनयः' एतस्योत्तरमाह—

स्थावरो जङ्गमश्चैव द्वियोनिः स्नेह उच्यते ।

वरावरत्वमाह—

तिलतैलं स्थावरेषु जङ्गमेषु घृतं वरम् ॥ २ ॥

Snehas (oleating materials) have two sources,—sthāvara (vegetable) and jaṅgama (animal); oil of tila (sesamum) and ghṛta (ghee) are best from sthāvara and jaṅgama sources respectively (2).

मिलितस्नेहनामान्याह—

द्वाभ्यां त्रिभिश्चतुर्भिस्तैर्यमकस्त्रिवृतो महान् ।

If two oleating substances are mixed and taken it is called yamaka sneha if three are added it is trivṛt sneha and if all the four it is called as mahān sneha (3).

स्नेहसात्म्ये कालावधिमाह—

पिबेत्र्यहं चतुरहं पञ्चाहं षडहं तथा ॥ ३ ॥

सप्तरात्रात्परं स्नेहः सात्मीभवति सेवितः ।

Sneha should be administered for three, four, five, six and seven days continuously and after the seventh day, it becomes accustomed (will have no effect) (3–4).

अथ स्नेहपानमात्राविषयमाह—

दोषकालाग्निवयसां बलं दृष्ट्वा प्रयोजयेत् ॥ ४ ॥
हीनां च मध्यमां ज्येष्ठां मात्रां स्नेहस्य बुद्धिमान् ।

The dose of oleating materials should be decided as hīna (minimum) madhyama (medium) or jyeṣṭha (maximum) depending upon the condition of doṣa (humors), kāla (season), agni (digestive capacity), vaya (age), and balā (strength) of the patient (4–5).

अमात्रादिसेवितस्य स्नेहस्य दोषमाह—

अमात्रया तथाऽकाले मिथ्याहारविहारतः ॥ ५ ॥
स्नेहः करोति शोफार्शस्तन्द्रानिद्राविसंज्ञताः ।
प्रकुर्याल्लङ्घनं तत्र स्वेदं ज्ञात्वा विरेचनम् ॥ ६ ॥

Sneha used in unsuitable dose, improper time, with improper foods and habits produces śopha (oedema), arśa (haemorrhoids), tandrā (drowsiness), nidrā (excessive sleep) and visanjñatā (unconciousness), If such a thing happens the patient should be advised a fast and given sweda (sudation) and virecana (purgation) therapies (5–6).

इदानीं स्नेहपानमात्रामाह—

देया दीप्ताग्नये मात्रा स्नेहस्य पलसंमिता । मध्यमाय त्रिकर्षा स्याज्जघन्याय द्विकार्षिकी ॥ ७ ॥

The dose of sneha for persons of good digestive capacity is one pala, for persons of medium capacity it is three karṣas and for persons of poor capacity it will be two karshas (7).

अथ विकल्पान्तरविहितां मात्रां दर्शयन्नाह—

अथवा स्नेहमात्राः स्युस्तिस्रोऽन्याः सर्वसंमताः । अहोरात्रेण महती जीर्यत्यह्नि तु मध्यमा ॥ ८ ॥
जीर्यत्यल्पा दिनार्धेन सा विज्ञेया सुखावहा ।

Another method of determining the dose approved by all is "that quantity of sneha wich gets digested well in one full day (24 hours) is mahatīmātrā (maximum dose) that which gets digested within a day time only (12 hours) is madhyama mātrā (medium dose) and that within half the day time (6 hours) is hina mātrā (minimum dose) (8–9).

अल्पादीनां गुणानाह—

अल्पा स्याद्दीपनी वृष्या स्वल्पदोषेषु पूजिता ॥ ९ ॥
मध्यमा स्नेहनी ज्ञेया बृंहणी भ्रमहारिणी । ज्येष्ठा कुष्ठविषोन्मादग्रहापस्मारनाशिनी ॥ १० ॥

The sneha of minimum dose is dīpana (improves appetite), vṛṣya (aphrodisiac) and suitable when the morbidity of the doṣas is least, the madhyamamātrā (medium dose) is bṛṃhaṇa (strengthening) and bhramahara (relieves giddiness) while the uttama mātrā (maximum dose) is beneficial in diseases like kuṣṭha (leprosy and other skin diseases), viṣa (poisons), unmāda (insanity) graha (seizure by evil spirits) and apasmāra (epilepsy) (9-10).

अथ दोषविशेषेण स्नेहविषयमाह—

केवलं पैत्तिके सर्पिर्वातिके लवणान्वितम् । पेयं बहुकफे चापि व्योषक्षारसमन्वितम् ॥ ११ ॥

येषां सर्पिर्दीयते तानाह—

रूक्षक्षतविषार्तानां वातपित्तविकारिणाम् । हीनमेधास्मृतीनां च सर्पिष्पानं प्रशस्यते ॥ १२ ॥

Sarpi (ghee) alone is ideal in disorders of pitta; with lavaṇa (salt) especially saindhava (rocksalt) in disorders of vāta and with vyoṣa (trikaṭu) and kṣāras in disorders of kapha. Sarpi pāna (ghee drinking) is best for persons who are suffering from rūkṣa (dryness), kṣata (lung disorders), viṣa (poisons), diseases of vāta and pitta; of poor intellegence and memory (11-12).

तैलयोग्यानाह—

क्रिमिकोष्ठानिलाविष्टाः प्रवृद्धकफमेदसः । पिबेयुस्तैलसात्म्या ये तैलं दार्ढ्यार्थिनस्तु ये ॥ १३ ॥

Taila (oil) is best for persons who have kṛmi (worms) in their koṣṭha (intestines), disorders of vāta, increase of kapha and medas (fat), who desire strength and those accustomed to taila in their food habits (13)

वसायोग्यानाह—

व्यायामकर्षिताः शुष्करेतोरक्ता महारुजः । महाग्निमारुतप्राणा वसायोग्या नराः स्मृताः ॥ १४ ॥

Vasā (muscle fat) is ideal for persons who have become weak by over exertion, loss of semen, blood, incurable diseases and in whom the digestive capacity is profound and vāta is powerful (14).

मज्जायोग्यानाह—

क्रूराशयाः क्लेशसहा वातार्ता दीप्तवह्नयः । मज्जानं च पिबेयुस्ते सर्पिर्वा सर्वतो हितम् ॥ १५ ॥

Majjā (marrow) is ideal for persons who have very hard bowels (constipation), of good stamina and powerful digestive capacity. Sarpi or ghee is suitable for all generally (15).

स्नेहपानकालः—

शीतकाले दिवा स्नेहमुष्णकाले पिबेन्निशि । वातपित्ताधिके रात्रौ वातश्लेष्माधिके दिवा ॥ १६ ॥

Snehapāna (drinking of sneha) should be done at day time during winter and in disorders due to increase of vāta and kapha; while it should be done at nights during summer and in disorders due to increase of vāta and pitta (16).

अथ तैलघृतयोर्विशिष्टकर्म दर्शयन्नाह—

नस्याभ्यञ्जनगण्डूषमूर्धकर्णाक्षितर्पणैः । तैलं घृतं वा युञ्जीत दृष्ट्वा दोषबलाबलम् ॥ १७ ॥

Taila (oil) or ghṛta (ghee) whichever is suitable can also be used as nāsya (nasal drops), abhyaṅga (external massage and bath), gaṇḍūṣa (mouthgargle), mūrdha tarpaṇa (application to the head), karṇa tarpaṇa (filling into the ear) and akṣi tarpaṇa (application to the eyes) (17).

इदानीं स्नेहानामनुपानान्याह—

घृते कोष्णं जलं पेयं तैले यूषः प्रशस्यते । वसामज्ज्ञोः पिबेन्मण्डमनुपानं सुखावहम् ॥ १८ ॥

Warm water is ideal as an anupāna (after drink) for ghee; yūṣa (decoction of grains) for oil; maṇḍa (thin gruel) for vasā (fat) and majjā (marrow) (18).

सान्नस्नेहस्य विषयमाह—

स्नेहद्विषः शिशून्वृद्धान्सुकुमारान् कृशानपि । उष्णकामानुष्णकाले सह भक्तेन पाययेत् ॥ १९ ॥

Snehas can be given mixed with food and given to persons who have an aversion to snehas, children, the aged, those of tender constitution, the emaciated, those desiring hot drinks and for others also during summer (19).

इदनीं स्नेहं विनापि यवाग्वा स्नेहनमाह—

सर्पिष्मती बहुतिला यवागूः स्वल्पतण्डुला । सुखोष्णा सेव्यमाना तु सद्यः स्नेहनकारिणी ॥ २० ॥

Yavāgū (gruel) prepared with little quantity of rice and more quantity of tila (sesamum) added with plenty of ghṛta (ghee) and taken hot acts as sadyaḥ sneha (immediate oleation) (20).

शर्कराचूर्णसंघृष्टे दोहनस्थे घृते तु गाम् । दुग्ध्वा क्षीरं पिबेदुष्णं सद्यःस्नेहनमुच्यते ॥ २१ ॥

Fresh milk, got directly from the udder of the cow into a vessel containing sugar and ghee and drinking it immediately will also act the same manner (21).

अथ स्नेहाजीर्णे चिकित्सामाह—

मिथ्याचाराद्बहुत्वाद्वा यस्य स्नेहो न जीर्यति । विष्टभ्य वापि जीर्येत वारिणोष्णेन वामयेत् ॥ २२ ॥

स्नेहस्य चतुःषष्टिविचारणाः ।

If the sneha does not get digested either due to excess quantity or inadvertant use or gets delayed digestion causing pain in the abdomen, such a person should be given hot water to drink so as to cause vomitting (22).

स्नेहाजीर्णे अन्यदपि प्रतीकारमाह—

स्नेहस्याजीर्णशङ्कायां पिबेदुष्णोदकं नरः । तेनोद्गारे भवेच्छुद्धो भक्तं प्रति रुचिस्तथा ॥ २३ ॥

If the person who has drunk the sneha doubts its good digestion, he should drink warm water often which helps digestion and creates good erectations and relish for food (23).

स्नेहोपद्रवभूतायास्तृष्णायाश्चिकित्सामाह—

स्नेहेन पैत्तिकस्याग्निर्यदा तीक्ष्णतरीकृतः । तदास्योदीरयेत्तृष्णां विषमां तस्य वामयेत् ॥ २४ ॥
शीतं जलं पाययेच्च पिपासा तेन शाम्यति ।

If the person develops severe thirst due to the increase of agni (digestive activity) by the action of sneha, he should be treated with drinks of cold water (24–25).

अथ स्नेहाऽयोग्यानाह—

अजीर्णी वर्जयेत्स्नेहमुदरी तरुणज्वरी ॥ २५ ॥
दुर्बलोऽरोचकी स्थूलो मूर्च्छार्तो मदपीडितः । दत्तबस्तिर्विरक्तश्च वान्तस्तृष्णाश्रमान्वितः ॥ २६ ॥
अकालप्रसवा नारी दुर्दिने च विवर्जयेत् ।

Snehapāna (drinking of ghee etc.) is contraindicated for persons suffering from ajirna (indigestion), udara (abdominal enlargemnet). tarunajwara (acute fevers), durbala (weakness), arocaka (anorexia), sthūla (obesity), mūrchā (fits), mada (intoxication); persons who have been treated just then with basti (enemata), virecana (purgation), vamana (emesis); persons who are thirsty and exhausted, women who had premature delevary. So also on a day when there is no sunlight (25–27).

येषां स्नेहपानं प्रशस्तं तानाह—

स्वेद्यसंशोध्यमद्यस्त्रीव्यायामासक्तमानसाः ॥ २७ ॥
वृद्धा बालाः कृशा रूक्षाः क्षीणास्राः क्षीणरेतसः । वातार्तास्तिमिरार्ता ये तेषां स्नेहनमुत्तमम् ॥२८॥

Snehapāna is indicated for and suitable to persons who are tobe given sweda (sudation), saṃśodhana (purificatory therapies), who are indulging in excessive alcohol, sex, exercise and worry; old people, adolescents, who are weak and dry, in whom blood and semen are decreased, those suffering from diseases of vāta, blindness and other eye troubles (27–28).

सम्यक् स्निग्धस्य लक्षणमाह—

वातानुलोम्यं दीप्तोऽग्निर्वर्चः स्निग्धमसंहतम् । मृदुस्निग्धाङ्गता ग्लानिः स्नेहोद्वेगोऽथ लाघवम् ॥२९॥
विमलेन्द्रियता सम्यक् स्निग्धे

रूक्षे लक्षणमाह—

—रूक्षे विपर्ययः ।

Downward movement of flatus, increased appetite, fatty stools, easy bowel movement, body becoming greasy and soft. slight weakness, lightness, increased clarity of the sensory perception are the effects of a good and samyak snehana (proper oleation therapy); qualities opposite of the above are the symptoms of rūkṣatā (dryness) (29).

अतिस्निग्धलक्षणमाह—

भक्तद्वेषो मुखस्रावो गुदे दाहः प्रवाहिका ॥ ३० ॥
तन्द्रातीसारपाण्डुत्वं भृशं स्निग्धस्य लक्षणम् ।

Aversion to food, excess watering of the mouth, burning sensation at the rectum, straining at stools, loose motions, drowsiness, whitish appearance of the skin are the symptoms of atisnehana (excess oleation) (30).

अथ हीनातिस्निग्धस्योपक्रममाह—

रूक्षस्य स्नेहनं स्नेहैरतिस्निग्धस्य रूक्षणम् ॥ ३१ ॥

रूक्षयोगमाह—

श्यामाकचणकाद्यैश्च तक्रपिण्याकसक्तुभिः ।

Snehana therapy is suitable for persons who are rūksa (dry all over) where as rūkṣaṇa (drying) therapy is to be done for persons who have had excess sneha therapy; with fried grains like shyamaka, caṇaka, takra (butter milk), piṇyāka (sesamum cake without oil) and saktus (dry flour) etc. (31½).

अथ स्नेहसेविनो लक्षणमाह—

दीप्ताग्निः शुद्धकोष्ठश्च पुष्टधातुर्दृढेन्द्रियः ॥ ३२ ॥
निर्जरो बलवर्णाढ्यः स्नेहसेवी भवेन्नरः ।

Persons who take snehana therapy regularly will obtain good digestive capacity, clean bowels, well nourished tissues, acuity of senses, good strength, complexion and can avoid oldage (32).

स्नेहसेवायां वर्ज्यान्याह—

स्नेहे व्यायामसंशीतवेगाघातप्रजागरान् ॥ ३३ ॥
दिवास्वप्नमभिष्यन्दि रूक्षान्नं च विवर्जयेत् ।

During sneha therapy, persons should avoid exertion, exposure to cold wind, cold foods and drinks, suppression of natural urges, keeping awake at nights, sleeping at day time, foods which are abhiṣyandi (causing too much moisture inside) and rūkṣa (dry) (33).

इति श्रीदामोदरसूनुना शार्ङ्गधराचार्येण प्रणीतायां शार्ङ्गधरसंहितायामुत्तरखण्डे
स्नेहविधिर्नाम प्रथमोऽध्यायः ॥ १ ॥

Thus ends the first chapter.

द्वितीयोऽध्यायः

CHAPTER II

अथ स्वेदविधिः

Swedavidhi (Sudation therapy)

तत्र तावत्पूर्वं स्वेदसंख्यामाह—

स्वेदश्चतुर्विधः प्रोक्तस्तापोष्मस्वेदसंज्ञकौ । उपनाहो द्रवः स्वेदः सर्वे वातार्तिहारिणः ॥ १ ॥

Sweda (sudation therapy) is of four kinds : viz. tāpa (fomentation), ūsmā (steam bath), upanāha (hot poultices) and drava (sudation by liquids), all are beneficial to relieve vāta disorders (nervous diseases) (1).

स्वेदौ तापोष्मजौ प्रायः श्लेष्मघ्नौ समुदीरितौ । उपनाहस्तु वातघ्नः पित्तसङ्गे द्रवो हितः ॥ २ ॥

Tāpa and ūṣma sweda relieve disorders of kapha, upanāha is specially beneficial in disorders of vāta while drava is useful in disorders of vāta mixed with pitta (2).

अथ त्रिविधस्वेदस्य विशेषमाह—

महाबले महाव्याधौ शीते स्वेदो महान्स्मृतः । दुर्बले दुर्बलः स्वेदो मध्ये मध्यतमो मतः ॥ ३ ॥

For persons who are strong and in severe diseases, swedana therapy can be of maximum intensity (degree); of moderate degree to persons and diseases of moderate strength and of minimum degree for persons and diseases of poor strength (3).

अथ दोषविशेषेण स्वेदविशेषमाह—

बलासे रूक्षणस्वेदो रूक्षस्निग्धं कफानिले । कफमेदोवृते वाते कोष्णं गेहं रवेः करान् ॥ ४ ॥

In disorders of only kapha, swedana therapy should be dry; in disorders of kapha and vāta dry and moist; if vāta is accompanied with kapha and medas (fat) the patient should be confined to a warm room or exposed to sunlight (4).

नियुद्धं मार्गगमनं गुरुप्रावरणं क्षुधः । चिन्ताव्यायामभारांश्च सेवेतामयमुक्तये ॥ ५ ॥

Basking in the sun, wrestling, brisk walking, covering the body with thick blankets, fasting, worry, strenuous excercise, carrying heavy loads all these subserve the purpose of swedana for relief from diseases (5).

प्राक्स्वेद्याः—

येषां नस्यं विधातव्यं बस्तिश्चापि हि प्लीहिनाम् । शोधनीयाश्च ये केचित्पूर्वं स्वेद्याश्च ते मताः ॥६॥

कालद्वयस्वेद्यानाह—

स्वेद्याः पूर्वं त्रयः प्लीहभगन्दरर्शसस्तथा । अश्मर्यश्चातुरो जन्तुः समये शस्त्रकर्मणः ॥ ७ ॥

Śwedana therapy is to be administered first for persons who are to be given nasya (errhines), basti (enemata) and other śodhana (purificatory) measures vamana (emisis), virecana (purgation) and persons who are suffering from plīhā (spleen enlargement), bhagandara (fistula in ano) arṣas (haemorrhoids) aśmarī, (renal caliculi) and others who are to undergo surgery (6–7).

पश्चात्स्वेद्याः—

पश्चात्स्वेद्या गते शल्ये मूढगर्भगदे तथा। काले प्रजाताऽकाले वा पश्चात्स्वेद्या नितम्बिनी ॥ ८ ॥

Swedana therapy should be given after the main operation to persons who had removal of a foreign body; cases of mūḍhagarbha (abnormal presentation of the foetus); premature or even normal delevary (8).

स्वेदकालः—

सर्वान्स्वेदान् निवाते च जीर्णाहारे च कारयेत्।

Sweda karma (sudation therapy) should be done in a closed room, devoid of breeze and after the food has been well digested (9).

स्वेदफलम्—

स्वेदाद्धातुस्थिता दोषाः स्नेहक्लिन्नस्य देहिनः ॥ ९ ॥
द्रवत्वं प्राप्य कोष्ठान्तर्गत्वा यान्ति विरेकताम्।

The doṣas (morbid humors) residing in the dhātus (tissues) get softened by sneha karma (oleation therapy) and become liquified by sweda (sudation). They then move into the koṣṭha (gastrointestinal tract) to be thrown out by virecana (purgation) and other śodhana therapies (9–10).

स्वेदितस्य रक्षा—

स्विद्यमानशरीरस्य हृदयं शीतलैः स्पृशेत् ॥ १० ॥
स्नेहाभ्यक्तशरीरस्य शीतैराच्छाद्य चक्षुषी।

During swedana therapy the patient should be anointed with oil all over the body and cold pack applied over the region of heart and eyes (10–11).

अस्वेदार्हाः—

अजीर्णी दुर्बलो मेही क्षतक्षीणः पिपासितः ॥ ११ ॥
अतिसारी रक्तपित्ती पाण्डुरोगी तथोदरी। मदार्तो गर्भिणी चैव नहि स्वेद्या विजानता ॥ १२ ॥
एतानपि मृदुस्वेदैः स्वेदसाध्यानुपाचरेत्।

केचिदत्रार्धं पठन्ति—

'मृदुस्वेदं प्रयुञ्जीत तथा हृन्मुष्कदृष्टिषु' ॥ १३ ॥

Swedana therapy is contraindicated for persons suffering from ajīrṇa (indigestion), durbala (debility), meha (diabetes), kṣata kṣīṇa (lung diseases), pipāsā (thirst), atisāra (diarrhoea), raktapitta (purpura), pāṇḍuroga (anaemia), udara (abdominal enlargement), mada (intoxication) and for the garbhiṇī (pregnant). If swedana becomes a necessity in such persons it should be given very mild. Similiarly mild swedana is to be given in diseases of heart, scrotum and eyes (11–13).

स्वेदातियोगजा रोगाः—

अतिस्वेदात्सन्धिपीडा दाहतृष्णा क्लमो भ्रमः । पित्तासृक्पिडकाकोपस्तत्र शीतैरुपाचरेत् ॥ १४ ॥

Excess swedana (sudation therapy) causes pain in the joints, burning sensation, thirst, weakness, giddiness, bleeding tendency and boils. These are to be treated with cold applications, cold drinks etc. (13–14).

तापस्वेदः—

तेषु तापाभिधः स्वेदो वालुकावस्त्रपाणिभिः । कपालकन्दुकाङ्गारैर्यथायोग्यः प्रयुज्यते ॥ १५ ॥

Tāpa sweda is done by touching the body parts with heated sand, cloth, palm of the hand, pot sherd, metal balls or by exposure to burning coal (15).

ऊष्मस्वेदः—

ऊष्मस्वेदः प्रयोक्तव्यो लोहपिण्डेष्टिकाश्मभिः । अततैरम्लसिक्तैश्च काये नक्तकवेष्टिते ॥ १६ ॥
अथवा वातनिर्नाशिद्रव्यकाथरसादिभिः । उष्णैर्घटं पूरयित्वा पार्श्वे छिद्रं विधाय च ॥ १७ ॥
विसृद्यास्यं त्रिखण्डां च धातुजां काष्ठवंशजाम् । षडङ्गुलास्यां गोपुच्छां नलीं युञ्ज्याद्द्विहस्तिकाम् ॥
सुखोपविष्टं स्वभ्यक्तं गुरुप्रावरणावृतम् । हस्तिशुण्डिकया नाड्यां स्वेदयेद्वातरोगिणम् ॥ १९ ॥

Uṣma sweda is done as follows :—the body part is tied with a poultice of vātahara leaves; a metal ball or brick is heated red hot and any sour liquid is poured over it. The fumes that emerge are made to touch the poultice and thus the part of the body gets sweated. Another method is to take a pot and make a hole by it's side just below it's neck. A metal tube or reed, two hastas in length and with an orifice of six aṅgulis wide is attached to the hole in the pot. Vātahara decoction or juice is put into the pot, covered with a lid, boiled till steam comes out of the tube. The person who is to be treated should be given an oil massage and made to sit or lie on a cot comfortably and a thick blanket covered over him. The fumes coming out of the tube is allowed over the patient from the bottom of the seat or cot. After he has perspired well the procedure is stopped (16–19).

पुरुषायाममात्रां वा भूमिमुत्कीर्य खादिरैः । काष्ठैर्दग्ध्वा तथाभ्युक्ष्य क्षीरधान्याम्लवारिभिः ॥ २० ॥
वातघ्नपत्रैराच्छाद्य शयानं स्वेदयेन्नरम् । एवं माषादिभिः स्विन्नैः शयानं स्वेदमाचरेत् ॥ २१ ॥

A pit of the length of a man is dug and filled with khadira wood, set fire and burning coals made. The flames are put out by sprinkling water, milk or any liquid. The black coal (hot of course) is covered over with a thick layer of leaves of vātahara properties. The patient covered with a thick blanket is to lie over these leaves till he perspires well (20–21).

उपनाहस्वेदमाह—

अथोपनाहस्वेदं च कुर्याद्वातहरौषधैः । प्रदिह्य देहं वातार्तं क्षीरमांसरसान्वितैः ॥ २२ ॥
अम्लपिष्टैः सलवणैः सुखोष्णैः स्नेहसंयुतैः । उपग्राम्यानूपमांसैर्जीवनीयगणेन च ॥ २३ ॥
दधि-सौवीरक-क्षीरैर्वीरतर्वादिना तथा । कुलत्थ-माष-गोधूमैरतसी-तिल-सर्षपैः ॥ २४ ॥
शतपुष्पा-देवदारु-शेफाली-स्थूलजीरकैः । एरण्डमूल बीजैश्च रास्ना-मूलक-शिग्रुभिः ॥ २५ ॥
मिशि-कृष्णा-कुठेरैश्च लवणैरम्लसंयुतैः । प्रसारिण्यश्वगन्धाभ्यां बलाभिर्दशमूलकैः ॥ २६ ॥
गुडूची-वानरीबीजैर्यथालाभं समाहृतैः । क्षुण्णैः स्विन्नैश्च वस्त्रेण बद्धैः संस्वेदयेन्नरम् ॥ २७ ॥
महाशाल्वणसंज्ञोऽयं योगः सर्वानिलार्तिहृत् ।

Now the upanāha sweda. Take vātahara drugs and prepare a paste with sour juices like kanji, add milk, meat juice and a little salt and boil the entire mass till it becomes a thick liquid, apply it warmly either to the whole body or to any of its parts which has earlier been anoninted with vātahara oil. Allow the paste over the body till it becomes cold and apply fresh warm paste, repeating the process many times

Meat of domestic animals or aquatic animals, drugs of jīvanīya gaṇa, curds, souvīraka (sour butter milk), milk, drugs of vīratarvādi gaṇa, kulattha (horse gram), māṣa (black gram), godhūma (wheat), atasī (linseed), tila (sesamum), sarṣapa (mustard), śatapuṣpa, devadāru, śephālī, sthūla jīraka, seeds and roots of eraṇda, rāsnā, mūlaka, śigru, miśi, kṛṣṇā, kuṭheraka, lavaṇas, amlas, prasāriṇī, aśwagandhā, the two balās, daśamūlas, guḍūcī, vānarībīja as many as can be gathered are made into small pieces and exposed to fumes. When they become hot, are put inside a bag af thick cloth (pinda) and applied over the affected part of the body. This recipe known as *Mahāśālvaṇa sweda,* cures all vāta rogas (nervous disorders) (22–28).

द्रवस्वेदविधिः—

द्रवस्वेदस्तु वातघ्नो द्रव्यक्वाथेन पूरितम् ॥ २८ ॥
कटाहं कोष्ठकं वाऽपि सूपविष्टोऽवगाहयेत् ।

Drava sweda is done by filling a bath tub with warm decoction of vātahara drugs and making the patient sit in it comfortably (28 29).

इदानीं द्रवस्य परिमाणमाह—

नाभेः षडङ्गुलं यावन्मग्नः क्वाथस्य धारया ॥ २९ ॥
कोष्णया स्कन्धयोः सिक्तस्तिष्ठेत् स्निग्धतनुर्नरः । एवं तैलेन, दुग्धेन, सर्पिषा स्वेदयेन्नरम् ॥ ३० ॥

Another type of drava sweda is done by making the patient sit comfortably in a bath tub and vātahara decoction being poured over the shoulders of the patient in a stream continuously till the decoction in the tub rises upto about six inches above the umbilicus of the patient. Then it is stopped. Such a dhāra (continuous stream of liquid) can be done with warm taila (oil), milk or ghee. (29-30)

अवगाहनकालनियमः—

एकान्तरोद्व्यन्तरो वा स्नेहयुक्तोऽवगाहने ।

अवगाहनफलम्—

सिरामुखै रोमकूपैर्धमनीभिश्च तर्पयेत् ॥ ३१ ॥

शरीरे बलमाधत्ते युक्तः स्नेहोऽवगाहने ।

धातुवर्धनमाह—

जलसिक्तस्य वर्धन्ते यथामूलेऽङ्कुरास्तरोः ॥ ३२ ॥

तथा धातुविवृद्धिर्हि स्नेहसिक्तस्य जायते । नातः परतरः कश्चिदुपायो वातनाशनः ॥ ३३ ॥

Avagāha sweda (tub bath) can be done with intervals of one or two days, this swedana therapy nourishes the openings of siras (veins), dhamanīs (arteris) and hair follicles and gives strength to the body. Just as a seed grows well if given sufficient water so also the dhātus grow when they are bathed with oil; there is no other method than swedana to mitigete the increased vāta. (31-33)

शीतशूलाद्युपरमे स्तम्भगौरवनिग्रहे । दीप्ताग्नौ मार्दवे जाते स्वेदनाद्विरतिर्मता ॥ ३४ ॥

Sweda karma (sudation therapy) should be stopped after relief from cold, pain, stiffness, heavyness and getting good appetite and softness of the parts. (34)

सुस्विन्नस्य पश्चात् कर्म दर्शयति—

सम्यक् स्विन्नं विमृदितं स्नानमुष्णाम्बुभिः शनैः । भोजयेच्चानभिष्यन्दि व्यायामं न च कारयेत् ॥ ३५ ॥

After proper swedana therapy, the patient is given a good massage, warm bath and nourishing foods. He should not be allowed to indulge in any kind of exertion (35).

इति श्रीदामोदरसूनुना शार्ङ्गधरेण विरचितायां शार्ङ्गधरसंहितायामुत्तरखण्डे स्वेदविधिर्नाम द्वितीयोऽध्यायः ॥ २ ॥

Thus ends the second chapter.

अथ तृतीयोऽध्यायः

CHAPTER III

अथ वमनविधिः—

Vamana Vidhi (Emesis therapy)

वमनप्रधानो विधिः वमनविधिः शोधनप्रकारः । अत एवाह—
शरत्काले वसन्ते च प्रावृट्काले च देहिनाम् । वमनं रेचनं चैव कारयेत्कुशलो भिषक् ॥ १ ॥

Vamana (emesis) and virecana (purgation) therapies should be done during śarat, vasanta or prāvṛṭ seasons (1).

वाम्याः—

बलवन्तं कफव्याप्तं हृल्लासादिनिपीडितम् । तथा वमनसात्म्यं च धीरचित्तं च वामयेत् ॥ २ ॥

Vamana should be administered to persons who are strong, suffering from too much accumilation of kapha, having hṛllāsa (nausea), who are strong of will (courageous) and who are accustomed to emesis (2).

वमनार्हा रोगाः—

विषदोषे स्तन्यदोषे मन्देऽग्नौ श्लीपदेऽर्बुदे । हृद्रोग-कुष्ठ-वीसर्प-मेहा-जीर्ण-भ्रमेषु च ॥ ३ ॥
विदारिका पची-कास-श्वास-पीनस-वृद्धिषु । अपस्मारे ज्वरो-न्मादे-तथा रक्तातिसारिषु ॥ ४ ॥
नासा-ताल्वोष्ठ-पाकेषु कर्णस्रावे द्विजिह्वके । गलशुण्ड्यामतीसारे पित्तश्लेष्मगदे तथा ॥ ५ ॥
मेदोगदेऽरुचौ चैव वमनं कारयेत् भिषक् ।

Vamana therapy (emesis) is indicated in viṣa (poisons), mandāgni (dyspepsia), ślīpada (filariasis), stanyaroga (disorders of breast milk), arbuda (cancer), hṛdroga (heart diseases), kuṣṭha (leprosy and other skin disorders), vīsarpa (erysepelas), meha (diabetes), ajīrṇa (indigestion), bhrama (giddiness), vidārikā (tumor inside the mouth), apacī (cervical gland) kāsa-swāsa (cough-dyspnoea), pīnasa (rhinitis), vṛddhi (scrotal enlargement), apasmāra (epilepsy) jwara (fever), unmāda (insanity), raktātisāra (bloody diarrhoea), pāka of nāsā, tālu-oṣṭha (ulcers of nose, palate and lips), karṇasrāva (discharge from the ear), dvijihwa (disease of epiglottis), galaśuṇḍi (enlargement of uvula), atisāra (diarrhoea), diseases of pitta, kapha and medas (fat) and aruci (anorexia) (3–5).

अथावाम्यानाह—

न वामनीयस्तिमिरी न गुल्मी नोदरी कृशः ॥ ६ ॥
नातिवृद्धो गर्भिणी च न स्थूलो न क्षुधातुरः । मदार्तो बालको रूक्षः क्षुधितश्च निरूहितः ॥ ७ ॥
उदावर्त्यूर्ध्वरक्ती च दुश्छर्दी केवलानिली । पाण्डुरोगी कृमिव्याप्तः पठनात्स्वरघातकः ॥ ८ ॥

Vamana is contraindicated in timira (blindness), gulma (abdominal tumors), udara (enlargement of abdomen), to persons who are weak, very aged, the pregnant, the obese; those suffering from kṣata (ulcers), mada (intoxication), children, the emaciated, hungry, persons who have been given an irūha vasti (decoction enema), those suffering from udāvarta (reverse peristalisis), urdhwa-rakta-pitta (bleeding from ear, nose, throat, eyes etc.), duśchardi (improper emesis), anila (diseases of vāta), pāṇḍu (anaemia), kṛmi (intestinal parasites), swaraghāta (loss of voice) due to excessive speech (6–8).

अथ यद्यप्येतेऽप्यजीर्णादिव्यापितास्तदा वामनीया इति विचार्याह—

एतेऽप्यजीर्णव्यथिता वाम्या ये विषपीडिताः । कफव्याताश्च ते वाम्या मधुकाथस्य पानतः ॥ ९ ॥

Decoction of madhuka (yaṣṭhī) is the ideal emetic recipe for those who are contraindicated for vamana, for persons suffering from viṣa (poison), ajīrṇa (indigestion) and diseases of kapha (9).

सुकुमारं कृशं बालं वृद्धं भीरुं च वामयेत् । पीत्वा यवागूमाकण्ठं क्षीरतक्रदधीनि वा ॥ १० ॥

For persons of tender constitution, the emaciated, children, the aged, and the frightful, it is better not to give any vamana (emetic drug), but make them drink yavāgū (thin gruel), kṣīra (milk), takra (buttermilk), or dadhi (curds) to their full capacity which alone gives them vamana (emesis) (10).

असात्म्यैः श्लेष्मलैर्भोज्यैर्दोषानुत्क्लिश्य देहिनः । स्निग्धस्विन्नाय वमनं दत्तं सम्यक् प्रवर्तते ॥ ११ ॥

Before administering of vamana, the person should be given an oil massage, sudation and unaccoustomed foods which increase the quantity of kapha in the body. These procedures help for proper emesis (11).

मधुसैन्धवयोः प्राधान्यम्—

वमनेषु च सर्वेषु सैन्धवं मधु वा हितम् ।

वमनार्हं द्रव्यम्—

बीभत्सं वमनं दद्यात् विपरीतं विरेचनम् ॥ १२ ॥

Saindhava and madhu (rock salt and honey) are ideal adjuvants for all vamanas; the vamana drug should be of the type which is repulsive in nature (offensive smell, unpleasant colour etc.), while a virecana drugs (purgative drug) should be pleasant and agreeable (12).

क्वाथ्यक्वाथयोर्मानम्—

क्वाथ्यद्रव्यस्य कुडवं श्रपयित्वा जलाढके । अर्धभागावशिष्टं च वमनेष्ववचारयेत् ॥ १३ ॥

One kuḍava of vamana drug is to be boiled in one āḍhaka of water and decoction reduced to half. This decoction is given to drink, for producing vomitting (13).

भेडमतेन वमने क्राथपानमात्रा—

क्राथपाने नवप्रस्था ज्येष्ठा मात्रा प्रकीर्तिता । मध्यमा षण्मिता प्रोक्ता त्रिप्रस्था च कनीयसी ॥ १४ ॥

Nine prasthas of decoction is the maximum dose, six prasthas medium and three prasthas is the minimum dose for vamana (14)

कल्कादिमानम्—

कल्कचूर्णावलेहानां त्रिपलं श्रेष्ठमात्रया । मध्यमां द्विपलां विद्यात्कनीया पलसंमिता ॥ १५ ॥

In case of cūrṇa (powders), kalka (paste) or avaleha (confection) three palas is the maximum dose, two palas medium and one pala the minimum dose (15).

वमनवेगाः—

वमने चाऽपि वेगाः स्युरष्टौ पित्तान्तमुत्तमाः । षड्वेगा मध्यमा वेगाश्चत्वारस्त्ववरे स्मृताः ॥ १६ ॥

Eight, six and four vomittings with pitta (bile) coming out at the end are the ideal (maximum) and moderate and least respectively (16).

प्रस्थमानम्—

वमने च विरेके च तथा शोणितमोक्षणे । सार्धत्रयोदशपलं प्रस्थमाहुर्मनीषिणः ॥ १७ ॥

One prastha is to be reckoned as equavalent to thirteen and a half palas in the context of vamana (emesis), virecana (purgation) and raktamokṣaṇa (blood letting) (17).

अथ दोषविशेषेण द्रव्यविशेषमाह—

कफं कटुकतीक्ष्णोष्णैः पित्तं स्वादुहिमैर्जयेत् । सुस्वादुलवणाम्लोष्णैः संसृष्टं वायुना कफम् ॥ १८ ॥

In diseases of kapha origin, the vamaka drugs (emetics) should be those possessing kaṭu (pungent), tīkṣṇa (penetrating) and uṣṇa (hot) properties, in diseases of pitta with swādu (sweet) and hima (cold) and in diseases of kapha accompanied with vāta with swādu (sweet), lavaṇa (salt), amla (sour) and uṣṇa (hot) properties (18).

कृष्णा राठफलं सिन्धु कफे कोष्णजलैः पिबेत् । पटोलवासानिम्बैश्च पित्ते शीतजलं पिबेत् ॥ १९ ॥
सश्लेष्मवातपीडायां सक्षीरं मदनं पिबेत् । अजीर्णे कोष्णपानीयैः सिन्धु पीत्वा वमेत्सुधीः ॥ २० ॥

In diseases of kapha; kṛṣṇā, (pippalī), rāṭhaphala and saindhava with warm water; in pitta diseases paṭola, vāsā and nimba with cold water and in diseases of vāta associated with kapha, madanaphala with milk and in cases of ajīrṇa (īndigestion), śaindhava with warm water—are best suited as emetics (19-20).

वमनविधिमाह—

वमनं पाययित्वा च जानुमात्रासने स्थितम् । कण्ठमेरण्डनालेन स्पृशन्तं वामयेद्भिषक् ॥ २१ ॥
ललाटं वमतः पुंसः पार्श्वे द्वे च प्रदापयेत् ।

The person who has been given the vamana drug (emetic) should be asked to sit on a stool and vomitting induced by tickling his throat with a reeds of eraṇḍa. His forehead and temporals are to be held tight during vomitting (21).

दुर्वान्तलक्षणमाह—

प्रसेको हृद्ग्रहः कोठः कण्डूर्दुश्छर्दिते भवेत् ॥ २२ ॥

Praseka (salivation), hṛdgraha (oppression in chest), koṭha (appearances of rashes) and kaṇḍū (itching) appear if vomittings are inadequate (22).

अतिवान्तेर्लक्षणमाह—

अतिवान्ते भवेत् तृष्णा हिक्कोद्गारौ विसंज्ञिता । जिह्वानिःसर्पणं चाक्ष्णोर्व्यावृत्तिर्हनुसंहतिः ॥ २३ ॥
रक्तच्छर्दिः ष्ठीवनं च कण्ठपीडा च जायते ।

Excessive vomitting produces tṛṣṇā (thirst), hikkā (hiccough), udgāra (erectation), visaṃjñatā (unconciousness), jihwā nissarpaṇa (indrawing of the tongue), cakṣu vyāvṛtti (changes in appearance of the eye), hanusaṃhati (lock-jaw), rakta chardi (vomitting of blood), rakta ṣṭhīvana (spitting of blood) and kaṇṭha pīḍa (pain in the throat) (23–24).

वमनोत्पन्नरोगचिकित्सामाह—

वमनस्यातियोगे तु मृदु कुर्याद्विरेचनम् ॥ २४ ॥
वमनान्तः प्रविष्टायां जिह्वायां कवलग्रहः । स्निग्धाम्ललवणैर्हृद्यैर्घृतक्षीररसैर्हितः ॥ २५ ॥
फलान्यम्लानि खादेयुस्तस्य चान्येऽग्रतो नराः । निःसृतां तु तिलद्राक्षाकल्कं लिप्त्वा प्रवेशयेत् ॥२६॥
व्यावृत्तेऽक्षिण घृताभ्यक्ते पीडयेच्च शनैः शनैः । हनुमोक्षे स्मृतः स्वेदो नस्यं च श्लेष्मवातहृत् ॥ २७ ॥
रक्तपित्तविधानेनरक्तच्छर्दिमुपाचरेत् । धात्रीरसाञ्जनोशीरलाजाचन्दनवारिभिः ॥ २८ ॥
मन्थं कृत्वा पाययेच्च सघृतक्षौद्रशर्करम् । शाम्यन्त्यनेन तृष्णाद्या पीडाश्छर्दिसमुद्भवाः ॥ २९ ॥

If vomitting becomes excessive the patient should be administered a mild virecana (purgative), quickly. A mouth gargle with liquid materials which are snigdha, amla (sour), lavaṇa (salt) and hṛdya (of pleasant smell) mixed with milk, ghee or meat juice will help to bring forward the indrawn tongue; this can also be achieved by making another person to chew sour fruits in front of the patient. When the tongue comes forward apply over it a paste of tila and drākṣā and keep it in position. For the eye trouble bathe it with ghee and gently massage it into position. If lower jaw has drooped down give it fermentation and do nasya karma (nasal drops) with drugs possessing vāta and kaphahara properties. Vomitting of blood should be treated as in the case of raktapitta (purpura). A thin drink, prepared with dhātrī, rasāñjana, uśīra, lājā and candana added with ghee, sugar or honey should be given in plenty. This will relieve thirst and other symptoms of excessive vomitting (24–29).

अथ सम्यग्वान्तलक्षणमाह—

हृत्कण्ठशिरसां शुद्धिर्दीप्ताग्नित्वं च लाघवम् । कफपित्तविनाशश्च सम्यग्वांतस्य लक्षणम् ॥ ३० ॥

If vomitting has been properly done, the throat, chest and head become cleared of accumilation of kapha, with increase of appetitc, lightness of the body and decrease of over accumulation of kapha and pitta (30).

अथ वान्तस्य पथ्यमाह—

ततोऽपराह्ने दीप्ताऽग्निं मुद्गषष्टिकशालिभिः । हृद्यैश्च जाङ्गलरसैः कृत्वा यूषं च भोजयेत् ॥ ३१ ॥

After the therapy the person should he given a light diet of ṣaṣṭika rice and soup prepared with mudga (green gram) or juice of meat of wild beasts (31).

सुवान्तस्यैते पीडाद्यर्थं न भवन्ति इत्याह—

तन्द्रा निद्रास्यदौर्गन्ध्यं कण्डूश्च ग्रहणी विषम् । सुवान्तस्य न पीडायै भवन्त्येते कदाचन ॥ ३२ ॥

Tandrā (drowsiness), nidrā (sleep), asyadourgandhya (bad smell in the mouth), kaṇḍū (itching), grahaṇī (sprue) and viṣa (poison) will not affect a person who has had a good emesis therapy (32).

वमने यन्निषिद्धं तदाह—

अजीर्णं शीतपानीयं व्यायामं मैथुनं तथा । स्नेहाभ्यङ्गं प्रकोपं च दिनैकं वर्जयेत्सुधीः ॥ ३३ ॥

Persons who have had emesis therapy should avoid ajīrṇa (indigestion), śītapāna (cold drinks), vyāyāma (exercise), maithuna (sexual intercourse), sneha—abhyaṅga (oil massage and bath) and prakopa (anger) at least for one day.

इति श्रीदामोदरसूनुना शार्ङ्गधराचार्येण प्रणीतायां शार्ङ्गधरसंहितायामुत्तरखण्डे वमनविधिर्नाम तृतीयोऽध्यायः ॥ ३ ॥

Thus ends the third chapter.

चतुर्थोऽध्यायः

CHAPTER IV

अथ विरेचनविधिः—

Virecana Vidhi (Purgation therapy)

विरेचनविषयमाह—

स्निग्धस्विन्नस्य वान्तस्य दद्यात्सम्यग् विरेचनम् ।

Purgation therapy is given to a person who has undergone snehana (oleation), swedana (sudation) and vamana (emesis) (1).

वमनेऽप्यकृते सति दोषमाह—

अवान्तस्य त्वधः स्रस्तो ग्रहणीं छादयेत्कफः ॥ १ ॥

मन्दाग्निं गौरवं कुर्याज्जनयेद्वा प्रवाहिकाम् । अथवा पाचनैरामं बलासं च विपाचयेत् ॥ २ ॥

स्निग्धस्य स्नेहनैः कार्यं स्वेदैः स्विन्नस्य रेचनम् ।

If given to a person who has had no emesis earlier, kapha will accumulate in grahaṇī (deodenum) and cause mandāgni (poor digestive power), gourava (heavyness), pravāhikā (dysentery) and produces āma (products of improper digestion). For such a person sneha (oleation) and sweda (sudation) therapies should be done first and then virecana (purgation) is administered (2–3).

विरेचनकालमाह—

शरद्दतो वसन्ते च देयं शुद्धौ विरेचनम् ॥ ३ ॥

अन्यदात्ययिके कार्यं स्वेदनं शीलयेद्बुधः ।

Purgation therapy for the healthy should be resorted to either in śarat or vasanta ṛtus for cleaning the body and at other times in cases of emergency during diseased states (3–4).

शरीरशुद्धौ शोधनमुक्तं तस्य फलमाह—

दोषाः कदाचित्कुप्यन्ति जिता लङ्घनपाचनैः ॥ ४ ॥

ये तु संशोधनैः शुद्धा न तेषां पुनरुद्भवः ।

Doṣas which are mitigated by śamana therapies (palliative measures) are likely to get aggravated again but those which are expelled out of the body by śodhanas (purificatory therapies) do not reccur at all (4–5).

अथ पित्तादौ विरेचनम्—

पित्ते विरेचनं युञ्ज्यादामोद्भूते गदे तथा ॥ ५ ॥

उदरे च तथाऽध्माने कोष्ठशुद्धयै विशेषतः ॥

Virecana (purgation) is indicated in diseases arising from increased pitta, and āma, in diseases like udara (abdominal enlargement), ādhmāna (tympanitis) and in others also for clearing the koṣṭha (gastro intestinal tract) (5–6).

इदानीं ये विरेचने निषिद्धास्तानाह—

बालवृद्धावतिस्निग्धः क्षतक्षीणो भयान्वितः ॥ ६ ॥

श्रान्तस्तृषार्तः स्थूलश्च गर्भिणी च नवज्वरी । नवप्रसूता नारी च मन्दाग्निश्च मदात्ययी ॥ ७ ॥

शल्यार्दितश्च रूक्षश्च न विरेच्या विजानता ।

Young children, old persons, persons who have had too much of snehana (oleation) therapy, the frightful, the exhausted, stricken with thirst, the obese, the pregnant, persons who have caught fever recently, woman who has just delevered, those having mandāgni (poor digestion), the intoxicated, those suffering from foreign bodies and other surgical conditions, and those who are dry in their tissues should not be given virecana (purgation) therapy (6-8).

विरेचनयोग्यानाह—

जीर्णज्वरी गरव्याप्तो वातरक्ती भगन्दरी ॥ ८ ॥
अर्शः पाण्डूदरग्रन्थिहृद्रोगारुचिपीडिताः । योनिरोगप्रमेहार्ता गुल्मप्लीहव्रणार्दिताः ॥ ९ ॥
विद्रधिच्छर्दिविस्फोटविसूचीकुष्ठसंयुताः । कर्णनासाशिरोवक्त्रगुदमेढ्रामयान्विताः ॥ १० ॥
प्लीहशोथाक्षिरोगार्ताः क्रिमिक्षीणानिलार्दिताः । शूलिनो मूत्रघातार्ता विरेकार्हा नरा मताः ॥ ११ ॥

The following persons need purgation therapy; persons suffering from chronic fevers, gara (artificial poisons), vātarakta (gout), bhagandara (fistula), arśas (piles), pāṇḍu (anaemia), udara (abdominal enlargement), granthi (tumors), hṛdroga (heart diseases), aruci (anorexia), yoniroga (vaginal and uterine disorder), prameha (diabetes), gulma (abdominal tumors), plīha (splenic enlargement), vraṇa (ulcers), vidradhi (abscess) chardi (vomitting), visphoṭa (small pox), visūcī (bad diarrhoeas), kuṣṭha (leprosy and other skin diseases), diseases of ear, nose, head, mouth, rectum, and penis, plīhā (splenic disorders), śotha (oedema), akṣirogas (eye diseases), kṛmi (parasites), kṣīṇa (emaciation), diseases of nerves, śūla (pain in the abdomen) and mūtrāghāta (suppression of urine) (8-11).

अथ विरेचनज्ञानार्थं कोष्ठभेदानाह—

बहुपित्तो मृदुः कोष्ठो बहुश्लेष्मा च मध्यमः । बहुवातः क्रूरकोष्ठो दुर्विरेच्यः स कथ्यते ॥ १२ ॥

Persons having pitta predominance in their constitution will have mṛdukoṣṭha (soft bowel movements), with kapha predominance madhyama koṣṭha (moderate movements) and with vāta predominance krūra koṣṭha (very hard bowel movements); the last responding to purgation with great difficulty (12).

कोष्ठानुरूपां मात्रामाह—

मृद्वी मात्रा मृदुकोष्ठे मध्यकोष्ठे च मध्यमा । क्रूरे तीक्ष्णा मता द्रव्यैर्मृदुमध्यमतीक्ष्णकैः ॥ १३ ॥

For person of mṛdukoṣṭha (soft bowel movements) purgative drugs must be mild and their dose minimum; for the moderate, medium dose and for hard boweled persons the drug should be powerful and its dose maximum (13).

मृद्वादिद्रव्याणिं कानि तानि इत्यत आह—

मृदुर्द्राक्षापयश्चाम्बुतैलैरपि विरिच्यते । मध्यमस्त्रिवृतातिक्ताराजवृक्षैर्विरिच्यते ॥ १४ ॥
क्रूरः स्नुक्पयसाहेमक्षीरीदन्तीफलादिभिः ।

Drākṣā, payas (milk), ambu (warm water), taila (castor oil) produce purgation in mṛdu koṣṭha persons; trivṛt, kirātatiktā, rājavṛkṣa are suitable for the moderate boweled while the hard boweled require milky sap of snuhī, hemakṣīrī, dantīphala etc. (14–15).

विरेकस्योत्तमादिमात्रायै वाङ्कैलिङ्गकपरिमाणमाह—

मात्रोत्तमा विरेकस्य त्रिंशद्वेगैः कफान्तगा ॥ १५ ॥
वेगैर्विंशतिभिर्मध्या हीनोक्ता दशवेगकैः ।

Thirty, twenty and ten purgations are the best, moderate and least respectively or till kapha comes out (15–16).

इदानीं कषायगुटिकाचूर्णात्मकानां विरेचनद्रव्याणां परिमाणमाह—

द्विपलं श्रेष्ठमाख्यातं मध्यमं च पलं भवेत् ॥ १६ ॥
पलार्धं च कषायाणां कनीयस्तु विरेचनम् । कल्कमोदकचूर्णानां कर्षं मध्वाज्यलेहतः ॥ १७ ॥
कर्षद्वयं पलं वाऽपि वयोरोगाद्यपेक्षया ।

For a purgative decoction, two palas, one pala and half pala are the maximum, moderate and minimum dosage; for powders, pills or confections one karṣa, along with honey, ghee and avaleha. Depending upon age and diseases the dose may even be two karṣas or one pala (16–18).

त्रिवृताचूर्णम्—

अथ वातादीनां कोष्ठमात्रादिभेदेन कतिपययोगान् दर्शयन्नाह—

पित्तोत्तरे त्रिवृच्चूर्णं द्राक्षाक्वाथादिभिः पिबेत् ॥ १८ ॥
त्रिफलाक्वाथगोमूत्रैः पिबेद्व्योषं कफार्दितः । त्रिवृत्सैन्धवशुण्ठीनां चूर्णमम्लैः पिबेन्नरः ॥ १९ ॥
वातार्दितो विरेकाय जाङ्गलानां रसेन वा ।

In diseases of pitta, powder of trivṛt is given with decoction of drākṣā; in diseases of kapha decoction of triphalā with gomūtra (cow's urine) and vyoṣa (trikaṭu) and in diseases of vāta powder of trivṛt, saindhava, śuṇṭhī to be given with any sour liquid or juice of meat of wild animals (18–20).

एरण्डतैलप्रयोगः—

एरण्डतैलं त्रिफलाक्वाथेन द्विगुणेन च ॥ २० ॥
युक्तं पीतं पयोभिर्वा नचिरेण विरिच्यते ।

Eraṇḍa taila (castor oil) with twice it's quantity of decoction of triphalā or milk gives quick purgations (20–21)

षड्ऋतुविरेचनम्—

त्रिवृता कौटजं बीजं पिप्पली विश्वभेषजम् ।
समृद्वीकारसक्षौद्रं वर्षाकाले विरेचनम् । त्रिवृद्दुरालभा मुस्ता शर्करोदीच्यचन्दनम् ॥ २२ ॥
द्राक्षाम्बुना सयष्ट्याह्वं शीतलं च घनात्यये । पिप्पली नागरं सिन्धु श्यामा च त्रिवृता सह ॥ २३ ॥
लिहेत्क्षौद्रेण शिशिरे वसन्ते च विरेचनम् । त्रिवृता शर्करा तुल्या ग्रीष्मकाले विरेचनम् ॥ २४ ॥

Trivṛt, kuṭajabīja, pippalī, viśwabheṣaja (śunṭhī) with juice of mṛdwīka and honey form a good purgative recipe in varṣā ṛtu; trivṛt, durālabhā, musta, udīcya, candana,—taken with sugar or cold infusion of drākṣā, yaṣṭi is good in ghana (śarat ṛtu); trivṛt, citraka, pāṭhā, ajājī, sarala, vaca and hemakṣīrī with warm water is suitable in hemanta ṛtu; pippalī, nāgara, saindhava and śyāma with honey is best in śiśira and vasanta ṛtus; trivṛt with equal quantity of sugar is ideal in grīṣma ṛtu (21–24).

तद्यथा—

त्रिवृतां हपुषां दन्तीं सप्तलां कटुरोहिणीम् । स्वर्णक्षीरीं च संचूर्ण्य गोमूत्रे भावयेत्त्र्यहम् ॥ २५ ॥
एष सर्वर्तुको योगः स्निग्धानां मलदोषहा ।

Trivṛt, hapuṣa, dantī, saptalā, kaṭurohiṇī and swarṇa kṣīrī are powdered and kept immersed in cow's urine for three days. This recipe is suitable for all seasons and removes the doṣas (25).

अभयादिमोदकाः—

अभया मरिचं शुण्ठीविडङ्गामलकानि च ॥ २६ ॥
पिप्पली पिप्पलीमूलं त्वक्पत्रं मुस्तमेव च । एतानि समभागानि दन्ती च द्विगुणा भवेत् ॥ २७ ॥
त्रिवृदष्टगुणा ज्ञेया षड्गुणा चात्र शर्करा । मधुना मोदकान्कृत्वा कर्षमात्रप्रमाणतः ॥ २८ ॥
एकैकं भक्षयेत्प्रातः शीतं चानु पिबेज्जलम् । तावद्विरिच्यते जन्तुर्यावदुष्णं न सेवते ॥ २९ ॥
पानाहारविहारेषु भवेन्नियन्त्रणः सदा । विषमज्वरमन्दाग्निपाण्डुकासभगन्दरान् ॥ ३० ॥
दुर्नामकुष्ठगुल्मार्शोगलगण्डभ्रमोदरान् । (विदाहप्लीहमेहांश्च यक्ष्माणं नयनामयान् ॥ ३१ ॥
वातरोगांस्तथाध्मानं मूत्रकृच्छ्राणि चाश्मरीम् ।) पृष्ठपार्श्वोरुजघनजङ्घोदररुजो जयेत् ॥ ३२ ॥
सततं शीलनादेषां पलितानि प्रणाशयेत् । अभयामोदका ह्येते रसायनवराः स्मृताः ॥ ३३ ॥

Abhaya, marica, śunṭhī, vidaṅga, āmalaka, pippalī, pippalīmūla, twak, patra and musta—each equal part and dantī double the total quantity of the above, trivṛt eight times, sugar six times are to be made into pills of one karṣa each with honey. One pill to be taken in the morning followed by cold water gives purgations till the person uses hot water. No restrictions need be followed in food or other activities. This pill known as *Abhaya modaka*, cures, by long use, diseases such as viṣama jwara (malarial, remittant fevers), mandāgni (dyspepsia), pāṇḍu (anaemia), kāsa (cough), bhagandara (fistula in ano), durnāma (piles), kuṣṭha (leprosy and other skin diseases), gulma (abdominal tumors), galagaṇḍa (lymph glands of neck), bhrama (giddiness), udara (abdominal enlargement), vidāha (heart burn) plīhā (splenic enlargement), meha (diabetes), yakṣmā (consumption), nayanāmayas (diseases of the eye), vāta rogas (nervous diseases), ādhmāna (tympanitis), mūtrakṛchra (dysuria), aśmarī (calculii), pain of back, flanks, chest, waist and hips; This is good rasāyana when used for long periods, wards off greying of hairs (26–33).

विरेचनं पीत्वा किं कुर्यात्तदाह—

पीत्वा विरेचनं शीतजलैः संसिच्य चक्षुषी । सुगन्धि किञ्चिदाघ्राय ताम्बूलं.शीलयेद्वरम् ॥ ३४ ॥
निवातस्थो न वेगांश्च धारयेन्न स्वपेत्तथा । शीताम्बु न स्पृशेत् क्वापि कोष्णनीरं पिबेन्मुहुः ॥ ३५ ॥

Having taken a purgativc ricipe, the person should wash his eyes with cold water, smell some fragrant substances, chew a tāmbūla (betal leaves) remain inside a room which is not having heavy breeze, he should not sleep, not touch cold water, but drink warm water often and await the urges of purgations and not suppressing them (34–35).

सम्यग्वान्तलक्षणेन सम्यग्विरेकलक्षणमाह—

बलासौषधपित्तानि वायुर्वान्ते यथा व्रजेत् । रेकात्तथा मलं पित्तं भेषजं च कफो व्रजेत् ॥ ३६ ॥

Just as balāsa (kapha), ouṣadha (emetic drug) and pitta comesout one after the other in vamana therapy (emesis); mala (faeces), pitta, ouṣadha and kapha will come out one after the other in virecana (purgation) (36).

अथ दुर्विरिक्तलक्षणमाह—

दुर्विरिक्तस्य नाभेस्तु स्तब्धत्वं कुक्षिशूलता । पुरीषवातसंगश्च कण्डूमण्डलगौरवः ॥ ३७ ॥
विदाहोऽरुचिराध्मानं भ्रमश्छर्दिश्च जायते ।

अथास्य दुर्विरिक्तस्य पुनः चिकित्सामाह—

तं पुनः पाचनैः स्नेहैः पक्त्वा संस्नेह्य रेचयेत् ॥ ३८ ॥
तेनाऽस्योपद्रवा यान्ति दीप्ताग्नेर्लघुता भवेत् ।

If purgations do not occur properly, the person develops stiffness round the umbilicus, pain in the abdomen, non-movement of faeces and flatus, itching, skin, rashes, heavyness, burning sensation, anorexia, tympanitis, giddiness and vomittings. He should be given pācana drugs (digestive) and snehana (oleating therapy) and later on another purgative drug. By this he will be relieved of all his troubles, gets appetite and lightness of the body (37–38).

इदानीं विरेकातिशयस्य लक्षणमाह—

विरेकस्यातियोगेन मूर्च्छा भ्रंशो गुदस्य च ॥ ३९ ॥
शूलं कफातियोगः स्यान्मांसधावनसंनिभम् । मेदोनिभं जलाभासं रक्तं वाऽपि विरिच्यते ॥ ४० ॥

अथ विरेकातियोगचिकित्सामाह—

तस्य शीताम्बुभिः सिक्त्वा शरीरं तण्डुलाम्बुभिः । मधुमिश्रैस्तथा शीतैः कारयेद्वमनं मृदु ॥ ४१ ॥

If purgations become excessive, the person may get mūrchā (unconciousness), gudabhraṃśa (prolapse of rectum), śūla (colic), expulsion of kapha (mucous), and rakta (blood) resembling meat broth and fatty matter. Such a person should be given a bath with cold water or rice wash and administered a mild emetic with honey to produce vomittings (39–41).

सहकारत्वचः कल्को दध्ना सौवीरकेण वा। पिष्ट्वा नाभिप्रलेपेन हन्त्यतीसारमुल्बणम् ॥ ४२ ॥

Bark of sahakāra (mango tree) is made into a paste with curds or souvīraka (sour gruel) and applied over the umbilicus stops excessive purgations quickly (42).

अजाक्षीरं रसं वाऽपि वैष्किरं हारिणं तथा। शालिभः षष्टिकैः स्वल्पं मसूरैर्वापि भोजयेत् ॥ ४३ ॥
शीतैः संग्राहिभिर्द्रव्यैः कुर्यात् संग्रहणं भिषक्।

Little quantity of ṣaṣṭika rice, soup of masūra dall, goats milk or meat broth of goat, deer or vaiṣkira birds (birds which find their food by scratching the earth) may be taken after purgation.

Drugs possessing śita guna and saṅgrāhī properties (binding the bowels) should be used afterwards for controlling the purgations (43–44).

सम्यग्विरिक्तस्य पाचनादिप्रकारमाह—

लाघवं मनसस्तुष्टिरनुलोमं गतेऽनिले ॥ ४४ ॥
सुविरिक्तं नरं ज्ञात्वा पाचनं पाययेन्निशि।

When symptoms like lightness of the body, calmness of mind, downward movement of flatus appear, it is known that purgations have been enough and the patient should be given digestive drinks at nights (44–45).

विरेचनस्य फलमाह—

इन्द्रियाणां बलं बुद्धेः प्रसादं वह्निदीपनम् ॥ ४५ ॥
धातुस्थैर्यं वयःस्थैर्यं भवेद्रेचनसेवनात्।

Increase of sensory acuity, freshness of mind, increase of digestive capacity, strength of the tissues, and slowing of senility are the benefits accruing from purgation therapy (45–46).

कृतविरेचनस्य प्रवातादीन् निषेधयति—

प्रवातसेवाशीताम्बुस्नेहाभ्यङ्गमजीर्णताम् ॥ ४६ ॥
व्यायामं मैथुनं चैव न सेवेत विरेचितः।

अथ विरिक्तस्य पथ्यार्थं पेयादि द्रव्याण्याह—

शालिषष्टिकमुद्गाद्यैर्यवागूं भोजयेत्कृताम् ॥ ४७ ॥
जङ्गालविष्किराणां वा रसैः शाल्योदनं हितम्।

Persons who have just undergone purgation therapy should avoid heavy breeze, cold water, oil bath, indigestion, exercise and sexual act. They should use ṣaṣtika rice with yavāgū (porridge) of mudga (green gram) and other grams; or broth of meat of wild animals and viṣkira birds (47–48).

इति श्रीदामोदरसूनुना शार्ङ्गधरप्रणीतायां शार्ङ्गधरसंहितायामुत्तरखण्डे विरेचनविधिर्नाम चतुर्थोऽध्यायः ॥ ४ ॥

Thus ends the fourth chapter.

पञ्चमोऽध्यायः

CHAPTER 5

Basti Vidhi (Enemata-oil enema therapy)

अथ बस्तिविधिः—

तत्राऽयं सम्बन्धः—'पञ्चकर्म वमी, रेको, निरूहोऽन्वास-नावनम्' इति। वमनविरेकयोरुक्तत्वात्पारिशेष्याद्बस्तिविधिमाह—

बस्तिर्द्विधानुवासाख्यो निरूहश्च ततः परम्। बस्तिभिर्दीयते यस्मात्तस्माद्बस्तिरिति स्मृतः ॥ १ ॥

Basti (enemata) are of two kinds viz.—anuvāsana and nirūha. Basti is so called because it is administered with a basti (urinary bladder of animals like ox, buffallo etc.) being used as an enema can (1).

तयोर्लक्षणमाह—

यः स्नेहैर्दीयते स स्यादनुवासननामकः। कषाय-क्षीर-तैलैर्यो निरूहः स निगद्यते ॥ २ ॥

Anuvāsana is the one which contains only sneha (fatty materials like oil, ghee, etc.), whereas nirūha has decoction of drugs, milk and oil together (2).

अथानुवासनादीनामनुक्रमविधानमाह—

तत्रानुवासनाख्यो हि बस्तिर्यः सोऽत्र कथ्यते। एवमेव ततो बस्तिर्निरूहाख्यो भविष्यति ॥ ३ ॥

निरूहादुत्तरं चैव बस्तिः स्यादुत्तराभिधः।

अथवा कथनक्रमेणैव बस्तिरनुवासनभेद एव इत्यत आह—

अनुवासनभेदश्च मात्रा बस्तिरुदीरितः ॥ ४ ॥

तस्य मात्रामाह—

पलद्वयं तस्य मात्रा तस्मादर्धोऽपि वा भवेत्।

In this chapter, shall be described the anuvāsana basti because it is given first, then the nirūha and it's other kind—the uttara basti. I shall now describe mātrābasti a variety of anuvāsana basti. The quantity of oil in mātrā basti is two palas or even half of it (3–4).

अनुवासनयोग्याः—

अनुवास्यस्तु रूक्षः स्यात्तीक्ष्णाग्निः केवलानिली ॥ ५ ॥

Anuvāsana basti (oil enemata) is indicated for those who are having rūkṣatā (dryness of the tissues and organs), tīkṣṇāgni (hyper activity of digestive functions) and those suffering from vāta vyādhis (nervous diseases) (5–6).

अथानुवासने ये त्याज्यास्तानाह—

नानुवास्यस्तु कुष्ठी स्यान्मेही स्थूलस्तथोदरी । नास्थाप्या नानुवास्याश्चाजीर्णोन्मादतृडर्दिताः ॥६॥
शोकमूर्च्छारुचिभयश्वासकासक्षयातुराः ।

Anuvāsana basti is contraindicated for persons suffering from kuṣṭha (leprosy and other skin diseases), meha (diabetes), sthūla (obesity) and udara (abdominal enlargement) (6).

Those unsuitable for both anuvāsana or nirūha bastis are those suffering from ajīrṇa (indigestion), unmāda (insanity), tṛṣṇā (thirst), śhoka (grief), mūrchā (convulsions), aruci (anorexia), bhaya (freight), swāsa (dyspnoea). kāsa (cough) and kṣaya (consumption) (7).

बस्तिकरणद्रव्याणि—

नेत्रं कार्यं सुवर्णादिधातुभिर्वृक्षवेणुभिः ॥ ७ ॥
नलैर्दन्तैर्विषाणाग्रैर्मणिभिर्वा विधीयते । एकवर्षात्तु षड्वर्षं यावन्मानं षडङ्गुलम् ॥ ८ ॥
ततो द्वादशकं यावन्मानं स्यादष्टसंमितम् । ततः परं द्वादशभिरङ्गुलैर्नेत्रदीर्घता ॥ ९ ॥

The netra (nozzle) of the basti yantra can be made from metals like gold; wood, bamboo, reed, tusks or horns of animals or even of mani (crystals, beads, glass etc.). It should be six aṅgulīs long for use in children of one to six years of age, eight aṅgulis for children of six to twelve years and twelve aṅgulis for persons above that age (7–9).

मुद्गच्छिद्रं कलायाभं छिद्रं कोलास्थिसंनिभम् । यथासंख्यं भवेन्नेत्रं श्लक्ष्णं गोपुच्छसन्निभम् ॥१०॥
आतुराङ्गुष्ठमानेन मूले स्थूलं विधीयते । कनिष्ठिकापरीणाहमग्रे च गुटिकामुखम् ॥ ११ ॥
तन्मूले कर्णिके द्वे च कार्ये भागाच्चतुर्थकात् । योजयेत्तत्र बस्तिं च बन्धद्वयविधानतः ॥ १२ ॥
मृगाजशूकरगवां महिषस्यापि वा भवेत् । मूत्रकोषस्य बस्तिस्तु तदलाभेन चर्मजः ॥ १३ ॥
कषायरक्तः सुमृदुर्बस्तिः स्निग्धो दृढो हितः । व्रणबस्तेस्तु नेत्रं स्यात् श्लक्ष्णमष्टाङ्गुलोन्मितम् ॥१४॥
मुद्गच्छिद्रं गृध्रपक्षनलिकापरिणाहि च ।

The netra (nozzle) should be like cow's tail in resemblance (cylindrically tapering) having the thickness of the thumb at the base and of the little finger at the tip, the tip resembling a round pill; at each quarter of it's length two karṇikā

(ridge) are to be made. The basti (bag like bladder) is to be tied firmly in between these ridges. The front orifice varies in size from that of a mudga (green gram) kalāya (pea) or kolāsthi (stone of the fruit of jujube). The basti (bag) can be made out of the urinary bladder of animals like deer, sheep, pig, cow or buffallo, or prepared with leather made soft, smooth and strong.

The length of the nozzle for use in vraṇas (ulcers) should be eight angulis with a small opening as would permit a green gram, and it's thickness, the size of a feather of a hawk (10–15).

बस्तिसेवागुणानाह—

शरीरोपचयं वर्णं बलमारोग्यमायुषः ॥ १५ ॥

कुरुते परिवृद्धिं च बस्तिः सम्यगुपासितः ।

Bastis (enema therapy) used for long periods bestows nourishment to the body, complexion, strength, health and long life (15–16).

अथ बस्तेः कालनियममाह—

दिवा शीते वसन्ते च स्नेहबस्तिः प्रदीयते ॥ १६ ॥

ग्रीष्मवर्षाशरत्काले रात्रौ स्यादनुवासनम् । न चातिस्निग्धमशनं भोजयित्वाऽनुवासयेत् ॥ १७ ॥

मदं मूर्च्छां च जनयेद्द्विधिस्नेहः प्रयोजितः । रूक्षं भुक्तवतोऽत्यन्नं बलं वर्णं च हीयते ॥ १८ ॥

Anuvāsana basti is given during day in śita kāla (cold season) and vasanta ṛtu (spring) while it is to be given at nights during grīṣma (summer), varṣā (rainy) and śarat ṛtus (winter). It should be given after a meal of not too much of fatty substances (a little quantity of fat may be allowed) because too much of sneha (fatty materials) from both directions (with food and also with enema) will cause mada (intoxication) and mūrchā (convulsions) and loss of strength and complexion, (taking large quantities of rūkṣa foods will lead to loss of strength and complexion) (16–18).

अथ बस्तेर्हीनातिमात्रयोर्निषेधमाह—

हीनमात्रावुभौ बस्ती नातिकार्यकरौ स्मृतौ । अतिमात्रौ तथाऽनाहक्लमातीसारकारकौ ॥ १९ ॥

Both the bastis (anuvāsana and nirūha) with inadequate dosage do not give the desired effect where as in heavy doses they produce anāha (enlargement of abdomen), klama (debility) and atisāra (diarrhoea) (19).

बस्तिमात्रा—

उत्तमस्य पलैः षड्भिर्मध्यमस्य पलैस्त्रिभिः । पलस्यार्धेन हीनस्य युक्ता मात्राऽनुवासने ॥ २० ॥

For Anuvāsana basti, six palas, three palas and one and half pala of sneha (oil) are the maximum, medium and minimum doses respectively (20).

सच स्नेहः केनोपहितो देयः ? इत्याह—

शताह्वा सैन्धवाभ्यां च देयं स्नेहे च चूर्णकम् । तन्मात्रोत्तममध्यान्ता षट्चतुर्द्वयमाषकैः ॥ २१ ॥

Shatāhwa and Saindhava are to be added to the oil of Anuvāsana basti in the proportion of six, four or two māṣas for maximum, medium and minimum quantities of taila (oil) (21).

अनुवासनविषयमाह—

विरेचनात्सप्तरात्रे गते जातबलाय च । भुक्तान्नायानुवास्याय बस्तिर्देयोऽनुवासनः ॥ २२ ॥

Anuvāsana basti (oil enema) is to be administered to the suitable person when the person has gained strength, after a lapse of seven days after purgation therapy and after feeding him with good food (22).

अथानुवास्यं स्वभ्यक्तमुष्णाम्बुस्वेदितं शनैः । भोजयित्वा यथाशास्त्रं कृतचङ्क्रमणं ततः ॥ २३ ॥
उत्सृष्टानिलविण्मूत्रं योजयेत्स्नेहबस्तिना । सुप्तस्य वामपार्श्वेन वामजङ्घाप्रसारिणः ॥ २४ ॥
कुञ्चितापरजङ्घस्य नेत्रं स्निग्धगुदे न्यसेत् । बद्ध्वा बस्तिमुखं सूत्रैर्वामहस्तेन धारयेत् ॥ २५ ॥
पीडयेद्दक्षिणेनैव मध्यवेगेन धीरधीः । जृम्भाकासक्षवादींश्च बस्तिकाले न कारयेत् ॥ २६ ॥
त्रिंशन्मात्रामितः कालः प्रोक्तो बस्तेस्तु पीडने । ततः प्रणिहितः स्नेह उत्तानो वाक्शतं भवेत् ॥२७॥
जानुमण्डलमावेष्ट्य कुर्याच्छोटिकया युतम् । एका मात्रा भवेदेषा सर्वत्रैष विनिश्चयः ॥ २८ ॥
प्रसारितैः सर्वगात्रैर्यथावीर्यं विसर्पति । ताडयेत्तलयोरेनं त्रीन्वारांश्च शनैः शनैः ॥ २९ ॥
स्फिजोश्चैवं ततः श्रोणीं शय्यां चैवोत्क्षिपेत्ततः । जाते विधाने तु ततः कुर्यान्निद्रां यथासुखम् ॥३०॥

On the day of anuvāsana, a good oil massage and warm bath should be given to the person in the morning ofter he has attended to his calls of nature and taken a little walk. In the afternoon, after he has finished his meals, he should be made to lie on a comfortable cot, on his left side folding his right leg at the knee and extending his left leg to its full length, The basti (enema bag) tied well with the nozzle should be held firmly by the physician in his left hand and the lubricated nozzle is to be inserted into the rectum of the patient slowly with the help of the right hand. Then the physician should squeeze the bag courageously with moderate speed. The patient should be warned not to sneeze, yawn or cough during the process. Thirty matras is the time for pressing the bag and the patient should retain for one hundred mātrākālas.

A mātrā kāla is the time required for making a round (at a moderate speed) of the knee joint by the hand, the gesture started with the sound of the thumb and middle finger.

After administering the basti (enema) the physician should pat the buttocks, back and pelvis of the patient with his palms and ask him to sleep comfortably stretching in limbs freely (22–30).

सम्यगनुवासितलक्षणमाह—

सानिलः सपुरीषश्च स्नेहं प्रत्येति यस्य वै। उपद्रवं विना शीघ्रं स सम्यगनुवासितः ॥ ३१ ॥

After some reasonable time (about an hour) the enema material will come out, preceeded by flatus and faeces and finally the oil (31).

स्नेहागते विधिमाह—

जीर्णान्नस्त्वथ सायाह्ने स्नेहे प्रत्यागते पुनः। लघ्वन्नं भोजयेत् कामं दीप्ताग्निस्तु नरो यदि ॥ ३२ ॥

If the oil comes out immediately or late in the evening after the noon meal is digested and if the patient is having good appetite, he should be given light food which he likes (32).

अनुवासनव्यापत्तौ प्रतीकारमाह—

अनुवासिताय दातव्यमितरेऽह्नि सुखोदकम्। धान्यशुण्ठीकषायं वा स्नेहव्यापत्तिनाशनम् ॥ ३३ ॥

The person who has been given anuvāsana basti should be given warm water or a decoction of dhānya and śunṭhī, the next day in order to prevent the bad effect of oleation therapy (33).

अथोक्तप्रकारमुपसंहरन् बस्तिदानसंख्यामाह—

अनेन विधिना सप्त चाष्टौ वाथ नवाऽपि वा। विधेया बस्तयस्तेषामन्तरा तु निरूहणम् ॥ ३४ ॥

In this manner six, seven, eight or nine anuvāsanas can be given intersperced with nirūha basti (decoction enema) (34).

(दत्तस्तु प्रथमो बस्तिः स्नेहयेत् बस्तिवंक्षणौ। सम्यग्दत्तो द्वितीयस्तु मूर्धस्थमनिलं जयेत् ॥३५॥
बलं वर्णं च जनयेत्तृतीयस्तु प्रयोजितः। चतुर्थपञ्चमौ दत्तौ स्नेहयेतां रसासृजी ॥ ३६ ॥
षष्ठो मांसं स्नेहयति सप्तमो मेद एव च। अष्टमो नवमश्चापि मज्जानं च तथाक्रमम् ॥ ३७ ॥
एवं शुक्रागतान्दोषान्द्विगुणः साधु साधयेत्।

The first anuvāsana basti (oil enema) lubricates the area of urinary bladder and the groins, the second brings control over vāta is the head (nervous activity), the third one confers strength and complexion, the fourth and fifth oleate the rasa and rakta dhātus (blood), the sixth oleates the māṃsa dhātu (muscle tissue), the seventh the medas (adipose tissue), the eighth and ninth, the majjā (marrow) and śukra (reproductive tissues) dhātus respectively (35–38).

अष्टादशाष्टादशकान्बस्तीनां यो निषेवते ॥ ३८ ॥
स कुञ्जरबलोऽश्वं जयेत्तुल्योऽमरप्रभः। रूक्षाय बहुवाताय स्नेहबस्तिं दिने दिने ॥ ३९ ॥
दद्याद्वैद्यस्तथान्येषामन्यां बाधामपाहरेत्। स्नेहोऽल्पमात्रो रूक्षाणां दीर्घकालमनत्ययः ॥ ४० ॥
तथा निरूहः स्निग्धानामल्पमात्रः प्रशस्यते।)

He who receives one or two courses of eighteen enemas will attain the strength of an elephant, can over power a horse and equals the king of the heavens. Anuvāsana basti (oil enema) is to be administered daily for persons who are very dry and suffering from severe vāta disorders (nervous affections) and for others only for that period as required by the disease, small quantities of oil does not cause harm to the persons who are dry, in the same way as nirūha basti (decoction enema) for persons who are having too much of oilyness in their body (39–40).

निवृत्तेऽनुवासने स्नेहे पुनरपि अनुवासनमाह—

अथवा यस्य तत्कालं स्नेहो निर्याति केवलः ॥ ४१ ॥

तस्यान्योऽल्पतरो देयो न हि स्निह्यत्यतिष्ठति । अशुद्धस्य मलोन्मिश्रः स्नेहो नैति यदा पुनः ॥४२॥
तदा शैथिल्यमाध्यानं शूलं श्वासश्च जायते । पक्वाशये गुरुत्वं च तत्र दद्यान्निरूहणम् ॥ ४३ ॥
तीक्ष्णं तीक्ष्णौषधैर्युक्ता फलवर्तिर्हिता तथा । यथानुलोमनं वायुर्मलं स्नेहश्च जायते ॥ ४४ ॥
यथा विरेचनं दद्यात्तीक्ष्णं नस्यं च शस्यते । यस्य नोपद्रवं कुर्यात्स्नेहवस्तिरनिःसृतः ॥ ४५ ॥
सर्वोल्पो वा वृते रौक्ष्यादुपेक्ष्यः स विजानता ।

If the oil of the enema comes out immediatly after administration, he should be given another dose quickly, for oleation will not have taken place if it comes out soon. It the oil does not come out even after a long time, it produces śaithilya (weakness), ādhmāna (tympanitis), śūla (colic), swāsa (dyspnoea) and gurutwa of pakwāśaya (heaviness of the large intestine). For such a condition immediate administration of a nirūhabasti (decoction enema) or a phala varti (suppositories) prepared with powerful drugs should be administered to move the bowels down or a powerful purgative may also be given. A tīkṣna nasya (nasal medication) will also be ideal (41–45).

अहोरात्रादनिःसृते प्रतीकारमाह—

अनायातं त्वहोरात्रे स्नेहं संशोधनैर्हरेत् । स्नेहवस्तावनायाते नान्यः स्नेहो विधीयते ॥ ४६ ॥

If for a person who is very dry inside, the oil of the enema does not come out nor cause any trouble, no further intervention is necessary.

If it does not come out even after twenty four hours, it should be removed by śodhana measure (purgation) but the second oil enema should not be given (46).

अथानुवासनार्थं गुडूच्यादितैलमाह—

गुडूच्येरण्डपूतीकभार्ङ्गीवृषकरोहिषम् ॥ ४७ ॥

शतावरीं सहचरं काकनासां पलोन्मिताम् । यवमाषातसीकोलकुलत्थान्प्रसृतोन्मितान् ॥ ४८ ॥
चतुर्द्रोणेऽम्भसः पक्त्वा द्रोणशेषेण तेन च । पचेत्तैलाढकं पेष्यैर्जीवनीयैः पलोन्मितैः ॥ ४९ ॥
अनुवासनमेतद्धि सर्ववातविकारनुत् ।

Gudūcī, eraṇḍa, pūtika, bhārṅgī, vṛsaka, rohiṣa, śatāvarī, sahacara and kākanāsā—each one pala; yava, māṣa, atasī, kola and kulattha—each one prasṛta are boiled in four droṇas of water and decoction reduced to quarter; to it one āḍhaka of taila (sesemum oil) is added and a paste of drugs of jīvanīyagaṇa is added. Oil is then cooked in the usual way and used for anuvāsana basti in all vāta diseases (nervous disorders) with great benefit (47–49).

इदानीं स्नेहव्यापत् चिकित्सामाह—

षट्सप्ततिव्यापदस्तु जायन्ते बस्तिकर्मणा । दूषितात् समुदायेन ताश्चिकित्स्यास्तु सुश्रुतात् ॥५०॥

Seventysix errors arising from various kinds of improper procedures of anuvāsana vasti (oil enema) are described in the cikitsā section of Suśruta saṃhitā (all these are to be avoided) (50).

अनुवासने पानदिपथ्यमाह—

पानाहारविहारश्च परिहारश्च कृत्स्नशः । स्नेहपानसमाः कार्या नात्रकार्या विचारणा ॥ ५१ ॥

The regimen regarding food and other habits are the same as those prescribed for snehapana (drinking of oil) therapy and there need not be any rethinking over it (51).

इति श्रीदामोदरसूनुशार्ङ्गधराचार्यप्रणीतशार्ङ्गधरसंहितायामुत्तरखण्डे स्नेहबस्तिविधिर्नाम पञ्चमोऽध्यायः ॥ ५ ॥

Thus ends the fifth chapter.

षष्ठोऽध्यायः

CHAPTER 6

Nirūha Basti Vidhi (Decoction enemata)

अथ (परिशेष्यात्) निरूहबस्तिविधिमाह—

तत्र तद्भेदानाह—

निरूहबस्तिर्बहुधा भिद्यते कारणान्तरैः । तैरेव तस्य नामानि कृतानि मुनिपुङ्गवैः ॥ १ ॥
निरूहस्यापरं नाम प्रोक्तमास्थापनं बुधैः । स्वस्थानास्थापनाद्दोषधातूनां स्थापनं मतम् ॥ २ ॥

Nirūha basti (decoction enema) has many synonyms due to different reasons. It is popularly known as asthāpana because it promotes the health of the healthy and gives strength to the tissues of the sick (1–2).

अथ दोषाद्यपेक्षया मात्रामाह—

निरूहस्य प्रमाणं च प्रस्थं पादोत्तरं परम् । मध्यमं प्रस्थमुद्दिष्टं हीनं च कुडवास्त्रयः ॥ ३ ॥

The quantity of decoction for the enema is one and a quarter prasthas, one prastha and three kuḍavas respectively for maximum, medium and minimum dosages (3).

अथानास्थापनीयानाह—

अतिस्निग्धोत्क्लिष्टदोषौ क्षतोरस्कः कृशस्तथा । आध्मानच्छर्दिहिक्कार्शः कासश्वासप्रपीडितः ॥ ४ ॥
गुदशोफातिसारार्तो विषूचीकुष्ठसंयुतः । गर्भिणी मधुमेही च नास्थाप्यश्च जलोदरी ॥ ५ ॥

Persons who are having too much of oilyness in their body, who have started vomitting, who are suffering from urakṣata (pain in the chest), kṛśa (emaciation), ādhmāna (tympanitis), chardi (vomitting), hikkā (hiccough), arśa (piles), kāsa (cough), swāsa (dyspnoea), gudaśopha (oedema of the rectum), atisāra (diarrhoea), viṣūcī (gastroenterits), kuṣṭha (leprosy and skin diseases), madhumeha (diabetes mallitus), jalodara (ascitis) and pregnant women are not to be given nirūha basti (4–5).

अथ निरूह्यानाह—

वातव्याधावुदावर्ते वातासृग्विषमज्वरे । मूर्च्छातृष्णोदरानाहमूत्रकृच्छ्राश्मरीषु च ॥ ६ ॥
वृद्धासृग्दरमन्दाग्निप्रमेहेषु निरूहणम् । शूलेऽम्लपित्ते हृद्रोगे योजयेद्विधिवद्बुधः ॥ ७ ॥

Nirūha basti is indicated to persons suffering from vāta vyādhi (nervous diseases), udāvarta (reverse peristalisis), vātāsṛk (gout), viṣamajwara (intermittant fevers), mūrchā (convulsions), tṛṣṇā (thirst), udara (abdominal enlargement), ānāha (enlargement of abdomen by gas), mūtrakṛchra (dysuria), aśmarī (urinary calculus), vṛddhi (hernia), asṛkdara (menorrhagia), mandāgni (dyspepsia), prameha (diabetes), śūla (colic), amlapitta (hyper-acidity) and hṛdroga (heart diseases) (6–7).

येन प्रकारेण निरूहणं कर्तव्यं कदाह—

उत्सृष्टानिलविण्मूत्रं स्निग्धस्विन्नमभोजितम् । मध्याह्ने गृहमध्ये च यथायोग्यं निरूहयेत् ॥ ८ ॥
स्नेहबस्तिविधानेन बुधः कुर्यान्निरूहणम् । जाते निरूहे च ततो भवेदुत्कटकासनः ॥ ९ ॥
तिष्ठेन्मुहूर्तमात्रं तु निरूहागमनेच्छया । अनायातं मुहूर्तं तु निरूहं शोधनैर्हरेत् ॥ १० ॥
निरूहैरेव मतिमान्क्षारमूत्राम्लसैन्धवैः ।

The person who would receive the nirūha basti (decoction enema) should empty his bowels and get snigdha (oil massage) and sweda (sudation) therapies done earlier. In the afternoon, he should abstain from food and confine himself to a room. The procedure of administration is similar to that of the anuvasana basti (oil enema). Having taken the decoction enema he should sit on his heels for one muhurta in expectation of evacuation of bowels. If it does not come out, he should be given another enema containing the decoction of a purgative drug, along with alkalies, cow's urine, saindhava anb some sour substances (8–10).

अथ सुनिरूढलक्षणमाह—

यस्य क्रमेण गच्छन्ति विट्पित्तकफवायवः । लाघवं चोपजायेत सुनिरूढं तमादिशेत् ॥ ११ ॥

Vit (faeces), pitta (bile), kapha (mucous), and vāyu (flatus) come out in successive order after the decoction comes out. Afterwards the patient feels light in his body (11).

अथ दुर्निरूहलक्षणमाह—

यस्य स्याद्बस्तिरल्पावेगो हीनमलानिलः। मूर्च्छार्तिजाड्यारुजिमान् दुर्निरूहं तमादिशेत्॥ १२॥

If evacuation does not occur due to small quantity of the decoction used or scanty faeces or other defects inside, and the person goes in for mūrchā (convulsion), ārti (restlessness), jāḍyā (uneasiness) and ruja (pains), it is then to be understood as improper nirūha therapy (12).

निरूहस्य बस्तिदानवद्देयतामाह—

अनेन विधिना युञ्ज्यान्निरूहं बस्तिदातवत्। द्वितीयं वा तृतीयं वा चतुर्थं वा यथोचितम्॥ १३॥

Two, three or four nirūha basti (decoction enemata) can be given continuosly as required adopting proper procedure (13).

अथ भोजनक्रममाह—

पित्तश्लेष्मनिलाविष्टं क्षीरयूषरसैः क्रमात्। निरूहं भोजयित्वा च ततस्तमनुवासयेत्॥ १४॥

If there is doubt of obstruction to the pitta, kapha or vāta even after a nirūha basti, the patient should be given a meal of milk, soup of grains (like mudga or māṣā) or mutton broth and a anuvāsana basti (oil enema) administered later in the evening (14).

इदानीं बालवृद्धयोर्मृदुबस्तिमाह—

सुकुमारस्य वृद्धस्य बालस्य च मृदुर्हितः। बस्तिस्तीक्ष्णः प्रयुक्तस्तु तेषां हन्याद्बलायुषी॥ १५॥

For persons of tender constitution, children and the aged, nirūha basti should be mild. A powerful basti deprives them of strength and span of life (15).

इदानीं बस्तीनां दानक्रममाह—

दद्यादुत्क्लेशनं पूर्वं मध्ये दोषहरं ततः। पश्चात् संशमनीयं च दद्याद्बस्तिं विचक्षणः॥ १६॥

During a course of nirūha bastis (a series of enemas) the first one is to be prepared with utkleśana drugs (aggravating the doṣas), in the middle with of doṣahara drugs (reducing the doṣas) while at the end with śamana drugs (normalising the doṣas) (16).

अथ तेषां स्वरूपाण्याह—

उत्क्लेशनबस्ति—

एरण्डबीजं मधुकं पिप्पली सैन्धवं वचा। हपुषा फलकल्कं च बस्तिरुत्क्लेशनः स्मृतः॥ १७॥

Seeds of eraṇḍa, madhuka, pippalī, saindhava, vaca, hapuṣa and madanaphala—all these form a utkleśaka basti (17).

अथ दोषहरबस्तिमाह—

शताह्वा मधुकं बिल्वं कौटजं फलमेव च। सकाञ्जिकः सगोमूत्रो बस्तिर्दोषहरो मतः॥ १८॥

Śatāhwa, madhuka, bilwa, kuṭajaphala, with kāñjika and gomūtra is a doṣhara basti (18).

अथ तेषां दोषहरमाह—

प्रियङ्गु मधुकं मुस्तं तथैव च रसाञ्जनम् । सक्षीरः शस्यते बस्तिदोषाणां शमनः स्मृतः ॥ १९ ॥

शोधनबस्तिमाह—

शोधनद्रव्यनिःक्वाथैस्तत्कल्कैः स्नेहसैन्धवैः । युक्त्या खजेन मथिता बस्तयः शोधनाः स्मृताः ॥२०॥

Priyaṅgu, madhuka, musta, rasāñjana and milk is a śamana basti (palliative enema). Decoction of purgative drugs, their paste, small quantity of oil and saindhava—all mixed well by churning them together acts as a śodhana basti (purificatory enemata) (19–20).

लेखनबस्तिमाह—

त्रिफलाक्वाथगोमूत्रक्षौद्रक्षारसमायुतः । उषकादिप्रतीवापा बस्तयो लेखनः स्मृताः ॥ २१ ॥

Decoction of triphalā, gomūtra, honey, kṣāras and drugs of uṣakādi gana act as lekhana bastis (remover of doṣas) (21).

अथ बृंहणबस्तीनाह—

बृंहणद्रव्यनिष्क्वाथाः कल्कैर्मधुरकैर्युताः । सर्पिर्मांसरसोपेता बस्तयो बृंहणाः स्मृताः ॥ २२ ॥

Decoction of drugs which are bṛṃhana (strengthening), with paste of substances which are sweet, with ghee and mutton broth—form bṛṃhana vasti (bestower of strength) (22).

पिच्छिलबस्तिमाह—

बदर्यैरावती शेलु-शाल्मली-धन्वनागराः ।
क्षीरसिद्धाः क्षौद्रयुक्ता नाम्ना पिच्छिलसंज्ञिताः । अजोरभ्रेणरुधिरैर्युक्ता देया विचक्षणैः ॥ २३ ॥
मात्रा पिच्छिलबस्तीनां पलैर्द्वादशभिर्मता ।

Decoction of badara, irāvatī (nagabala), śelu, śālmali, dhanwa and nāgara, with milk and honey forms a pichila basti (unctous, sticky) which should be given mixed with the blood of goat, sheep or deer. The dose of this basti is twelve palas (23–24).

अथ निरूहार्थं द्रव्याणां परिमाणपूर्वकं विधानमाह—

दत्त्वादौ सैन्धवस्याक्षं मधुनः प्रसृतिद्वयम् ॥ २४ ॥
विनिर्मथ्य ततो दद्यात्स्नेहस्य प्रसृतित्रयम् । एकीभूते ततः स्नेहे कल्कस्य प्रसृति क्षिपेत् ॥ २५ ॥
संमूर्च्छिते कषायं तु चतुःप्रसृतिसंमितम् । क्षिप्त्वा विमथ्य दद्याच्च निरूहं कुशलो भिषक् ॥ २६ ॥
वाते चतुष्पलं क्षौद्रं दद्यात्स्नेहस्य षट्पलम् । पित्ते चतुष्पलं क्षौद्रं स्नेहं दद्यात्पलत्रयम् ॥ २७ ॥
कफे च षट्पलं क्षौद्रं क्षिपेत्स्नेहं चतुष्पलम् ।

Basti material is to be prepared in the following manner—saindhava lavaṇa one akṣa in measure is put into a vessel and two prasṛtis of honey is added and mixed well. Then three prasṛtis of sneha (oil) is added along with one prasṛti of kalka (paste) and mixed well. Later four prasrutas of kaṣāya (decoction) is added and the entire mass churned with a churner to form a homogenous mixture and filled into the enema bag.

In diseases of vāta, four palas of honey and six of oil; in diseases of pitta four palas of honey and three of oil; while in diseases of kapha six palas of honey and four[1] palas of oil are advocated (25-28).

मधुतैलिकसंज्ञं बस्तिविधानमाह—

एरण्डक्काथतुल्यांशं मधुतैलं पलाशकम् ॥ २८ ॥

शतपुष्पापलार्धेन सैन्धवार्धेन संयुतम् । मधुतैलकसंज्ञोऽयं बस्तिः खजविलोडितः ॥ २९ ॥

मेदोगुल्मकृमिप्लीहमलोदावर्तनाशनः । बलवर्णकरश्चैव वृष्यो दीपनबृंहणः ॥ ३० ॥

Decoction of eraṇḍa, honey and oil each one pala and half pala each of paste of śatapuṣpā and saindhava are mixed well and enema given. This recipe known as *Madhutailika basti* is effective in diseases like medoroga (obesity), gulma (abdominal tumor), kṛmi (intestinal worms), plihā (splenic enlargement), mala bandha (constipation), udāvarta (reverse peristalisis). It bestows strength, complexion, virility, digestive capacity and good physique (29-30).

अथ यापनबस्तिमाह—

क्षौद्रा-ऽज्य-क्षीर-तैलानां प्रसृतं भवेत् । हपुषासैन्धवाक्षांशो बस्तिः स्याद्दीपनः परः ॥ ३१ ॥

Honey, ghee, milk, oil each one prasruta, saindhava and hapuṣa each one akṣa put together forms a *Dīpana basti* (appetiser enema) (31).

अथ युक्तरथबस्तिमाह—

एरण्डमूलनिष्काथो मधुतैलं ससैन्धवम् । एष युक्तरथो बस्तिः सवचापिप्पलीफलः ॥ ३२ ॥

Decoction of roots of eraṇḍa, honey, oil, saindhava, vaca, pippalī and madana phala forms a *Yuktaratha-basti* (32).

अथ सिद्धबस्तिमाह—

पञ्चमूलस्य निष्काथस्तैलं मागधिका मधु । ससैन्धवः समधुकः सिद्धबस्तिरिति स्मृतः ॥ ३३ ॥

Decoction of pañcamūlas, oil, pippalī, honey, saindhava, and madhuyaṣṭi form a *Siddha basti* (33).

पथ्यापथ्यमाह—

स्नानमुष्णोदकैः कुर्यात् दिवा स्वप्नमजीर्णताम् । वर्जयेदपरं सर्वं, आचरेत्स्नेहबस्तिवत् ॥ ३४ ॥

1. The quantity of sneha in disorders of kapha should be less, the quantity mentioned here seems to be in appropriate.

The person who has been given an enema should take bath in warm water avoid day sleep, indigestion and observe other rules as prescribed under snehabasti (oil enema) (34).

इति श्रीदामोदरसूनुना श्रीशार्ङ्गधरेण विरचितायां शार्ङ्गधरसंहितायामुत्तरखण्डे निरूहबस्तिविधिरध्यायः समाप्तः ॥ ६ ॥

Thus ends the sixth chapter.

सप्तमोऽध्यायः

CHAPTER 7

Uttara Basti Vidhi (Urethral and Vaginal douches)

परिशेष्यादुत्तरबस्तिमाह—

अतः परं प्रवक्ष्यामि बस्तिमुत्तरसंज्ञितम् । द्वादशाङ्गुलकं नेत्रं मध्ये च कृतकर्णिकम् ॥ १ ॥
मालतीपुष्पवृन्ताभं छिद्रं सर्षपसन्निभम् ।

I shall now describe the uttara basti (enema administered into the urinary bladder and uterus).

The nozzle should be twelve aṅgulis long, with a single karṇikā (ridge) in its middle, resembling the stalk of a mālatī flower (jasmine) with its orifice of the size of a mustard (1–2).

स्नेहमात्रामाह—

पञ्चविंशतिवर्षाणामधो मात्रा द्विकार्षिका ॥ २ ॥
तदूर्ध्वं पलमात्रा च स्नेहस्योक्ता भिषग्वरैः ।

The quantity of oil (enema material) should be two karṣas for persons below twentyfive years of age and for those above that age one pala is the dose (2–3).

अथोत्तरबस्तेर्विधानमाह—

अथास्थापनशुद्धस्य तृप्तस्य स्नानभोजनैः ॥ ३ ॥
स्थितस्य जानुमात्रे च पीठेऽन्विष्य शलाकया । स्निग्धया मेढ्रमार्गं च ततो नेत्रं नियोजयेत् ॥ ४ ॥
शनैः शनैर्घृताभ्यक्तं मेढ्ररन्ध्रेऽङ्गुलानि षट् । ततोऽवपीडयेद्बस्तिं शनैर्नेत्रं च निर्हरेत् ॥ ५ ॥
ततः प्रत्यागते स्नेहे स्नेहबस्तिक्रमो हितः ।

The person who has been administered asthāpana basti (decoction enema) earlier and given good nutrient foods and bath later on, should be made to sit comfortably on a stool of the height of one's knee. The nozzle should be smeared with ghee or oil (lubricant) all over and slowly introduced into the urethral passage to a length of six aṅgulīs. The enema bag is then squeezed gently to push in the oil and the nozzle drawn out slowly and gently (3–6).

पुंसामुत्तरबस्तिनेत्रमुक्त्वा स्त्रीणामुत्तरबस्तिमाह—

स्त्रीणां कनिष्ठिकास्थूलनेत्रं कुर्याद्दशांगुलम् ॥ ६ ॥

मुद्गप्रवेशयोग्यं च योन्यन्तश्चतुरङ्गुलम् । व्यङ्गुलं मूत्रमार्गे च सूक्ष्मं नेत्रं नियोजयेत् ॥ ७ ॥

बालानामपि नेत्रपरिमाणमाह—

मूत्रकृच्छ्रविकारेषु बालानां त्वेकमङ्गुलम् । शनैर्निष्कम्पमाधेयं सूक्ष्मनेत्रं विचक्षणः ॥ ८ ॥

In case of women the nozzle should be ten aṅgulīs long, of the size of the little finger in thickness and it's orifice of the size of a green gram. If enema is to be given to the uterus, the nozzle should be introduced to a length of four aṅgulīs into the uterine orifice and if into the urinary bladder to a length of two aṅglīs. In case of children suffering from mūtrakṛchra (dysuria) the nozzle should go in for about one aṅgulī, and the bag squeezed firmly (6–8).

अथापत्यमूत्रमार्गयोर्विषयप्वात् स्नेहपरिमाणमाह—

योनिमार्गेषु नारीणां स्नेहमात्रा द्विपालिकी । मूत्रमार्गे पलोन्माना बलानां च द्विकार्षिकी ॥ ९ ॥

The prescribed dose of oil for uterine enema is two palas, for enema of urinary bladder one pala and for children two karṣas (9).

अथ स्त्रीणामुत्तरबस्तिः कथं योज्यः ? इत्याह—

उत्तानायै स्त्रियै दद्यादूर्ध्वजान्वै विचक्षणः । अप्रत्यागच्छति भिषग्वस्तावुत्तरसंज्ञिते ॥ १० ॥

भूयो बस्तिं निदध्याच्च संयुक्तैः शोधनैर्गणैः । फलवर्तिं निदध्याद्वा योनिमार्गे दृढां भिषक् ॥ ११ ॥

सूत्रैर्विनिर्मितां स्निग्धां शोधनद्रव्यसंयुताम् । दह्यमाने तथा बस्तौ दद्याद्‌बस्तिं विशारदः ॥ १२ ॥

If the oil given into the uterus does not comeout soon, another basti prepared with decoction of drugs of śodhana group should be given or a phala varti (suppositary) prepared with the same kind of drugs is placed in the vaginal orifice; if there is complaint of burning sensation inside the uterus a decoction enema prepared with drugs of kṣīra vṛkṣa group mixed with milk is administered cold (10–12).

क्षीरवृक्षकषायेण पयसा शीतलेन वा । बस्तिः शुक्ररुजः पुंसां स्त्रीणामार्तवजां रुजम् ॥ १३ ॥

हन्यादुत्तरबस्तिस्तु नोचितो मेहिनां क्वचित् ।

Uttara basti is beneficial in disorders of śukra and ārtava (reproductive elements of man and woman respectively) but it should not be given to persons suffering from prameha (diabetes) (13–14).

उत्तरबस्तेः स्नेहबस्तिसमानायाः गुणदोषनाह—

सम्यग्दत्तस्य लिङ्गानि व्यापदः क्रम एव च ॥ १४ ॥
बस्तेरुत्तरसंज्ञस्य समानं स्नेहबस्तिना ।

The signs and symptoms of a properly administered uttarabasti are similar to those of a sneha basti (oil enema per rectum) (14–15).

अथ पूर्वोद्दिष्टां फलवर्तिमाह—

घृताभ्यक्ते गुदे क्षेप्या श्लक्ष्णा स्वाङ्गुष्ठसन्निभा ॥ १५ ॥
मलप्रवर्तनी वर्तिः फलवर्तिश्च सा स्मृता ।

A wick like stick (prepared with paste of purgative drugs smeared over layers of cloth and rolled like a stick) of the size of a thumb, smeared over with ghee and introduced into the rectum in order to remove the accumilated mala (faeces) is called a phala varti (suppository) (15–16).

इति श्रीदामोदरसूनुशार्ङ्गधराचार्यप्रणीतशार्ङ्गधरसंहितायामुत्तरखण्डे उत्तरबस्तिविधिर्नाम सप्तमोऽध्यायः ॥ ७ ॥

Thus ends the seventh chapter.

अष्टमोऽध्यायः

CHAPTER 8

अथ नस्यविधिः—

Nasya Vidhi (Nasal medication)

नस्यस्य निरुक्तिमाह—

नस्यं तत्कथ्यते धीरैर्नासाग्राह्यं यदौषधम् । नावनं नस्यकर्मेति तस्य नामद्वयं मतम् ॥ १ ॥

Administration of medicines through the nose is called nasya. It is also known as nāvana and nasya karma (1).

नस्यभेदानाह—

नस्यभेदो द्विधा प्रोक्तो रेचनः स्नेहनस्तथा । रेचनं कर्षणं प्रोक्तं स्नेहनं बृंहणं मतम् ॥ २ ॥

It is of two kinds—recana (purgative to the head, purificatory) and snehana (oleating, palliative); the former is karṣaṇa (reducing) while the later is bṛṃhaṇa (strengthening) (2).

नस्यकर्मकालमाह—

कफपित्तानिलध्वंसे पूर्वमध्यापराह्णके । दिने तु गृह्यते नस्यं रात्रावप्युत्कटे गदे ॥ ३ ॥

Nasya is administered in the morning, afternoon and evening of the daytime for diseases of kapha, pitta and vāta respecsively; it is administered at nights only in emergency (3).

नस्यं यस्मिन्काले त्याज्यं यैश्च त्याज्यं तानाह—

नस्यं त्यजेद्भोजनान्ते दुर्दिने चापतर्पिते । तथा नवप्रतिश्यायी गर्भिणी गरदूषितः ॥ ४ ॥
अजीर्णी दत्तबस्तिश्च पीतस्नेहोदकासवः । क्रुद्धः शोकाभिभूतश्च तृषार्तो वृद्धबालकौ ॥ ५ ॥
वेगावरोधी स्नातश्च स्नातुकामश्च वर्जयेत् ।

Nasya is not to be administered after the midday meal, on a cloudy day, after fasting, and for those suffering from recent attack of cold, pregnancy, homicidal poisoning, indigestion; who has taken as enema, or oleation therapy; who has drunk too much water or alcoholic beverages, who are in fits of anger, sorrow and thirst; old people, young boys, those who are suppressing their body urges and who have taken bath or wish to take bath immediately (4–6).

नस्यार्हानर्हानाह—

अष्टवर्षस्य बालस्य नस्यकर्म समाचरेत् ॥ ६ ॥
अशीतिवर्षादूर्ध्वं च नावनं नैव दीयते ।

Nasya, can be administered from the age of eight to the age of eighty years after which it is not done (6-7).

अथ वैरेचनं नस्यमाह—

अथ वैरेचनं नस्यं ग्राह्यं तैलैः सुतीक्ष्णकैः ॥ ७ ॥
तीक्ष्णभेषजसिद्धैर्वा स्नेहैः क्वाथै रसैस्तथा ।

Virecana nasya (purgative) consists of a strong oil as such or a medicated oil prepared with pungent drugs, or decoction or fresh juice of such drugs (7–8).

विरेचनस्य मात्रामान—

नासिकारन्ध्रयोरष्टौ षट् चत्वारश्च बिन्दवः ॥ ८ ॥
प्रत्येकं रेचने योज्या मुख्यमध्यान्त्यमात्रया ।

Eight, six and four bindus (drops, minims) of the liquid poured into each nostril are the maximum, medium and minimum dosage of a purgative nasya (8–9).

नस्यार्थं द्रव्याणां परिमाणमाह—

नस्यकर्मणि दातव्यं शाणैकं तीक्ष्णमौषधम् ॥ ९ ॥
हिङ्गु स्याद्यवमात्रं तु माषैकं सैन्धवं मतम् । क्षीरं चैवाष्टशाणं स्यात्पानीयं च त्रिकार्षिकम् ॥१०॥
कार्षिकं मधुरं द्रव्यं नस्यकर्मणि योजयेत् ।

In preparing the recipe for nasal medication, the quantity of pungent drugs should be one śāṇa, hiṅgu one yava, saindhava one māṣā, eight śāṇas of milk;

water or decoction, three karṣas and sweet substances (like honey, sugar etc.) one karṣa (9–10).

अथ शिरोविरेचनभेदानाह—

अवपीडप्रधमनौ द्वौ भेदावपरौ स्मृतौ ॥ ११ ॥

शिरोविरेचनस्यात्र तौ तु देयं यथायथम् ।

अथावपीडप्रधमनयोः स्वरूपमाह—

कल्कीकृतादौषधाद्यः पीडितो निःसृतो रसः ॥ १२ ॥

सोऽवपीडः समुद्दिष्टस्तीक्ष्णद्रव्यसमुद्भवः । षडङ्गुला द्विवक्त्रा या नाडी चूर्णं तथा धमेत् ॥ १३ ॥

तीक्ष्णं कोलमितं वक्त्रवातैः प्रधमनं हि तत् ।

Virecana nasya (purgative medication) is of two kinds, avapīda and pradhamana (insuffulation); the fresh juice of pungent substances directly put into the nose is avapīda, whereas pradhamana is blowing one kola in quantity of a fine powder of pungent substances into the nose by means of a hollow tube of six aṅgulīs in length (11–14).

ऊर्ध्वजत्रुगते रोगे कफजे स्वरसंक्षये ॥ १४ ॥

अरोचके प्रतिश्याये शिरःशूले च पीनसे । शोफाऽपस्मारकुष्ठेषु नस्यं वैरेचनं हितम् ॥ १५ ॥

Purgative medication is indicated in diseases of organs above the shoulders, disorders of kapha, swara kṣaya (loss of voice), arocaka (anorexia), pratiśyāya (common-cold), śirahśūla (head ache), pīnasa (ch. rhinitis), śopha (oedema), apasmāra (epilepsy) and kuṣṭha (leprosy and other skin diseases) (14–15).

अथ बृंहणनस्यविषयमाह—

भीरुस्त्रीकृशबालानां नस्यं स्नेहेन शस्यते ।

येषु अवपीडनं युज्यते तानाह—

गलरोगे सन्निपाते निद्रायां विषमज्वरे ॥ १६ ॥

मनोविकारे कृमिषु युज्यते चावपीडनम् ।

For persons who are frightful, women, children and the weak, bṛṃhaṇa-nasya should be administered in the form of sneha (pure or medicated oil).

Avapīdana is indicated in diseases of the throat, sannipāta jwara (toxic fevers), atinidrā (excessive sleep), viṣama jwara (remittant fevers), manovikāras (mental disorders) and kṛmi (parasitic disorders) (16).

येषु प्रधमनं युज्यते तानाह—

अत्यन्तोत्कटदोषेषु विसंज्ञेषु च दीयते ॥ १७ ॥

चूर्णं प्रधमनं धीरैस्तद्धि तीक्ष्णतरं यतः ।

Pradhamana is indicated when the doṣas have attained profound disturbances, when the persons are unconcious, because it is very powerful than the former kind (17).

इदानीमवपीडनप्रधमनयोः कतिपययोगानाह—

गुडादिनस्यम्–पिप्पल्यादिनस्यम्—

नस्यं स्याद्गुडशुण्ठीभ्यां पिप्पल्याः सैन्धवेन वा ॥ १८ ॥

जलपिष्टेन तेनाक्षिकर्णनासाशिरोगदाः । मन्याहनुगलोद्भूता नश्यन्ति भुजपृष्ठजाः ॥ १९ ॥

Guda (jaggery) and śunṭhī or pippalī and saindhava—macerated well with water and put into the nose, cures diseases of eyes, ears, nose, head, neck, lower jaw, throat, shoulders and back (18–19).

मधूकसारादिनस्यम्—

मधूकसारकृष्णाभ्यां वचामरिचसैन्धवैः । नस्यं कोष्णजले पिष्टं दद्यात्संज्ञाप्रबोधनम् ॥ २० ॥

अपस्मारे तथोन्मादे सन्निपातेऽपतन्त्रके ।

Madhūkasāra (pith of madhūka tree), kṛṣṇā, vaca, marica and saindhava to be made into liquid with warm water and instilled into the nostrils restores conciousness in cases of apasmāra (epilepsy), unmāda (insanity), sannipāta (severe fevers) and apatantraka (tetanus) (20).

तन्द्रायां सैन्धवादिनस्यम्—

सैन्धवं श्वेतमरिचं सर्षपाः कुष्ठमेव च ॥ २१ ॥

बस्तमूत्रेण पिष्टानि नस्यं तन्द्रानिवारणम् ।

Saindhava, sweta marica, sarṣapa and kuṣṭha with goat's urine made into a nasal medication relieves excessive drowsiness (21).

मरिचादिनस्यम्—

रोहितमत्स्यपित्तेन भावितं सैन्धवं वचा ॥ २२ ॥

मरिचं पिप्पली शुण्ठी कङ्कोलं लशुनं पुरम् । कट्फलं चेति तच्चूर्णं देयं प्रधमनं बुधैः ॥ २३ ॥

Saindhava, vaca, marica, pippalī, śunṭhī, kaṅkola, laśuna, puram and kaṭphala mecerated with the bile of rohiṣa fiish and made into a fine powder forms a good pradhamana nasya (insuffulation) (22–23).

अथ बृंहणनस्यकल्पनामाह—

अथ बृंहणनस्य कल्पना कथ्यतेऽधुना । मर्शश्च प्रतिमर्शश्च द्वौ भेदौ स्नेहनौ मतौ ॥ २४ ॥

मर्शस्य तर्पणी मात्रा मुख्या शाणैः स्मृताऽष्टभिः । मध्यमा च चतुःशाणैर्हीना शाणमिता स्मृता ॥२५॥

एकैकस्मिंस्तु मात्रेयं देया नासापुटे बुधैः । मर्शस्य द्वित्रिवेलं वा वीक्ष्य दोषबलाबलम् ॥ २६ ॥

एकान्तरं द्व्यन्तरं वा नस्यं दद्याद्विचक्षणः । त्र्यहं पञ्चाहमथवा सप्ताहं वा सुयन्त्रितम् ॥ २७ ॥

मर्शे शिरोविरेके च व्यापदो द्विविधाः स्मृताः । दोषोत्क्लेशात्क्षयाच्चैव विज्ञेयास्ता यथाक्रमम् ॥२८॥

दोषोत्क्लेशनिमित्तासु युञ्ज्याद्वमनशोधनम् । अथ क्षयनिमित्तासु यथास्वं बृंहणं हितम् ॥ २९ ॥

Bṛṃhaṇa (sneha), nasya (oily errhines) is again of two kinds; marśa and pratimarśa. Eight, four and one śāṇas are the maximum, medium and minimum doses of marśa; put into each nostril twice or thrice a day, administered with intervals of one or two days continued for a period of three, five or seven days, marśa and purgations of the head produce many untoward symptoms by aggravation or diminishen of the doṣas; vamana (śirovirecana) should be administered when symptoms of aggravation manifest and when symptoms of diminishen appear, bṛṃhaṇa (bṛṃhaṇa nasya) should be administered (24–29).

शिरोनासाक्षिरोगेषु सूर्यावर्तार्धभेदके । दन्तरोगे बले हीने मन्याबाह्वंसजे गदे ॥ ३० ॥
मुखशोषे कर्णनादे वातपित्तगदे तथा । अकालपलिते चैव केशश्मश्रुप्रपातने ॥ ३१ ॥
युज्यते बृंहणं नस्यं स्नेहैर्वा मधुरद्रवैः ।

Bṛṃhaṇa nasya is indicated in diseases of the head, nose, eyes, sūryāvarta (migraine headache), ardhavabheda (hemicrania), dantarogas (dental diseases), for debilitated persons. In those suffering from diseases of neck, shoulders, and arms; mukhaśoṣa (dryness of mouth), karṇanāda (ringing in the ears), disorders of vāta and pitta, premature greying and falling of hairs and mustaches, medicated oil or liquid of sweet substances being used (30–32).

कुङ्कुमनस्यम्—

सशर्करं पयःपिष्टं भृष्टमाज्येन कुङ्कुमम् ॥ ३२ ॥
नस्य प्रयोगतो हन्याद्वातरक्तभवा रुजः । भ्रूशङ्खाक्षिशिरःकर्णसूर्यावर्तार्धभेदकान् ॥ ३३ ॥

Kuṅkuma kesara fried in ghee, macerated with milk and sugar applied to the nose relieves disorders arising from vāta and rakta, pain in the forehead, temples, head, ears, sūryāvarta (migrane) and ardhavabheda (hemicrania) (33).

अन्यबृंहणनस्यमाह—

नस्यं स्यादणुतैलेन यथा नारायणेन वा । माषादीना वा सर्पिर्भिस्तत्तद्भेषजसाधितैः ॥ ३४ ॥

दोषेषु स्नेहव्यवस्था—

तैलं कफे स्याद्वाते च केवले पवने वसाम् । दद्यान्नस्यं सदा पित्ते सर्पिर्मज्जानमेव च ॥ ३५ ॥

Anutaila, narāyaṇataila, māṣā taila or ghṛta prepared with appropriate drugs can also be used as bṛmhaṇa nasya; taila (oil) should be chosen in disorders of kapha and kaphavāta; vasa (muscle fat) in disorders of vāta; ghṛta (ghee) and majjā (marrow) in disorders of pitta (34–35).

माषादिनस्यम्—

माषाऽत्मगुप्तारास्नाभिर्बलारुबुकरोहिषैः । कृतोऽश्वगन्धया क्वाथो हिङ्गुसैन्धवसंयुतः ॥ ३६ ॥
कोष्णो नस्य प्रयोगेण पक्षाघातं सकम्पनम् । जयेदर्दितवातं च मन्यास्तम्भापबाहुकौ ॥ ३७ ॥

Māṣā, atmagupta, rāsnā, balā, rubuka, rohiṣa and aswagandhā are made into decoction; hiṅgu and saindhava added to it and applied warm to the nostrils relieves pakṣāghāta (hemiplegia) associated with kampa (tremors), ardita (facial paralysis), manyāstambha (wry neck) and apabāhuka (shoulder-hand syndrome). (36-37).

अथ प्रतिमर्शमाह—

प्रतिमर्शस्य मात्रा तु द्विद्विबिन्दुमिता मता । प्रत्येकशो नस्तकयोः स्नेहेति विनिश्चतम् ॥ ३८ ॥
स्नेहे ग्रन्थिद्वयं यावन्निमग्ना चोद्धृता ततः । तर्जनीयं स्रवेद्बिन्दुं सा मात्रा बिन्दुसंज्ञिता ॥ ३९ ॥
एवंविधैर्बिन्दुसंज्ञैरष्टभिः शाण उच्यते । स देयो मर्शनस्ये तु प्रतिमर्शो द्विबिन्दुकः ॥ ४० ॥
समयाः प्रतिमर्शस्य बुधैः प्रोक्ताश्चतुर्दश । प्रभाते दन्तकाष्ठान्ते गृहान्निर्गमने तथा ॥ ४१ ॥
व्यायामाध्वव्यवायान्ते विण्मूत्रान्तेऽञ्जने कृते । कवलान्ते भोजनान्ते दिवासुप्तोत्थिते तथा ॥ ४२ ॥
वमनान्ते तथा सायं प्रतिमर्शः प्रयुज्यते । ईषदुच्छिङ्कनात्स्नेहो यदा वक्त्रं प्रपद्यते ॥ ४३ ॥

Pratimarśa, is also oil errhine itself but its dose is only two bindus (drops) for each nostril. A bindu (drop) is that quantity of oil which drops from the index finger dipped into oil to the level of its first two phallanges. Eight times of this quantity is equivalent to one śāṇa which is the dose of marśa nasya (described earlier). Pratimarśa nasya can be administered at fourteen periods; such as early morning, after brushing the teeth; going out of the house, after exercise, after long walk, after sex act, after micturation, after defaecation, after applying collyrium to the eyes, after a mouth gargle, after meals, after midday nap, after emesis and in the evening (38-43).

नस्ये निषिक्तं तं विद्यात्प्रतिमर्शं प्रमाणतः । उच्छिन्दन्न पिबेच्चैतनिष्ठीवेन्मुखमागतम् ॥ ४४ ॥

The oil applied to the nostrils slowly reaching the throat is to be considered as ideal dose, it can be spit out when it comes to the throat fully (44).

क्षीणे तृष्णास्यशोषार्ते बाले वृद्धे च युज्यते । प्रतिमर्शेन शाम्यन्ति रोगाश्चैवोर्ध्वजत्रुजाः ॥ ४५ ॥
वलीपलितनाशश्च बलमिन्द्रियजं भवेत् ।

Pratimarśa nasya is advocated for the debilitated, young or old and for those suffering from thirst and diseases of mouth, head, of organs above the shoulders, premature greying and falling of hairs. It confers strength to the sense organs (45-46).

अथ पलिते नस्यम्—

बिभीतनिम्बकम्भारी शिवा शेलुश्च काकिनी ॥ ४६ ॥
एकैकतैलनस्येन पलितं नश्यति ध्रुवम् ।

Oil extracted from or prepared out of any one of vibhitaka, nimba, gambhārī, śiva, śelu, or kākinī—cures palita (greying of hairs) (46).

अथ नस्यग्रहणे नस्यविधिमाह—

अथ नस्यविधिं वक्ष्ये तस्यग्रहणहेतवे ॥ ४७ ॥

देशे वातरजोमुक्ते कृतदन्तनिघर्षणम् । विशुद्धं धूमपानेन स्विन्नभालगलं तथा ॥ ४८ ॥

उत्तानशायिनं किंचित्प्रलम्बशिरसं नरम् । आस्तीर्णहस्तपादं च वस्त्राच्छादितलोचनम् ॥ ४९ ॥

समुन्नमितनासाग्रं वैद्यो नस्येन योजयेत् । कोष्णमच्छिन्नधारं च हेमताराद्रिशुक्तिभिः ॥ ५० ॥

शुक्त्या वा यत्र युक्त्या वा प्लोतैर्वा नस्यमाचरेत्

The person to whom nasya karma is to be done should clean his mouth and teeth, have dhūmapāna (inhalation) and comfortably lie down on a cot with his face upwards, hands and legs stretched straight, head slightly bent back with a pillow supporting the neck. Oil is to be applied over the forehead and face and mild fomentation given. The eyes are covered with cloth, nostrils are uplifted and oil poured warm into them either with a spoon of gold, silver, shell or even with a pad of cotton, wool or cloth (47–50).

नस्येष्वासिच्यमानेषु शिरो नैव प्रकम्पयेत् ॥ ५१ ॥

न कुप्येन्न प्रभाषेत नोच्छिदेन्न हसेत्तथा । एतैर्हि विहितः स्नेहो नैवान्तः संप्रपद्यते ॥ ५२ ॥

ततः कासप्रतिश्यायशिरोऽक्षिगदसंभवः । शृङ्गाटकमभिप्लाव्य स्थापयेन्न गिलेद्द्रवम् ॥ ५३ ॥

अथ नस्यधारणार्थं मात्रासंख्यामाह—

पञ्च सप्त दशैव स्युर्मात्रा नस्यस्य धारणे ।

तस्यदानानन्तरं किं कर्तव्यं ? इत्यत आह—

उपविश्याथ निष्ठीवेन्नासावक्त्रगतं द्रवम् ॥ ५४ ॥

वामदक्षिणपार्श्वाभ्यां निष्ठीवेत्संमुखे न हि । नीते नस्ये मनस्तापं रजः क्रोधं च संत्यजेत् ॥ ५५ ॥

शयीत निद्रां त्यक्त्वा च प्रोत्तानो वा शतं नरः । तथा वैरेचनश्चान्ते धूमो वा कवलो हितः ॥५६॥

After application of nasya, the patient should not shake his head, talk, lough, sneeze, or yawn; which prevents the oil reaching the throat. Kāsa (cough), pratiśyāya (running in the nose), disorders of head and eyes will occur, if the oil does not reach the sṛṅgāṭaka (a vital spot just above the throat); five, seven or ten mātras are the duration of time for retaning the nasya. Afterwards, the nasya material can be spit out, sitting up or bending to either side. Later he should avoid worry and anger and comfortably lie down without sleeping for a duration of about one hundred syllables. Later he should take a dhūmapāna (inhalation) or a kavalagraha (mouth gargle) (51–56).

अथ नस्ये कति लक्षणानि भवन्ति ? इत्याह—

नस्ये त्रीण्युपदिष्टानि लक्षणानि प्रयोगतः । शुद्धिहीनातियोगानि विशेषाच्छास्त्रचिन्तकैः ॥ ५७ ॥

Nasya has three aspects śuddhi-(proper-therapy), hīna— (inadequate) and ati (excess) therapy (57).

नस्यशुद्धिलक्षणमाह—

लाघवं मनसः शुद्धिः स्रोतसां व्याधिसंक्षयः। चित्तेन्द्रियप्रसादश्च शिरसः शुद्धिलक्षणम् ॥ ५८ ॥

Feeling of lightness in the head, clearance of the passages, lessening of the symptoms, clarity of mind and senses are the signs of proper purification of the head (58).

अथ हीनशुद्धेर्लक्षणमाह—

कण्डूपदेहौ गुरुता स्रोतसां कफसंस्रवः। मूर्ध्नि हीनविशुद्धेस्तु लक्षणं परिकीर्तितम् ॥ ५९ ॥

अतिशयशुद्धस्य लक्षणमाह—

मस्तुलुङ्गागमो वातवृद्धिरिन्द्रियविभ्रमः। शून्यता शिरसश्चापि मूर्ध्नि गाढं विरेचिते ॥ ६० ॥

Irritation, viscidity, incresed secretions from the orifices, heavyness of the head are effects of inadequate therapy where as expulsion of mastubuṅga (brain or it's fluid) increase of vāta activity, disturbances of sense faculties and feeling of emptyness of the head are symptoms of excessive therapy (59=60).

हीनातिशुद्धौ चिकित्सामाह—

हीनातिशुद्धे शिरसि कफवातघ्नमाचरेत्। सम्यक् विशुद्धे शिरसि सर्पिर्नस्ये निषेचयेत् ॥ ६१ ॥

In case of inadequate therapy kaphahara measures are to be adopted while in case of excessive therapy the vātahara measures; ghee is to administered as nasya for the persons who got proper therapy (61).

अतिस्निग्धलक्षणचिकित्सामाह—

कफप्रसेकः शिरसो गुरुतेन्द्रियविभ्रमः। लक्षणं तदतिस्निग्धे तत्र रूक्षं प्रदापयेत् ॥ ६२ ॥
भोजयेच्चानभिष्यन्दि तस्याचारिकमादिशेत्।

If excessive oleation takes place, it manifests with running in the nose, heavyness of the head and disturbances of sense organs; for such persons rūkṣaṇā (drying) measures are to be adopted and anabhiṣyandi (foods causing dryness) are to be given (62).

प्रकरणार्थमुपसंहरति—

वमनं रेचनं नस्यं निरूहश्चानुवासनम्। एतानि पञ्च कर्माणि कथितानि मुनीश्वरैः ॥ ६३ ॥

Vamana (emesis), virecana (purgation), nasya (nasal medication), nirūha (decoction enema) and anuvāsana (oil enema)—these are designated by the great sages of the past as pañcakarmas—the five important therapies (63).

इति श्रीदामोदरसूनुना शाङ्गधराचार्येण विरचितायां शाङ्गधरसंहितायामुत्तरखण्डे
नस्यविधिर्नामाष्टमोऽध्यायः ॥ ८ ॥

Thus ends the eighth chapter.

नवमोऽध्यायः

CHAPTER 9

अथ धूमपानविधिः—

Dhūmapāna Vidhi (*Inhalation, Fumigation therapy*)

धूमसंख्या—

धूमस्तु षड्विधः प्रोक्तः शमनो बृंहणस्तथा । रेचनः कासहा चैव वामनो व्रणधूपनः ॥ १ ॥

Dhūma (inhalation) is of six kinds; viz., Śamana (palliative), bṛṃhaṇa (strengthening), recana (purgative), kāsaghna (anti tussive), vamana (emetic) and vraṇadhūpana (fumigation of ulcers) (1)

शमस्य तु पर्यायौ मध्यः प्रयोगिकस्तथा । बृंहणस्यापि पर्यायौ स्नेहिको मृदुरेव च ॥ २ ॥
रेचनस्यापि पर्यायौ शोधनस्तीक्ष्ण एव च ।

Śamana has two synonyms, madhya and prāyogika; bṛṃhaṇa has snehana and mṛdu as synonyms, while śodhana and tīkṣṇa are the synonym of recana (2).

येषां धूमो न विहितस्तानाह—

अधूमार्हाश्च खल्वेते श्रान्तो भीतश्च दुःखितः ॥ ३ ॥
दत्तबस्तिर्विरिक्तश्च रात्रौ जागरिस्तथा । पिपासितश्च दाहार्तस्तालुशोषी तथोदरी ॥ ४ ॥
शिरोऽभितापी तिमिरी छर्द्याध्मानप्रपीडितः । क्षतोरस्कः प्रमेहार्तः पाण्डुरोगी च गर्भिणी ॥ ५ ॥
रूक्षः क्षीणोऽभ्यवहृतक्षीरक्षौद्रघृतासवः । भुक्तान्नदधिमत्स्यश्च बालो वृद्धः कृशस्तथा ॥ ६ ॥

The following persons are unsuitable for inhalation of smoke; the exhausted, the frieghtened, the sorrowful, those who have taken basti (enema) and virecana (purgative); who have been awake all night, who are thirsty, feeling burning sensation in the throat or dryness of ṭhroat, those suffering from udara (abdominal enlargement), śirobhitāpa (headache), timira (blindness), chardi (vomitting). ādhmāna (tympanitis), urakṣata (ulcers of the lungs), prameha (diabetes), pāṇḍuroga (anaemia), garbhiṇī (pregnant), rūkṣa (those who are dry), kṣiṇa (emaciated), who have consumed milk, honey, ghee and alcoholic beverages; boiled rice, curds and fish; young children, old people and the weak (3–6).

अकाले धूमपाने दोषं तत्प्रतीकारं चाह—

अकाले चातिपीतश्च धूमः कुर्यादुपद्रवान् । तत्रेष्टं सर्पिषः पानं नावनाञ्जनतर्पणम् ॥ ७ ॥
सर्पिरिक्षुरसं द्राक्षां पयो वा शर्कराम्बु वा । मधुराम्लौ रसौ वापि शमनाय प्रदापयेत् ॥ ८ ॥

Dhūma (inhalation) taken in improper time or in excess quantity produces complications. Such persons should be given a little ghee to drink, as well as to be put into nose; añjanas (collyriums) and tarpaṇa done to the eyes; ghee, sugar cane juice, drākṣā, milk, sugar water, sour and sugared beverages are to be given to reduce the irritation (7–8).

धूमः कदा गृह्यते को वा गुण इत्याह—

धूमस्तु द्वादशाद्वर्षाद्गृह्यतेऽशीतिकान्न च । कासश्वासप्रतिश्यायान्मन्याहनुशिरोरुजः ॥ ९ ॥
वातश्लेष्मविकारांश्च हन्याद्धूमः सुयोजितः । धूमप्रयोगात्पुरुषः प्रसन्नेन्द्रियवाङ्मनाः ॥ १० ॥
दृढकेशद्विजश्मश्रुः सुगन्धिवदनो भवेत् ।

Dhūma is indicated between the ages of twelve and eighty years; it is advocated in diseases like kāsa (cough), swāsa (dyspnoea), pratiśyāya (running in the nose), pain in the neck; lower jaw and head and diseases arising from vāta and kapha. Proper usage of dhūma confers clarity of sense faculties, speech and mind, firm teeth, mustaches and hairs and plessant odour to the mouth (9–10).

यथा नाड्या धूमो गृह्यते तद्विधानमाह—

धूमनाडी भवेत्तत्र त्रिखण्डा च त्रिपर्विका ॥ ११ ॥
कनिष्ठिकापरीणाहा राजमाषागमान्तरा । धूमनाडी भवेद्दीर्घा शमने रोगिणोऽङ्गुलैः ॥ १२ ॥
चत्वारिंशन्मितैस्तद्वद्द्वात्रिंशद्भिर्मृदौ मता । तीक्ष्णे चतुर्विंशतिभिः कासघ्नी षोडशोन्मितैः ॥ १३ ॥
दशाङ्गुलैर्वामनीये तथा स्याद्व्रणनाडिका । कलायमण्डलस्थूला कुलित्थागमरन्ध्रका ॥ १४ ॥

The tube for fumigation consists of three peices (tubes which can be fixed to one another forming three knots) of the thickness of the little finger, the lumen permitting a rājamāṣā (black gram) to pass freely through. Its length should be forty aṅgulīs in case of śamana dhūma; thirty-two aṅgulīs in cases of mṛdu dhūma (snehana); twentyfour aṅgulīs for tīkṣṇa (śodhana), sixteen aṅgulī for kāsaghna; twelve aṅgulīs for vamana. The tube for vraṇa dhūma, should have a passage permitting a pea and a mouth permitting a horsegram to pass through freely (11–14).

इदानीं धूमपानार्थं ईषिकाविधानमाह—

अथेषिकां प्रलिम्पेच्च सुश्लक्ष्णां द्वादशाङ्गुलाम् । धूमद्रव्यस्य कल्केन लेपक्ताष्टाङ्गुलः स्मृतः ॥१५॥
कल्कं कर्षमितं लिप्त्वा छायाशुष्कं च कारयेत् । ईषिकामपनीयाथ स्नेहाक्तां वर्तिमादरात् ॥ १६ ॥
अङ्गारैर्दीपितां कृत्वा धृत्वा नेत्रस्य रन्ध्रके । वदनेन पिबेद्धूमं वदनेनैव संत्यजेत् ॥ १७ ॥
नासिकाभ्यां ततः पीत्वा मुखेनैव वमेत्सुधीः ।

A hollow reed of twelve aṅgulīs long is covered over with one karṣa of a nice paste of drugs of fumigation to a length of ten aṅgulīs leaving bare a space two aṅgulīs at any one end. It should be dried well in shade and the reed removed carefully. The roll of the paste is smeared with a little ghee and fixed to the nozzle without breaking it. It is lit at one end and smoke drawn into the mouth. The smoke is later left out through the mouth itself, or drawn through the nose and left out through the mouth (15–17).

शरावसंपुटे क्षिप्त्वा कल्कमङ्गारदीपितम् ॥ १८ ॥
छिद्रे नेत्रं निवेश्याथ व्रणं तेनैव धूपयेत् ।

In case of fumigation of ulcers, the paste of drugs is put on a plate containing burning coal, covered with another plate containing a hole in its centre for the tube to be fixed and the outgoing fumes are lead over to the ulcer (18).

शमनधूमादौ यद्द्रव्यकल्को धूमार्थं देयस्तदाह—

एलादिकल्कं शमने स्निग्धं सर्जरसं मृदौ ॥ १९ ॥

रेचने तीक्ष्णकल्कं च कासघ्नं क्षुद्रिकोषणम् । वामने स्नायुचर्माद्यं दद्याद्धूमस्य पानकम् ॥ २० ॥

व्रणे निम्बवचाद्यं च धूपनं संप्रशस्यते ।

Drugs of elādi gana (as told by Sushruta) are best for śamana, sarjarasa mixed with ghee or oil for mṛdu (bṛṃhaṇa); paste of drugs possessing tīkṣṇa properties for recana; the root of kṣudra (kanṭakāri) and marica for kāsaghna dhūma; paste of skin, tendons and hoofs of animals for vamana dhūma and the powder of nimba, vaca etc. for vraṇadhūpana (fumigation of ulcers) (19-20).

बालग्रहादौ धूमपानमाह—

अन्येऽपि धूमा गेहेषु कर्तव्या रोगशान्तये ॥ २१ ॥

मयूरपिच्छं निम्बस्य पत्राणि बृहतीफलम् । मरिचं हिङ्गु मांसी च बीजं कार्पाससंभवम् ॥ २२ ॥

छागरोमाहिनिर्मोकं विष्ठा बैडलिकी तथा । गजदन्तश्च तच्चूर्णं किंचिद्घृतविमिश्रितम् ॥ २३ ॥

गेहेषु धूपनं दत्तं सर्वान्बालग्रहाञ्जयेत् । पिशाचान्राक्षसाञ्जित्वा सर्वज्वरहरं भवेत् ॥ २४ ॥

Dhūma can also be done with many other substances as for example, the plumes of peacock, leaves of nimba, fruits of bṛhatī, marica, hiṅgu, māṃsī, seeds of karpasa, hairs of goat, the skinpeel of the snake, the excreta of cat, powder of elephants tusk or tooth—each one mixed with a little ghee. These fumes ward off all bālagrahas, piśācas and rākṣasas (evil spirits, germs and bacteria) if allowed in to dwelling places and prevent all kinds of diseases (21-24).

धूमपाने पथ्यं, नेत्रद्रव्याण्याह—

परिहारस्तु धूमेषु कार्यो रेचननस्यवत् । नेत्राणि धातुजान्याहुर्नलवंशादिजान्यपि ॥ २५ ॥

The after care of dhūmapana is similar to those adopted for recana nasya; The tube can be made out of metals or reeds of bamboo (25).

इति श्रीदामोदरसूनुना शार्ङ्गधरेण विरचितायां शार्ङ्गधरसंहितायामुत्तरखण्डे धूमपानविधिर्नाम नवमोऽध्यायः ॥ ९ ॥

Thus ends the ninth chapter

दशमोऽध्यायः

CHAPTER X

(*Gaṇḍūṣa, Kavala, Pratisāraṇa Vidhi* (*Mouth gargles*)

अथ गण्डूषकवलप्रतिसारणविधिः—

चतुर्विधः स्याद्गण्डूषः स्नैहिकः शमनस्तथा । शोधनो रोपणश्चैव कवलश्चापि तद्विधः ॥ १ ॥

Gaṇḍūṣa (mouth gargle) is of four kinds viz., snaihika (oleating), śamana (palliative), śodhana (purificatory) and ropaṇa (healing), like wise is kavala (another type of gargling) (1).

स्निग्धैस्तु स्नैहिको वाते स्वादुशीतैः प्रसादनः । पित्ते कट्वम्ललवणैरुष्णैः संशोधनः कफे ॥ २ ॥
कषायतिक्तमधुरैः कदुष्णो रोपणो व्रणे । चतुष्प्रकारो गण्डूषः कवलश्चापि कीर्तितः ॥ ३ ॥

Snaihika is done in diseases of vāta with drugs possessing snigdha and uṣṇa properties, in diseases of pitta with drugs possessing swādu and śita; for kapha śodhana with drugs possessing kaṭu, amla, lavaṇa and uṣṇa; for healing of ulcers with drugs possessing kaṣāya, tikta and madhura; and used warm :—these are the four modes of using gaṇḍūṣa and kavala (2–3).

असंचारी मुखे पूर्णे गण्डूषः कवलश्चरः । तत्र द्रवेण गण्डूषः कल्केन कवलः स्मृतः ॥ ४ ॥
दद्याद्द्रवेषु चूर्णं च गण्डूषे कोलमात्रकम् । कर्षप्रमाणः कल्कश्च दीयते कवले बुधैः ॥ ५ ॥

Gaṇḍūṣa is holding any liquid in the mouth to its full capacity without any movement inside, whereas kavala is that which allows movement of the liquid. Gaṇḍūṣa is usually done with liquids and kavala with kalka (paste of drugs mixed with a little water). One kola by measure is the dose of either a liquid or a powder for gaṇḍūṣa; while for kavala the dose of kalka (paste) is one karṣa (4–5)

कस्मिन् वयसि गण्डूषो धार्यते कियत्परिमिता गण्डूषः कार्या इत्याह

धार्यन्ते पञ्चमाद्वर्षाद्गण्डूषकवलादयः । गण्डूषान्सुस्थितः कुर्यात्स्विन्नभालगलादिकः ॥ ६ ॥
मनुष्यस्त्रींस्तथा पञ्च सप्त वा दोषनाशनात् । कफपूर्णास्यता यावच्छेदो दोषस्य वा भवेत् ॥ ७ ॥
नेत्रघ्राणस्रुतिर्यावत्तावद्गण्डूषधारणम् ।

Gaṇḍūṣa and kavala are advocated after the age of five years. The person to be given this therapy should be seated comfortably, his forehead, neck and shoulders given mild fomentation, asked to take the liquid into the mouth and hold it till his mouth gets cleared of accumilated kapha or other doṣas (excretions) or till he gets secretions inside his nostrils. At a stretch, three, five or seven gargles can be done to get rid of the dosas (5–7).

वाते स्नैहिकगण्डूषमाह—

तिलकल्कोदकं क्षीरं स्नेहो वा स्नैहिके हितः ॥ ८ ॥

For snaihika gaṇḍūṣa, a paste of tila, with water or milk and oil is ideal (8).

तिला नीलोत्पलं सर्पिः शर्करा क्षीरमेव च । सक्षौद्र हनुवक्त्रस्थो गण्डूषो दाहनाशनः ॥ ९ ॥

Tila, nīlotpala, ghee, sugar, milk and honey together forms a good gargle for burning of the mouth and throat (9).

वैशद्यं जनयत्यास्ये संदधाति मुखव्रणान् । दाहतृष्णाप्रशमनं मधुगण्डूषधारणम् ॥ १० ॥

Honey alone used as gaṇḍūṣa clears the mouth, heals ulcers, alleviates burning and thirst (10).

विषक्षाराग्निदग्धे च सर्पिर्धार्यं पयोऽथवा । तैलसैन्धवगण्डूषो दन्तचाले प्रशस्यते ॥ ११ ॥

Ghee is to be used as gargle in cases of poisoning and scalds by alkalies or fire. In cases of shaky teeth, gargle with taila (sesame oil) mixed with saindhava is ideal (11).

शोषं मुखस्य वैरस्यं गण्डूषः काञ्जिको जयेत् । सिन्धुत्रिकटुराजीभिरार्द्रकेण कफे हितः ॥ १२ ॥
त्रिफलामधुगण्डूषः कफास्रकपित्तनाशनः ।

Gargle with kāñjika (sour gruel) is good for dryness of mouth and vairasya (bad taste); mixed with saindhava, trikaṭu, rājika, ārdraka it is effective in disorders of kapha, gargle of triphalā and honey mitigate kapha, rakta and pitta (12-13).

अथ मुखपाके गण्डूषः—
(प्रतिसारणचूर्णम्)

दार्वी गुडूची त्रिफला द्राक्षा जात्याश्च पल्लवाः ॥ १३ ॥
यवासश्चेति तत्क्वाथः षडंशक्षौद्रसंयुः । शीतो मुखे धृतो हन्यान्मुखपाकं त्रिदोषजम् ॥ १४ ॥

Darvi, guḍūci, triphalā, drākṣā, tender leaves of jati and yavasa made into a decoction, mixed with one sixth part of honey and held in the mouth cold, heals ulcers of the mouth caused by all the three doṣas (13–14).

यस्योषधस्य गण्डूषस्तस्य वै प्रतिसारणम् । कवलश्चापि तस्यैव ज्ञेयोऽत्र कुशलैर्नरैः ॥ १५ ॥

Pratisāraṇa (application of pastes or powders into the mouth) is done with the same drugs as indicated for gaṇḍūṣa and kavala (15).

केशरं मातुलुङ्गस्य सैन्धवोषणसंयुतम् । हन्यात्कवलतो जाड्यमरुचिं कफवातजाम् ॥ १६ ॥

Kesara of matulinga (fimbriae of the fruit), saindhava, uṣaṇa (marica) used as kavala relieves diseases of kapha and vāta and cures aruchi (anorexia) (16).

कल्कोऽवलेहश्चचूर्णं च त्रिविधं प्रतिसारणम् । अङ्गुल्यग्रगृहीतं च यथास्वं मुखरोगिणम् ॥ १७ ॥

Pratisāraṇa is of three kinds, kalka (paste), avaleha (confection) and cūrṇa (powder) and used by the tip of the finger in all diseases of the mouth (17).

कुष्ठं दार्वी समङ्गा च पाठा तिक्ता च पीतिका । तेजनी मुस्तलोध्रे च चूर्णं स्यात्प्रतिसारणम् ॥१८॥
रक्तस्रुतिं दन्तपीडां शोथं दाहं च नाशयेत् ।

Kuṣṭha, dārvī, samaṅga, pāṭhā, tikta, pītika (haridrā), tejanī, musta and lodhra-all equal parts made into nice powder applied to mouth stops bleeding, pain, swelling and tooth ache (18).

हीनयोगानाह—

हीनयोगात्कफोत्क्लेशो रसाज्ञानारुची तथा ॥ १९ ॥
अतियोगान्मुखे पाकः शोषस्तृष्णा क्लमो भवेत् ।

In adequate gargling therapy causes profuse salivation, loss of taste perception and anorexia, whereas excessive therapy produces ulcers, dryness, thirst and exhaustion (19).

शुद्धगण्डूषलक्षणमाह—

व्याधेरपचयस्तुष्टिर्वैशद्यं वक्त्रलाघवम् ॥ २० ॥
इन्द्रियाणां प्रसादश्च गण्डूषे शुद्धिलक्षणम् ।

A proper therapy of gandhūṣa brings about alleviation of diseases, cleanses the mouth and stimulates the sense organs (20).

इति श्रीदामोदरसूनुना शार्ङ्गधरेण विरचितायां शार्ङ्गधरसंहितायामुत्तरखण्डे गण्डूषादिविधिनाम दशमोऽध्यायः ॥ १० ॥

Thus ends the tenth chapter.

एकादशोऽध्यायः

CHAPTER 11

Lepa, Mūrdha Taila, Karṇapūraṇa Vidhi (Topical applicatian, Oletation of head, ears etc.)

तत्र तावत्प्रलेपनामाह—

आलेपस्य च नामानि लिप्तो लेपश्च लेपनम् । दोषघ्नो विषहा वर्ण्यो मुखलेपस्त्रिधा मतः ॥ १ ॥

Ālepana (topical application) also known as lipta, lepa or lepana is of three kinds, viz., doṣaghna (anti-doshic), viṣaghna (anti-poisonous) and varṇya mukha-lepa (cosmetic application over the face to improve colour and complexion) (1).

त्रिप्रमाणश्चतुर्भागत्रिभागाऽर्धाङ्गुलोन्नतः । आर्द्रो व्याधिहरः स स्याच्छुष्को दूषयति च्छविम् ॥२॥

One fourth, one third and half aṅgulīs is the thickness of the paste respectively for doṣaghna, viṣaghna and varṇya lepas. They are effective so long as they are moist and once they dry up they will harm the skin (2).

दोषघ्नो लेपो यथा—

पुनर्नवां दारु शुण्ठीं सिद्धार्थं शिग्रुमेव च। पिष्ट्वा चैवारनालेन प्रलेपः सर्वशोथजित् ॥ ३ ॥

Punarnavā, dāru, śuṇṭhī, siddhārtha and śigru made into a paste with ricewash and applied relieves all kinds of śotha (oedema) (3).

अथ दाहे लेपः

बिभीतफलमज्जाया लेपो दाहार्तिनाशनः।

Paste of marrow of vibhītakī fruit relieves burning sensation of the skin (4).

अथ दशाङ्गलेपो विसर्पशोथव्रणादौ—

शिरीषं मधुयष्टी च तगरं रक्तचन्दनम ॥ ४ ॥

एला मांसी निषायुग्मं कुष्ठं वालकमेव च। इति संचूर्ण्य लोपोऽयं पञ्चमांशघृतप्लुतः ॥ ५ ॥

जलेन क्रियते सुज्ञैर्दशाङ्ग इति संज्ञितः। विसर्पान्विषविस्फोटाञ्शोथान्दुष्टव्रणाञ्जयेत् ॥ ६ ॥

Śirīṣa madhuyaṣṭī, tagara, raktacandana, elā, māṃsī, the two niśās, kuṣṭha and vālaka made into paste with water and one fifth part of ghee added and applied over the skin. This recipe known as *Daśāṅga lepa* is effective in visarpa (erysepelas) viṣa (poison), visphoṭa (boils), śotha (oedema, tumors) and duṣṭa vraṇa (bad ulcers) (5–6).

विषघ्नो लेपो यथा—

अजादुग्धतिलैर्लेपो नवनीतेन संयुतः। शोथमारुष्करं हन्ति लेपो वा कृष्णमृत्तिकैः ॥ ७ ॥

Paste of tila with goat's milk and butter or a paste of black clay will be effective against oedema caused by contact of aruṣkara (bhallātaka) (7).

अथ कीटघ्नलेपः—

लाङ्गल्यतिविषालाबुजालिनीमूलबीजकैः। लेपो धान्याम्बुसंपिष्टः कीटविस्फोटनाशनः ॥ ८ ॥

Lāṅgalī, ativiṣa, alābu, jalinī and seeds of mūlaka made into a paste with sour gruel is effective against insect stings (8).

वर्ण्यो लेपो यथा—

रक्तचन्दनमञ्जिष्ठालोध्रकुष्ठप्रियङ्गवः। व्रटाङ्कुरा मसूराश्च व्यङ्गघ्ना मुखकान्तिदाः ॥ ९ ॥

Rakta candana, mañjiṣṭhā, lodhra, kuṣṭha, priyaṅgu, vaṭāṅkura and masūra is a good application for vyaṅga (pigmented patch over the face, acne) and confers fair complexion to the face (9).

मातुलुङ्गजटा सर्पिः शिला गोशकृतो रसः। मुखकान्तिकरो लेपः पिटिकाव्यङ्गकालजित् ॥ १० ॥

Root of mātuluṅga; ghee, manaśila, rubbed with juice of cowdung applied to the face removes pimples, black spots and patches (10).

लोध्रधान्यवचालेपस्तारुण्यपिटिकापहः । तद्वद्गोरोचनायुक्तं मरिचं मुखलेपनम् ॥ ११ ॥
सिद्धार्थकवचालोध्रसैन्धवैश्च प्रलेपनम् ।

Paste of either lodhra, dhānya, vaca; or gorocana and marica; or siddārtaka, vaca, lodhra and saindhava makes effective application for pimples of adolescents (11).

व्यङ्गेषु चार्जुनत्वग्वा मञ्जिष्ठा वा समाक्षिका ॥ १२ ॥
लेपः सनवनीतो वा श्वेताश्वखुरजा मषी ।

Arjuna twak (bark of Arjunatree) or mañjiṣṭhā or ashes of hoofs of a white horse mixed with honey or butter forms a good paste for vyaṅga (dark patches on the face) (12).

अर्कक्षीरहरिद्राभ्यां मर्दयित्वा विलेपनात् ॥ १३ ॥
मुखकार्ष्ण्यं शमं याति चिरकालोद्भवं ध्रुवम् ।

Sap of arka and the two haridrās mixed and applied to the face is effective in removin the black patches of the face however old it night be (13).

वटस्य पाण्डुपत्राणि मालती रक्तचन्दनम् ॥ १४ ॥
कुष्ठं कालीयकं लोध्रमेभिर्लेपं प्रयोजयेत् । तारुण्यपिटिकाव्यङ्गनीलिकादिविनाशनम् ॥ १५ ॥

Ripened leaves of vāta, mālatī, raktachandana, kuṣṭha, kālīyaka and lodhra made into a paste removes pimples, black spots, patches on the face etc. (14–15).

अथारुंषिकायां लेपः—

पुराणमथ पिण्याकं पुरीषं कुक्कुटस्य च । मूत्रपिष्टः प्रलेपोऽयं शीघ्रं हन्यादरुंषिकाम् ॥ १६ ॥

Old tila (sesamum) from which oil has been taken out and excreta of the cock made into a paste with cow's urine and applied destroys arūṃṣikās (pustular ulcers on the head) (16).

खदिरारिष्टजम्बूनांत्वग्भिर्वा मूत्रसंयुतैः । कुटजत्वक्सैन्धवं च लेपो हन्यादरुंषिकाम् ॥ १७ ॥

A paste of barks of khadira, ariṣṭa, jambū, kuṭaja and saindhava prepared with cow's urine cures arūṃṣikā (pustules on the head) (17).

दारुणे लेपः—

प्रियालबीजमधुककुष्ठमाषैः ससैन्धवैः । कार्यो दारुणके मूर्ध्नि प्रलेपो मधुसंयुतः ॥ १८ ॥

Priyālabīja, madhuka, kuṣṭha, māṣa and saindhava made into a paste with honey and applied to the head removes dāruṇaka (dandruf) (18).

दुग्धेन खाखसं बीजं प्रलेपाद्दारुणं जयेत् । आम्रबीजस्य चूर्णं तु शिवाचूर्णसमं द्वयम् ॥ १९ ॥
दुग्धपिष्टः प्रलेपोऽयं दारुणं हन्ति दारुणम् ।

Seeds of khākhasa made into paste with milk, or āmrabīja (kernal of mango stone) and powder of śiva (haritaki) each equal parts made into a paste with milk and applied relieves even severe dāruṇaka (dandruff) (19).

अथेन्द्रलुप्ते—

रसस्तिक्तपटोलस्य पत्राणां तद्विलेपनात् ॥ २० ॥
इन्द्रलुप्तं शमं याति त्रिभिरेव दिनैर्ध्रुवम् ।

Juice of leaves of tikta paṭola applied to the head cures indralupta (alopacia) within three days (20).

इन्द्रलुप्तापहो लेपो मधुना बृहतीरसः ॥ २१ ॥
गुञ्जामूलं फलं वापि भल्लातकरसोऽपि वा ।

Juice of bṛhatī with honey or juice of roots of guñjā or it's fruit or juice of bhallātaka relieves indralupta (alopacia) (21).

गोक्षुरस्तिलपुष्पाणि तुल्ये स मधुसर्पिषि ॥ २२ ॥
शिरःप्रलेपनं तेन केशसंवर्धनं परम् ।

Gokṣura, flowers of tila (sesamum) with eqal parts of honey and ghee applied to the head promotes growth of hair (22).

हस्तिदन्तमषीं कृत्वा छागीदुग्धं रसाञ्जनम् ॥ २३ ॥
रोमाण्यनेन जायन्ते लेपात्पाणितलेष्वपि ।

Ash of elephants tusk, goat's milk and rasañjana applied over the head helps growth of hair; even in the palms of hand (23).

यष्टीन्दीवरमृद्वीकातैलाज्यक्षीरलेपनैः ॥ २४ ॥

Yaṣṭī, indīvara, mṛdwika, oil, ghee and milk—all made into a paste and applied to the head not only relieves indralupta but also helps growth of thick and smooth hairs (24).

इन्द्रलुप्तं शमं याति केशाः स्युः सघना दृढाः । चतुष्पदानां त्वग्रोमनखश्रृङ्गास्थिभस्मभिः ॥ २५ ॥
तैलेन सह लेपोऽयं रोमसंजननः परः ।

Ash of the skin, hairs, hoofs, horns and bones of quadrupeds made into a paste with taila (oil) helps growth of hairs thick and firm (25).

पलित लेपाः—

इन्द्रवारुणिकाबीजतैलेनाभ्यङ्गमाचरेत् ॥ २६ ॥
प्रत्यहं तेन जायन्ते कुन्तला भृङ्गसंनिभाः ।

Seeds of indravāruṇī and taila used as an abhyaṅga (oil bath) makes the hairs black like the colour of the bees (26).

अयोरजो भृङ्गराजस्त्रिफला कृष्णमृत्तिका ॥ २७ ॥
स्थितमिक्षुरसे मासं लेपनात्पलितं जयेत् ।

Ayoraja (iron filings), bhṛṅgarāja, triphalā, kṛṣṇamṛttika (black clay) kept for one month in sugarcane juce and applied to the head relieves palita (grey hairs) (27).

धात्रीफलत्रयं पथ्ये द्वे तथैलं बिभीतकम् ॥ २८ ॥
पञ्चाभ्रमज्जा लोहस्य कर्षैकं च प्रदीयते । पिष्ट्वा लोहमये भाण्डे स्थापयेदुषितं निशि ॥ २९ ॥
लेपोऽयं हन्ति नचिरादकालपलितं महत् ।

Three karsas of dhātrīphala, two of pathya, one of vibhītaka, five of kernal of stones of āmra and one of loha (iron filings)—all made into a paste and kept over night inside an iron vessel and applied to the head relieves palita (premature grey hairs) quickly (28–29).

त्रिफला नीलिकापत्रं लोहं भृङ्गरजः समम् ॥ ३० ॥
अविमूत्रेण संपिष्टं लेपात्कृष्णीकरं स्मृतम् ।

Triphalā, leaves of nīlikā, loha and bhṛṅgarāja all equal parts made into a paste with sheep's urine and applied to the head makes the hair black (30).

त्रिफला लोहचूर्णं च दाडिमत्वग्बिसं तथा ॥ ३१ ॥
प्रत्येकं पञ्चपलिकं चूर्णं च कुर्याद्विचक्षणः । भृङ्गराजरसस्यापि प्रस्थषट्कं प्रदापयेत् ॥ ३२ ॥
क्षिप्त्वा लोहमये पात्रे भूमिमध्ये निधापयेत् । मासमेकं ततः कुर्याच्छागीदुग्धेन लेपनम् ॥ ३३ ॥
कूर्चे शिरसि रात्रौ च संवेष्ट्यैरण्डपत्रकैः । स्वपेत्प्रातस्ततः कुर्यात्स्नानं तेन च जायते ॥ ३४ ॥
पलितस्य विनाशश्च त्रिभिर्लेपैर्न संशयः ।

Triphalā, lohacūrṇa, dāḍima twak and bisa each five palas, juice of bhṛṅgarāja six prasthas are to be kept in an iron vessel and buried underground for one month. Later it is taken out mixed with goat's milk and to be applied to the hairs at nights and covered with leaves of eraṇḍa. Next day morning the person may take bath. The hairs will turn black without doubt within three such applications (31–34).

अथ रोमशातने—

शङ्खचूर्णस्य भागौ द्वौ हरितालं च भागिकम् ॥ ३५ ॥
मनःशिला चार्धभागा स्वर्जिका चैकभागिका । लेपोऽयं वारिपिष्टस्तु केशानुत्पाट्य दीयते ॥ ३६ ॥
अनया लेपयुक्त्या च सप्तवेलं प्रयुक्तया । निर्मूलं केशस्थानं स्यात्क्षपणस्य शिरो यथा ॥ ३७ ॥

Two parts of powder of śaṅkha, one part of haritāla, half part of manaśila and one of swarjika made into a paste with water and applied to the shaven head prevents hair growth within about seven applications making the head resemble that of a monk (35–37).

तालकं शाणयुग्मं स्यात्षट्शाणं शङ्खचूर्णकम् । द्विशाणिकं पलाशस्य क्षारं दत्त्वा प्रमर्दयेत् ॥ ३८ ॥
कदलीदण्डतोयेन रविपत्ररसेन वा । अस्यापि सप्तभिर्लेपै रोम्णां शातनमुत्तमम् ॥ ३९ ॥

Two śāṇas of tālaka, six śāṇas of śaṅkha cūrṇa, two śāṇas of kṣāra of palaśa are made into a paste with juice of banana stem and leaves of ravi (arka) and applied to the head acts as a good depilatory within seven applications (38-39).

श्वित्रे लेपाः—

सुवर्णपुष्पी कासीसं विडङ्गानि मनःशिला । रोचना सैन्धवं चैव लेपनाच्छ्वित्रनाशनम् ॥ ४० ॥

Suvarṇapuṣpī, kāsīsa, viḍaṅga, manaśila, gorocana and saindhava made into an application cures śvitra (leucoderma) (40).

वायस्येडगजाकुष्ठकृष्णाभिर्गुटिका कृता । बस्तमूत्रेण संपिष्टा प्रलेपनाच्छ्वित्रनाशिनी ॥ ४१ ॥

Vayasya (kākamācī), eḍagaja, kusṭha and kṛṣṇa made into paste with goat's urine, rolled into a pil', dried and applied over the body cures śvitra (leucoderma) (41).

तालकं शाणमात्रं स्याच्चतुःशाणा च बाकुची । गोमूत्रपिष्टं तच्चूर्णं लेपनाच्छ्वित्रनाशनम् ॥ ४२ ॥

One śāṇa of tālaka, four śāṇas of bākucī made into a paste with cow's urine cures śvitra (leucoderma) (42).

बाकुची वेतसो लाक्षा काकोदुम्बरिका कणा । रसाञ्जनमयश्चूर्णं तिलाः कृष्णास्तदेकतः ॥ ४३ ॥
चूर्णयित्वा गवां पित्तैः पिष्ट्वा च गुटिका कृता । अस्या प्रलेपाच्छ्वित्राणि प्रणश्यन्त्यतिवेगतः ॥४४॥

Bākucī, vetasa, lākṣā, kākodumbarikā, kaṇa, rasāñjana, ayascūrṇa and kṛṣṇatila all equal parts, mixed with ox-bile and applied cures śvitra (leucoderma) quikly (43-44).

अथ सिध्मे लेपः—

धात्री सर्जरसश्चैव यवक्षारस्य चूर्णितः । सौवीरेण प्रलेपोयं प्रयोज्यः सिध्मनाषने ॥ ४५ ॥

Dhātrī, sarjarasa, yavakṣāra, applied along with souvīra (sour gruel) cures sidhma (a kind of skin disease) (45).

दार्वी मूलकबीजानि तालकं सुरदारु च । ताम्बूलपत्रं सर्वाणि कार्षिकाणि पृथक्पृथक् ॥ ४६ ॥
शङ्खचूर्णं शाणमात्रं सर्वाण्येकत्र कारयेत् । लेपोऽयं वारिणा पिष्टः सिध्मनां नाशनः परः ॥ ४७ ॥

One karṣa each of dārvī, mūlaka bīja, tālaka, suradāru and tāmbūla patra, one śāṇa of śaṅkha cūrṇa are made into a paste with water and applied is effective against sidhma (a kind of leprosy) (46-47).

अथ नेत्ररोगे लेपः—

हरीतकी सैन्धवं च गैरिकं च रसाञ्जनम् । बिडालको जलैः पिष्टः सर्वनेत्रामयापहः ॥ ४८ ॥

Harītakī, saindhava, gairika and rasāñjana made into a paste with water and applied over the eyelids cures all diseases of the eyes (48).

रसाञ्जनं व्योषयुतं संपिष्टं वटकीकृतम् । कण्डूपाकान्वितां हन्ति लेपादनञ्जनामिकाम् ॥ ४९ ॥

Rasāñjana and vyoṣa (trikaṭu) are made into fine paste with water and rolled into small pills. Applied into the eyes like a collyrium it cures añjananāmikā (a kind of eye disease exuding pus and accompanied with itching) (49).

अथ कण्ड्वादौ लेपः—

प्रपुन्नाटस्य बीजानि बाकुची सर्षपास्तिलाः । कुष्ठं निशाद्वयं मुस्तं पिष्ट्वा तक्रेण चैकतः ॥ ५० ॥
प्रलेपादस्य नश्यन्ति दद्रुकण्डूविचर्चिकाः ।

Seeds of prapunnāṭa, bākucī, sarṣapa, tila, kuṣṭha, the two niśās and musta made into a paste with butter milk and applied over the skin cures skin diseases like dadru (ringworm), kaṇḍū (itching) and vicarcikā (eczema) (50-51).

हेमक्षीरी विडङ्गानि दरदं गन्धकस्तथा ॥ ५१ ॥
दद्रुघ्नः कुष्ठसिन्दूरे सर्वाण्येकत्र मर्दयेत् । धत्तूरनिम्बताम्बूलीपत्राणां स्वरसैः पृथक् ॥ ५२ ॥
अस्य प्रलेपमात्रेण पामादद्रूविचर्चिकाः । कण्डूश्च रकसश्चैव प्रशमं यान्ति वेगतः ॥ ५३ ॥

Hemakṣīrī, viḍaṅga, darada (hiṅgula), gandhaka, dadrughna (cakramarda) kuṣṭha and sindūra—each equal quantity is made into a paste with fresh juice of leaves of dhattūra, nimba and tāmbūlī separately. This recipe applied as a paste quickly removes pāmā (scabies), dadru (ringworm), vicarcikā (eczema), kaṇḍū (itching) and rasaka (a variety of leprosy) (51–53).

दूर्वाऽभया सैन्धवं चक्रमर्दः कुठेरकः । एभिस्तक्रयुतो लेपः कण्डूदद्रूविनाशनः ॥ ५४ ॥

Dūrva, abhaya, saindhava, cakramarda and kuṭeraka, made into a paste with buttermilk will cure kaṇḍū (itching) and dadru (ringworm) (54).

दूर्वानिशायुतो लेपः कण्डूपामाविनाशनः । कृमिदद्रूहरश्चैव शीतपित्तापहः स्मृतः ॥ ५५ ॥

Dūrvā and niśā, made into paste and applied to skin relieves kaṇḍū (itching), pāmā (scabies), kṛmi (bacteria), dadru (ringworm) and also eruptions of śītapitta (allergy) (55).

सिद्धार्थरजनीकुष्ठप्रपुन्नाटतिलैः सह । कटुतैलेन संमिश्रं दद्रुघ्नं च प्रलेपनम् ॥ ५६ ॥

Siddhārtha, rajanī, kuṣṭha, prapunnāṭa and tila made into a paste, mixed with kaṭu taila (mustard oil) and applied cures dadru (ringworm) (56).

अथ वातविसर्पादौ लेपाः –

रास्ना नीलोत्पलं दारु चन्दनं मधुकं बला । घृतक्षीरयुतो लेपो वातवीसर्पनाशनः ॥ ५७ ॥

Rāsnā, nīlotpala, daru, candan, madhuka and balā made into a thin paste with ghṛta (ghee) and kṣīra (milk) cures vātaja visarpa (erysepelas) (57).

मृणालं चन्दनं लोध्रमुशीरं कमलोत्पलम् । सारिवामलकी पथ्या लेपः पित्तविसर्पनुत् ॥ ५८ ॥

Mṛṇāla, candana, lodhra, uśīra, kamalotpala, sārivā, āmalakī and pathya—made into a paste relieves pitta visarpa (erysepelas) (58).

त्रिफला पद्मकोशीरं समङ्गा करवीरकम् । नलमूलमनन्ता च लेपः श्लेष्मविसर्पहा ॥ ५९ ॥

Triphalā, padmaka, uśīra, samaṅga, karavīra, nalamūla and ananta made into a paste relieves sleṣma visarpa (erysepalas) (59).

वातरक्ते पित्तरक्ते च योगः—

मांसी सर्जरसो लोध्रं मधुकं सहरेणुकम् । मूर्वा नीलोत्पलं पद्मं शिरीषकुसुमैः सह ॥ ६० ॥

Māṃsī, sarjarasa, lodhra, madhuka, hareṇuka, mūrvā, nīlotpala, padma and śirīṣakusuma are mixed with ghee, washed a thousand times forms an effective application in vātarakta (gout) and raktapitta (purpura) (60).

प्रलेपः पित्तवातास्रे शतधौतघृतप्लुतः । आमलं घृतभृष्टं तु पिष्टं काञ्जिकवारिभिः ॥ ६१ ॥
जयेन्मूर्ध्नि प्रलेपेन रक्तं नासिकया स्रुतम् ।

Āmalaka fruits fried in ghee is made into a paste with kāñjika (sour rice-wash) and applied over the head stops bleeding through nose (61–62).

शिरोरोगे योगाः—

कुष्ठमेरण्डतैलेन लेपात्काञ्जिकपेषितम् ॥ ६२ ॥
शिरोऽर्तिं वातजां हन्यात्पुष्पं वा मुचुकुन्दजम् ।

Kuṣṭha made into a paste with rice wash and applied to the head mixed with a little eraṇḍa taila (castor oil) relieves vātaja śirorti (head-ache due to preponderance of vāta). Flowers of mucukunda also acts like-wise (62–63).

देवदारु नतं कुष्ठं नलदं विश्वभेषजम् ॥ ६३ ॥
सकाञ्जिकः स्नेहयुक्तो लेपो वातशिरोऽर्तिनुत् ।

Devadāru, nata, kuṣṭha, nalada and viśvabheṣja—made into a paste with rice-wash and applied to the head with a little quantity of some sneha (oil) relieves vātaja śiraḥśūl (headache with preponderance of vāta) (63–64).

चन्दनोशीरयष्ट्याह्वबलाव्याघ्रनखोत्पलैः ॥ ६४ ॥
क्षीरपिष्टैः प्रलेपः स्याद्रक्तपित्तशिरोऽर्तिजित् ।

Candana, uśīra, yaṣṭī, balā, vyāghranakha and utpala—made into a paste with milk and applied over the head cures pittaja śiraḥśūla (headache with predominance of pitta) (64–65).

धात्रीकसेरुह्रीबेरपद्मपद्मकचन्दनैः ॥ ६५ ॥
दूर्वोशीरनलानां च मूलैः कुर्यात्प्रलेपनम् । शिरोऽर्तिं पित्तजां हन्याद्रक्तपित्तरुजं तथा ॥ ६६ ॥

Dhātrī, kaseru, hrībera, padma, padmaka, candana, uśīra, and nala—made into a paste and applied over the head relieves pittaja śirorti (headache with preponderance of pitta) and raktapitta (purpura) also (65–66).

हरेणुनतशैलेयमुस्तैलागरुदारुभिः । मांसीरास्नारुबूकैश्च कोष्णो लेपः कफार्तिनुत् ॥ ६७ ॥

Hareṇu, nata, śaileya, musta, elā, agaru, dāru, māṃsī, rāsnā and urubūka—made into a paste and applied warm over the head relieves kaphaja śirorti (headache with preponderance of kapha) (67).

शुण्ठीकुष्ठप्रपुनाटदेवकाष्ठैः सरोहिषैः । सुखोष्णैर्मूत्रपिष्टैश्च लेपः श्लेष्मशिरोऽर्तिनुत् ॥ ६८ ॥

Śuṇṭhī, kuṣṭha, prapunnāta, devakāṣṭha and rohiṣa, made into a paste with cow's urine and applied warm over the head with a little quantity of oil is effective in kaphaja śiroruja (headache) (68).

सारिवाकुष्ठमधुकवचाकृष्णोत्पलैस्तथा । लेपः सकाञ्जिकस्नेहः सूर्यावर्तार्धभेदयोः ॥ ६९ ॥

Sārivā, kuṣṭha, madhuka, vacā, kṛṣṇa utpala—made into a paste with rice-wash and applied with little oil cures sūryavarta (migraine) and ardhavabheda (hemicrania) (69).

वरी नोलोत्पलं दूर्वा तिलाः कृष्णाः पुनर्नवा । शङ्खकेऽनन्तवाते च लेपः सर्वशिरोऽर्तिजित् ॥७०॥

Varī, nīlotpala, dūrvā, black tila and punarnavā forms an effective application in cases of śaṅkhaka, anantavāta and all other types of śirorti (headache of different kinds) (70)

अथान्यो लेपविधिः कथ्यते—

अथ लेपविधिश्चान्यः प्रोच्यते सुज्ञसंमतः । द्वौ तस्य कथितौ भेदौ प्रलेपाख्यप्रदेहकौ ॥ ७१ ॥
चमार्द्रं माहिषं यद्वत्प्रोन्नतं सा मितिस्तयोः ।

Further on will be described the technique of application of lepa as approved by the experts: lepa is of two kinds, viz., pralepa and pradeha. The thickness of these applications on the skin should be equal to the thickness of a buffalos skin (71–72).

शीतस्तनुर्विशोषी च प्रलेपः परिकीर्तितः ॥ ७२ ॥
आर्द्रो घनस्तथोष्णः स्यात्प्रदेहः श्लेष्मवातहा ।

Pralepa is that which is applied cold, thin and which dries quickly; whereas pradeha is applied warm, thick and remains moist for a long time (72–73).

रोमाभिमुखमादेयौ प्रलेपाख्यप्रदेहकौ ॥ ७३ ॥
वीर्यं सम्यग्विशत्याशु रोमकूपैः शिरामुखैः ।

Both these applications should be gently rubbed in an upward or reverse direction as of the hair over the skin to make the action of the application quick and effective (73–74).

न रात्रौ लेपनं कुर्याच्छुष्यमाणं न धारयेत् ॥ ७४ ॥
शुष्यमाणमुपेक्षेत प्रदेहं पीडनं प्रति ।

Pralepa should not be applied at nights nor it should be allowed to stay on after it dries up; whereas pradehas can be allowed to stay on (even after drying) in order to cause constriction or pressure over the part of the body (74–75).

(तमसा पिहितो ह्यूष्मा रोमकूपमुखे स्थितः ॥ ७५ ॥
विना लेपेन निर्याति रात्रौ नो लेपयेदतः ।)

The heat of the body comes out through the skin pores at nights normally; if medicinal applications are done at nights the skin pores get blocked and obstruct the transfer of, body heat. So external applications should not be done at nights (75–76).

रात्रावपि प्रलेपादिविधिः कार्यो विचक्षणैः ॥ ७६ ॥
अपक्वशोथे गम्भीरे रक्तश्लेष्मसमुद्भवे ।

But in cases of apakva śotha (unripe abscess), gambhīra śotha (deep seated abscess) and śotha arising from rakta and sleṣmā (abscess with predominance of blood and kapha), applications can be made even at nights (76–77).

इदानीं व्रणविषयक्रममाह—
आदौ शोथहरो लेपो द्वितीयो रक्तसेचनः ॥ ७७ ॥
तृतीयश्चोपनाहः स्याच्चतुर्थः पाटनक्रमः । पञ्चमः शोधनो भूयात्षष्ठो रोपण इष्यते ॥ ७८ ॥
सप्तमो वर्णकरणो व्रणस्यैते क्रमान्मताः ।

In cases of vraṇaśothas (inflammatory abscess) the following seven kinds of cikitsā (therapeutics) are indicated; one after the other in succession. (1). Śothahara lepa (application of paste), (2). Rakta-secana (blood letting), (3). Upanāha (warm poultices), (4). Pāṭana (incision), (5). Śodhana (cleansing), (6). Ropaṇa (healing), (7). Varṇakaraṇa (procedure of imparting normal colour) (77–79).

इदानीं स यथेत्यनेन व्रणस्य सप्तविषयक्रमाणां प्रत्येकं योगानाह—
बीजपूरजटा हिंस्रा देवदारु महौषधम् ॥ ७९ ॥
रास्नाग्निमन्थो लेपोऽयं वातशोथविनाशनः ।

Roots of bījapūra, hiṃsrā, devadāru, mahouṣadhi, rāsnā and agnimantha made into a paste and applied relieves vāta-śotha (oedema of vāta predominance) (79-80).

मधुकं चन्दनं मूर्वा नलमूलं च पद्मकम् ॥ ८० ॥
उशीरं वालकं पद्मं पित्तशोथे प्रलेपनम् ।

Madhuka, candana, mūrvā, roots of nala, padmaka, uśira, vālaka and padma- made into a paste is useful in pitta śotha (oedema of pitta predominance) (80-81).

कृष्णा पुराणपिण्याकं शिग्रुत्वक्सिकता शिवा ॥ ८१ ॥
मूत्रपिष्टः सुखोष्णोऽयं प्रदेहः श्लेष्मशोथहा ।

Kṛṣṇa, old oil cake of tila, bark of śigru, śikatā (sand) and śiva made into a paste with cow's urine and applied warm is effective in cases of kaphaśotha (oedema of kapha predominance) (81–82).

द्वे निशे चन्दने द्वे च शिवा दूर्वा पुनर्नवा ॥ ८२ ॥
उशीरं पद्मकं लोध्रं गैरिकं च रसाञ्जनम् । आगन्तुजे रक्तजे च शोथे कुर्यात्प्रलेपनम् ॥ ८३ ॥

The two niśas, two candanas, śiva, dūrvā, punarnavā, uśira, padmaka, lodhra, gairika and rasāñjana is an effective paste in āgantu śotha (traumatic oedema) and raktaja śotha (oedema where blood is predominant) (82–83).

शणमूलकशिग्रूणां फलानि तिलसर्षपाः । सवचः किण्वमतसी प्रदेहः पाचनः स्मृतः ॥ ८४ ॥

A pradeha prepared out of roots of śaṇa, seeds of śigru, tila, sarṣapa, vaca, kiṇva, (yeast) and atasī is efficacious in helping suppuration (84).

दन्ती चित्रकमूलत्वक्स्नुह्यर्कपयसी गुडः । भल्लातकास्थि कासीसं सैन्धवं दारणः स्मृतः ॥ ८५ ॥

A pradeha prepared out of dantī, bark of chitramūlaka, sap of snuhī and arka, jaggery, seeds of bhallātaka, kāsīsa and saindhava is effective in bursing of abscesses (85).

चिरिबिल्वोऽग्निको दन्ती चित्रको हयमारकः । कपोतकङ्कगृध्राणां मलं लेपेन दारणम् ॥ ८६ ॥

Cirabilva, agnika (bhallātaka), dantī, citraka, hayamāraka, excreta of pigeon, crow and hawk made into a paste and applied also helps in bursting of abscesses (86).

स्वर्जिकायावशूकाद्याः क्षारा लेपेन दारणाः । हेमक्षीर्यास्तथा लेपो व्रणे परमदारणः ॥ ८७ ॥

Svarjikā and kṣāra of yāvaśūka (barley husk) also act similarly; milky sap of hemakṣīrī likewise is a good burster of abcesses (87).

तिलसैन्धवयष्ट्याह्वनिम्बपत्रनिशायुगैः । त्रिवृद्धृतयुतैः पिष्टैः प्रलेपो व्रणशोधनः ॥ ८८ ॥

Tila, saindhava, yaṣṭi, leaves of nimba, the two niśas and trivṛt made into a paste and mixed with ghee and applied to wounds acts as a good cleanser (88),

निम्बपत्रघृतक्षौद्रदार्वीमधुकसंयुतः । तिलैश्च सह संयुक्तो लेपः शोधनरोपणः ॥ ८९ ॥

Leaves of nimba, ghee, honey, dārvī, madhuka and tila made into a paste and applied to wounds cleanses them and helps healing (89).

करञ्जारिष्टनिर्गुण्डी लेपो हन्याद्व्रणक्रिमीन् । लशुनस्याथवा लेपो हिङ्गुनिम्बभवोऽथवा ॥ ९० ॥

Paste of karañja, ariṣṭa and nirguṇḍī—removes the krimis (maggots etc.) from the wounds; the paste of laśuna. or of hiṅgu and nimba leaves act likewise (90).

निम्बपत्रं तिला दन्ती त्रिवृत्सैन्धवमाक्षिकम् । दुष्टव्रणप्रशमनो लेपः शोधनरोपणः ॥ ९१ ॥

Leaves of nimba, tila, dantī, taivṛt, saindhava and mākṣika (honey) made into a paste and applied to bad ulcers cleanses them and helps healing (91).

अथोदरशूलादौ लेपः—

मदनस्य फलं तिक्तां पिष्ट्वा काञ्जिकवारिणा । कोष्णं कुर्यान्नाभिलेपं शूलशान्तिर्भवेत्ततः ॥ ९२ ॥

Madanaphala and tikta, made into a paste with rice wash and applied warm over the umbilical region relieves abdominal pain (92).

इदानीं व्रणरोपणक्रमद्वारेण सर्वेषां व्रणजातीनां शमनयोगानाह तत्र तावत्पूर्वं विद्रधौ—

शिग्रुशेफालिकैरण्डयवगोधूममुद्गकैः। सुखोष्णो बहलो लेपः प्रयोज्यो वातविद्रधौ ॥ ९३ ॥

Śigru, śephālika, eraṇḍa, yava, godhūma and mudga made into a paste and applied warm and thick is effective in vātaja vidradhi (abscesses) (93).

पैत्तिके सर्पिषा लाजामधुकैः शर्करान्वितैः। प्रलिम्पेत्क्षीरपिष्टैर्वा पयस्योशीरचन्दनैः ॥ ९४ ॥

Paste prepared with sarpi (ghee), lājā, madhuka and śarkarā (sugar) or payasya, uśīra and candana with milk is effective in pitta vidradhi (abscess where pitta is predominant) (94).

इष्टिका सिकता लोहकिट्टं गोशकृता सह। सुखोष्णः स्यात्प्रदेहोऽयं मूत्रैः स्याच्छ्लेष्मविद्रधौ ॥९५॥

Powder of brick, sikatā (sand), lohakiṭṭa (iron rust) and cowdung made into paste with cow's urine applied as a pradeha is beneficial in kaphaja vidradhi (abscess where kapha is predominant) (95).

रक्तचन्दनमञ्जिष्ठानिशामधुकगैरिकैः। क्षीरेण विद्रधौ लेपो रक्तागन्तुनिमित्तजे ॥ ९६ ॥

Rakta candana, mañjiṣṭhā, niśā, madhuka and gairika made into a paste with milk is beneficial in abscesses which is due to injury or in which rakta is predominant (96).

अथ गलगण्डे—

निचुलः शिग्रुबीजानि दशमूलमथापि वा। प्रदेहो वातगण्डेषु सुखोष्णः संप्रदीयते ॥ ९७ ॥

Nicula, śigrubīja and daśamūlas made into a paste and applied warm helps in bursting the vātaja galagaṇḍa (scrofula) (97).

देवदारु विशाला च कफगण्डे प्रदेहकः।

Devadāru and viśālā, made as a pradeha acts on kaphaja galagaṇḍa (scrofula) (98).

सर्षपारिष्टपत्राणि दग्ध्वा भल्लातकैः सह ॥ ९८ ॥
छागमूत्रेण संपिष्टमपचीघ्नं प्रलेपनम्।

Sarṣapa, leaves of ariṣṭa and bhallātaka are burnt together, the ash thus obtained applied mixed with goats urine and applied over apacī (goitre) helps to reduce them (98–99).

सर्षपाः शिग्रुबीजानि शणबीजातसीयवाः ॥ ९९ ॥
मूलकस्य च बीजानि तक्रेणाम्लेन पेषयेत्। गण्डमालार्बुदं गण्डं लेपेनानेन शाम्यति ॥ १०० ॥

Sarṣapa, seeds of śigru, śāṇa, atasī, yava, mūlaka seeds made into a paste with sour buttermilk and applied over gaṇḍamāla (multiple srofula), arbuda (cancer), gaṇḍa (adenoma) helps their reduction (99–100).

अथ गृध्रस्यादिषु लेपः—

तक्षयित्वा क्षुरेणाङ्गं केवलानिलपीडितम् । तत्र प्रदेहं दद्याच्च पिष्टं गुञ्जाफलैः कृतम् ॥ १०१ ॥
तेनापबाहुजा पीडा विश्वाची गृध्रसी तथा । अन्यापि वातजा पीडा प्रशमं याति वेगतः ॥ १०२ ॥

Such of the parts of the body which have severe pain are incised slightly with a sharp knife and a paste of guñjā is applied warm as a pradeha. This method is beneficial in cases of apabāhuka (loss of function of arms), viśvācī (severe pain in the arms), gṛdhrasī (sciatica) and many other kinds of vāta diseases causing pain (101–102).

अथ श्लीपदे—

धत्तूरैरण्डनिर्गुण्डीवर्षाभूशिग्रुसर्षपैः । प्रलेपः श्लीपदं हन्ति चिरोत्थमपि दारुणम् ॥ १०३ ॥

Dhattūra, eraṇḍa, nirguṇḍī, varṣābhū, śigru and sarṣapa made into a paste and applied is effective in ślīpada (filariasis) however old it might be (103).

अथ अण्डवृद्धौ लेपः—

अजाजीहपुषाकुष्ठमेरण्डबदरान्वितम् । काञ्जिकेन तु संपिष्टं कुरण्डघ्नं प्रलेपनम् ॥ १०४ ॥

Ajājī, hapuṣā, kuṣṭha, eraṇḍa and badara made into a paste with sour rice-wash is useful in kuraṇḍa (hydrocele) (104).

अथोपदंशे—

करवीरस्य मूलेन परिपिष्टेन वारिणा । असाध्यापि व्रजत्यन्तं लिङ्गोत्था रुक्प्रलेपनात् ॥ १०५ ॥

Paste of roots of karavīra applied over bad ulcers of the penis helps them to heal (105).

दहेत्कटाहे त्रिफलां सा मषी मधुसंयुता । उपदंशे प्रलेपोऽयं सद्यो रोपयति व्रणम् ॥ १०६ ॥

Ashes of triphalā and honey applied over ulcers of upadaṁśa (veneral ulcers) helps them to heal (106).

रसाञ्जनं शिरीषेण पथ्यया च समन्वितम् । सक्षौद्रं लेपनं योज्यमुपदंशगदापहम् ॥ १०७ ॥

Rasāñjana, śirīṣa and pathya made into a paste with honey is also beneficial in upadaṁśa (veneral ulcers) (107).

अथाग्निदग्धे—

अग्निदग्धे तुगाक्षीरीप्लक्षचन्दनगैरिकैः । सामृतैः सर्पिषा स्निग्धैरालेपं कारयेद्भिषक् ॥ १०८ ॥
तिन्दुकीत्वक्कषायैर्वा घृतमिश्रैः प्रलेपयेत् । यवान्दग्ध्वा मषी कार्या तैलेन युतया तया ॥ १०९ ॥
दद्यात्सर्वाग्निदग्धेषु प्रलेपो व्रणरोपणः ।

In cases of burns, a paste of tugākṣīrī, plakṣa, candana, gairika, amṛta and ghee; or a decoction of bark of tinduka tree with ghee or ashes of yava (barley) mixed with sesamum oil—applied over the skin helps to heal the ulcers due to burns (108–110).

इदानीं लेपप्रकरणत्वादन्यानपि लेपानाह तत्रादौ भगसंकोचः—
पलाशोदुम्बरफलैस्तिलतैलसमन्वितैः ॥ ११० ॥
मधुना योनिमालिम्पेद्गाढीकरणमुत्तमम् ।

Palāśa and udumbara phala made into a paste with taila (sesamum oil) and honey, applied into vagina helps it to become narrow (110–111).

माकन्दफलसंयुक्तमधुकर्पूरलेपनात् ॥ १११ ॥
गतेऽपि यौवने स्त्रीणां योनिर्गाढाऽतिजायते ।

Fruits of mākanda (māciphala) honey and karpūra (camphor) made into a paste and applied into the vagina of even old women helps it to become narrow (111–112).

अथ लिङ्गवृद्धौ योनिसंकोचे—
मरिचं सैन्धवं कृष्णा तगरं बृहतीफलम् ॥ ११२ ॥
अपामार्गस्तिलाः कुष्टं यवा माषाश्च सर्षपाः । अश्वगन्धा च तच्चूर्णं मधुना सह योजयेत् ॥ ११३ ॥
अस्य संततलेपेन मर्दनाच्च प्रजायते । लिङ्गवृद्धिः स्तनोत्सेधः संहतिर्भुजकर्णयोः ॥ ११४ ॥

Marica, saindhava, kṛṣṇa, tagara, bṛhatīphala, apāmārga, tila, kuṣṭha, yava, māṣa, sarṣapa and aśvagandhā are all made into a paste and applied with honey often helps to increase the size of the penis, breasts, shoulders and ears (112–114).

सिताश्वगन्धासिन्धूत्थछागक्षीरैर्घृतं पचेत् । तल्लेपान्मर्दनाल्लिङ्गवृद्धिः संजायते परा ॥ ११५ ॥

Sita (sugar), aśvagandhā, saindhava, goats milk and ghee arep repared into a medicated ghee. This applied over the penis helps it to increase in size and girth (115).

इन्द्रवारुणिकापत्ररसैः सूतं विमर्दयेत् । रक्तस्य करवीरस्य काष्ठेन च मुहुर्मुहः ॥ ११६ ॥
तल्लिप्तलिङ्गसंयोगाद्योनिद्रावोऽभिजायते ।

A little quantity of sūta (mercury) is placed in a morter, juice of leaves of indravāruṇī is added and rubbed for some time with paste made from roots of red variety of karavīra. This paste applied over the penis of men makes the vagina of women to become moist during coitus (116–117).

ताम्बूलपत्रचूर्णं तु चूर्णं कुष्ठशिवाभवम् ॥ ११७ ॥
वारिणा लेपनं कुर्याद्गात्रदौर्गन्ध्यनाशनम् ।

Powders of tāmbūlapatra, kuṣṭha and śiva made into a paste with water and applied removes the bad odour of perspiration (117–118).

कुलित्थसक्तवः कुष्टं मांसी चन्दनजं रजः ॥ ११८ ॥
सक्तवश्चणकस्यैव त्वक्चैवैकत्र कारयेत् । स्वेददौर्गन्ध्यनाशश्च जायतेऽस्यावधूलनात् ॥ ११९ ॥

Flour of kulattha, kuṣṭha, māṁsī, candana, caṇaka and tvak are all powdered nicely and used as dusting powder helps removal of bad smell of perspiration (118–119).

वचा सौवर्चलं कुष्ठं रजन्यौ मरिचानि च । एतल्लेपप्रभावेण वशीकरणमुत्तमम् ॥ १२० ॥

Vacā, souvarcala, kuṣṭha, the two rajanis and marica—made into paste and applied acts as a vaśikaraṇa (helps attract women) (120).

अथ मूर्धतैलम्—

अभ्यङ्गपरिषेकश्च पिचुर्बस्तिरिति क्रमात् । मूर्धतैलं चतुर्धा स्याद्बलवच्च यथोत्तरम् ॥ १२१ ॥
त्रयोऽभ्यङ्गादयः पूर्वं प्रसिद्धाः सर्वतः स्मृताः ।

Abhyaṅga, pariṣeka, picu and basti are the four kinds of mūrdha taila (anointing of the head) each one successively stronger.

The first three procedures being well known since long; only śirobasti will be described here as advocated by experts (121–122).

अथाभ्यङ्गबस्तिप्रकारमाह—

शिरोबस्तिविधिश्चात्र प्रोच्यते सुज्ञसंमतः ॥ १२२ ॥
शिरोबस्तिश्चर्मणः स्याद्द्विमुखो द्वादशाङ्गुलः । शिरः प्रमाणं तं बध्वा मस्तके माषपिष्टकैः ॥१२३॥
सन्धिरोधं विधायाशु स्नेहैः कोष्णैः प्रपूरयेत् । तावद्धार्यस्तु यावत्स्यान्नासाकर्णमुखस्रुतिः ॥१२४॥
वेदनोपशमो वापि मत्राणां वा सहस्रकम् । विना भोजनमेवात्र शिरोबस्ति प्रशस्यते ॥ १२५ ॥
प्रयोज्यस्तु शिरोबस्तिः पञ्चसप्ताहमेव वा । विमोच्य शिरसो बस्तिं गृह्णीयाच्च समन्ततः ॥ १२६ ॥
ऊर्ध्वकायं ततः कोष्णनीरैः स्नानं च कारयेत् । अनेन दुर्जया रोगा वातजा यान्ति संक्षयम् ॥ १२७ ॥
शिरःकम्पादयस्तेन सर्वकालेषु युज्यते ।

A piece of soft leather of twelve inches in height is tied round the head and the crevices are cemented with a paste of flour of black gram so as to prevent leakage of oil. Medicated oil is slightly warmed and poured into this cap (to a height of about two aṅgulīs over the scalp) and the patient is asked to sit straight up. It is to be retained till the person gets moisture in his mouth, nose and ears or relief from pain or for a duration of one thousand mātrās. This is best done before food and once in five or seven days. After the stipulated time, the oil is poured out and the patient given an abhyaṅga (oil bath) with warm water. By this procedure, intractiable vāta diseases (nervous disorders), śiraḥkampa (shaking of the head) etc. will be cured for ever (122–128).

पूर्वमुक्तं लेपमूर्धतैलकर्णपूरणं तदिदानीं कर्णपूरणमाह—

स्वेदयेत्कर्णदेशं तु किञ्चिन्नुः पार्श्वशायिनः ॥ १२८ ॥
मूत्रैः स्नेहै रसैः कोष्णैस्ततः श्रोत्रं प्रपूरयेत् । कर्णं च पूरितं रक्षेच्छतं पञ्च शतानि वा ॥ १२९ ॥
सहस्रं वापि मात्राणां श्रोत्रकण्ठशिरोगदे । स्वजानुनः करावर्तं कुर्याच्छोटिकया युतम् ॥ १३० ॥
एषा मात्रा भवेदेका सर्वत्रैवैष निश्चयः ।

The region round the ear is slightly fomented and ears filled with warm oils, juices of plants, or urine of animals while the patient retains this medication for a duration of 100 or 500 or 1000 mātrās. A mātrā is the time required to move the fist saround one's knee quickly (128–131).

रसाद्यैः पूरणं कर्णे भोजनात्प्राक्प्रशस्यते ॥ १३१ ॥
तैलाद्यैः पूरणं कर्णे भास्करेऽस्तमुपागते ।

Karṇa-pūraṇa is best done before food if juice of herbs is to be used and if oil is indicated it is to done after sunset (131–132).

कर्णशूले योगाः—

पीतार्कपत्रमाज्येन लिप्तं वह्नौ प्रतापयेत् ॥ १३२ ॥
तद्रसः श्रवणे क्षिप्तः कर्णशूलहरः परः ।

Ripened yellow leaves of arka smeared with ghee are warmed and juice expressed from them put into the ears relieves ear-aches quickly (132–133).

कर्णशूलातुरे कोष्णं बस्तमूत्रं ससैन्धवम् ॥ १३३ ॥
निक्षिपेत्तेन शाम्यन्ति शूलपाकादिका रुजः ।

In cases of severe pains due to ulcerations in the ears a little quantity of goat's urine mixed with saindhava is warmed and filled into the ear for quick relief (133).

शृङ्गबेरं च मधुकं मधु सैन्धवमामलम् ॥ १३४ ॥
तिलपर्णीरसस्तैलं टङ्कणं निम्बुकद्रवम् । कदुष्णं कर्णयोर्देयमेतद्वा वेदनापहम् ॥ १३५ ॥

Sṛṅgavera, madhuka, madhu (honey), saindhava, āmalaka, juice of tilaparṇī, taila, ṭaṅkaṇa, juice of nimbu (lemon) are mixed together, warmed and poured into the ears for relief of pain (134–135).

कपित्थमातुलुङ्गाम्लशृङ्गबेररसैः शुभैः । सुखोष्णैः पूरयेत्कर्णं कर्णशूलोपशान्तये ॥ १३६ ॥

Juice of leaves of kapittha, mātuluṅga fruit, āmlavetasa and śṛṅgavera warmed and instilled into ears relieves ear-aches quickly (136).

अर्काङ्कुरानम्लपिष्टांस्तैलाक्तांल्लवणान्वितान् । संनिदध्यात्स्नुहीकाण्डे कोरिते तच्छदावृते ॥१३७॥
पुटपाकक्रमं कृत्वा रसैस्तच्च प्रपूरयेत् । सुखोष्णैस्तेन शाम्यन्ति कर्णपीडाः सुदारुणाः ॥ १३८ ॥

Tender leaves of arka made into a paste with saindhava and a little quantity of oil rolled into a pill is kept inside the stem of snuhī and sealed up with a coating of mud as described under puṭapāka and baked well. After it cools, the juice expressed from the paste is poured into the ears for immediate relief of severe pain of the ears (137–138).

दीपिकातैलम्—

महतः पञ्चमूलस्य काण्डान्यष्टाङ्गुलानि च । क्षौमेणावेष्ट्य संसिच्य तैलेनादीपयेत्ततः ॥ १३९ ॥
यत्तलं च्यवते तेभ्यः सुखोष्णं तेन पूरयेत् । ज्ञेयं तद्दीपिकातैलं सद्यो गृह्णाति वेदनाम् ॥ १४० ॥
एवं स्याद्दीपिकातैलं कुष्ठे देवतरौ तथा ।

Stems of each of the Mahatpañcamūla (bilva, agnimantha, syonāka, kāśmarī, (pāṭalā) each eight aṅgulīs long are tied together with cloth and kept immerced in oil for some time. Later it is lit with fire and the oil exuding from the flame is collected into a vessel. This oil known as *Dīpikā taila* poured into ears warm, relieves ear-aches quickly. Kuṣṭha and devadāru wood may also be used for preparing dīpikā taila (139-141).

स्योनाकतैलम्—

तैलं स्योनाकमूलेन मन्देऽग्नौ परिपाचितम् ॥ १४१ ॥
हरेदाशु त्रिदोषोत्थं कर्णमूलं प्रपूरणात् ।

Oil of roots of syonāka taken out as described above and poured into ears relieves ear aches arising from all the three doṣas together (141-142).

यष्टीवसा—

कल्कक्वाथेन यष्ट्याह्वकाकोलीमाषधान्यकैः ॥ १४२ ॥
शूकरस्य वसां पक्त्वा कर्णनादार्तिनाशिनी ।

Yaṣṭī, kākolī, māṣa and dhānyaka are made into a decoction, muscle fat of pig is mixed and cooked. This fat instilled into ears relieves karṇarnāda (tinnitus) and ārti (pain) (142-143).

स्वर्जिकातैलम्—

स्वर्जिका मूलकं शुष्कं हिङ्गु कृष्णासमन्वितम् ॥ १४३ ॥
शतपुष्पा च तैस्तैलं पक्वं सूक्तचतुर्गुणम् । प्रणादं शूलबाधिर्यं स्रावं कर्णस्य नाशयेत् ॥ १४४ ॥

Svarjikā, dried mūlaka, hiṅgu, kṛṣṇā and śatapuṣpā each equal parts, taila (oil) and sūkta (sour greal) four parts are cooked into a medicated oil. This oil used constantly relieves karṇanāda (tinnitus), karṇaśūla (pain in the ears), bādhirya (deafness) and karṇasrāva (discharge from the ears) (143-144).

अपामार्गक्षारतैलं बाधिर्ये—

अपामार्गक्षारजले तत्क्षारं कल्कितं क्षिपेत् । तेन पक्वं जयेत्तैलं बाधिर्यं कर्णनादकम् ॥ १४५ ॥

Apāmārga kṣāra is made into a kalka with apāmārga juice, oil is added and cooked well. This will relieve bādhirya (deafness) and karṇanāda (tinnitus) (145).

शम्बूकतैलम्—

शम्बूकस्य तु मांसेन पचेत्तैलं तु सार्षपम् । तस्य पूरणमात्रेण कर्णनाडी प्रशाम्यति ॥ १४६ ॥

Taila is prepared cooking it with the flesh of śambūka (molluses) and instilled into ears relieves karṇanāḍī (discharge from the ears) (146).

कर्णस्रावे योगाः—

चूर्णं पञ्चकषायाणां कपित्थरसमेव च । कर्णस्रावे प्रशंसन्ति पूरणं मधुना सह ॥ १४७ ॥

Decoction of barks of the five kaṣāyas (refer next verse) and juice of kapittha leaves mixed with honey is effective in cases of discharge from the ears (147).

तिन्दुकान्यभया लोध्रः समङ्गा चामलक्यपि । ज्ञेयाः पञ्च कषायास्तु कर्मण्यस्मिन्भिषग्वरैः ॥१४८॥

Tinduka, abhaya, lodhra, samaṅga and āmalaka are the five kaṣāya vṛkṣas known to physicions for this purpose (148).

स्वर्जिकारसयोगः—

स्वर्जिकाच्चूर्णसंयुक्तं बीजपूररसं क्षिपेत् । कर्णस्रावरुजादाहाः प्रणश्यन्ति न संशयः ॥ १४९ ॥

Juice of bījapūra mixed with little of svarjikā kṣāra is effective in cases of discharges and pain of the ears (149).

आम्रादितैलम्—

आम्रजम्बूप्रवालानि मधुकस्य वटस्य च । एभिः संसाधितं तैलं पूतिकर्णोपशान्तिकृत् ॥ १५० ॥

Tender leaves of āmra, jambū, madhuka and vaṭa are cooked in oil and this oil put into the ears cureṣ pūtikarṇa (foul smell of ears) (150).

कर्णकीटे हरितालादियोगः—

पूरणं हरितालेन गवां मूत्रयुतेन च । अथवा सार्षपं तैलं कर्णकीटहरं परम् ॥ १५१ ॥

Filling the ears with cow's urine mixed with a little quantity of haritāla or with sarṣapa taila (mustard oil) is helpful in destroying krimis (bacteria) in the ears (151).

कर्णकीटे शिग्रुस्वरसादियोगः—

स्वरसं शिग्रुमूलस्य सूर्यावर्तरसं तथा । त्र्यूषणं चूर्णितं चैव कपिकच्छूजटारसम् ॥ १५२ ॥
कृत्वैकत्र क्षिपेत्कर्णे कर्णकीटहरं परम् ।

Juice of roots of śigru, sūryāvarta, tryūṣaṇa and roots of kapikachū mixed together and poured into ears destroys krimis (bacteria, worms) in the ears.

Similarly instilling madya (alcohol) or hiṅgu water into the ears removes the worms (152-153).

इति श्रीदामोदरसूनुना श्रीशार्ङ्गधराचार्येण विरचितायां श्रीशार्ङ्गधरसंहितायामुत्तरखण्डे
लेपादिविधिर्नामैकादशोऽध्यायः ॥ ११ ॥

Thus ends the eleventh chapter.

द्वादशोऽध्यायः

CHAPTER 12

अथ शोणितविस्रावविधिरधुना विधीयते

Soṇitasrāva Vidhi (Blood letting)

अतः शोणितस्रावणमाह—

शोणितं स्रावयेज्जन्तोरामयं प्रसमीक्ष्य च। प्रस्थं प्रस्थार्धकं वापि प्रस्थार्धार्धमथापि वा ॥ १ ॥

Blood letting should be resorted to after diagnosis of the disease; the quantity may be a prastha, half a prastha or quarter prastha (1).

शरत्काले स्वभावेन कुर्याद्रक्तस्रुतिं नरः। त्वग्दोषग्रन्थिशोथाद्या न स्यू रक्तस्रुतेर्यतः ॥ २ ॥

Even for healthy persons it can be resorted to during śaratkāla (autumn) to be free from skin diseases, granthi (tumors) and śotha (oedema) etc. (2).

आदौ रक्तस्य रसवर्णगुणादीनाह—

मधुरं वर्णतो रक्तमशीतोष्णं तथा गुरु। शोणितं स्निग्धविस्रं स्याद्विदाहश्चास्य पित्तवत् ॥ ३ ॥
विस्रता द्रवता रागश्चलनं विलयस्तथा। भूम्यादिपञ्चभूतानामेते रक्तगुणाः स्मृताः ॥ ४ ॥

Normal blood is madhura (sweet), red in colour, neither cold nor hot, heavy, slightly unctous, of unpleasant smell, and during vidāha (disordered state) produces symptoms like pitta. Visratā (slight unpleasant smell), dravatā (liquidity), rāga (redness), calana (movement), vilaya (pervasiveness every where in the body)—these properties of each of the pañcabhūtas starting with pṛthvī respectively are present in rakta (3-4).

दुष्टरक्तलक्षणे किं भवतीत्याह—

रक्ते दुष्टे वेदना स्यात्पाको दाहश्च जायते। रक्तमण्डलता कण्डूः शोथश्च पिटिकोद्गमः ॥ ५ ॥

If rakta becomes disordered, pain, suppuration, burning sensation, reddish rashes on the skin, itching, oedema and appearance of eruption on the skin will manifest (5).

वृद्धे रक्ताङ्गनेत्रत्वं सिराणां पूरणं तथा। गात्राणां गौरवं निद्रा मदो दाहश्च जायते ॥ ६ ॥
क्षीणेऽम्लमधुराकाङ्क्षा मूर्च्छा च त्वचि रूक्षता। शैथिल्यं च सिराणां स्याद्वातादुन्मार्गगामिता ॥७॥

If blood becomes increased (diseased state) it causes redness of eyes, skin, fullness of veins (and arteries), heavyness of the body, somnolence, intoxication and burning sensation all over the body and even bleeding from various part of the body. If blood becomes decreased, the person develops craving for sweet and sour foods, convulsions, dryness of the skin, thinness of veins (and arteries) and consequent increase of vāta (6-7).

अरुणं फेनिलं रूक्षं परुषं तनु शीघ्रगम् । अस्कन्दि सूचिनिस्तोदि रक्तं स्याद्वातदूषितम् ॥ ८ ॥
पित्तेन पीतं हरितं नीलं श्यावं च विस्रकम् । अस्कन्द्युष्णं मक्षिकाणां पिपीलानामनिष्टकम् ॥ ९ ॥
शीतलं बहलं स्निग्धं गैरिकोदकसंनिभम् । मांसपेशीप्रभं स्कन्दि मन्दगं कफदूषितम् ॥ १० ॥
द्विदोषदुष्टं संसृष्टं त्रिदुष्टं पूतिगन्धकम् । सर्वलक्षणसंयुक्तं काञ्जिकाभं च जायते ॥ ११ ॥

If blood becomes vitiated by vāta, it appears pink, frothy, dry (viscid), lustreless, thin, ffows quickly, does not get clotted and causes pricking pain inside the body; vitiated by pitta, it assumes yellow, green, blue or black colour, bad smell does not clot and becomes disagreeable to flies and ants; if vitiated be kapha, it is cold, thick, unctous, fainty red like gairika water, or mutton wash; clots quickly and flows out very slowly; if vitiated by any two doṣas together it will have mixed signs and vitiated by all the doṣas it appears like kāñjikā (sour gruel) (8–11).

विषदुष्टं भवेच्छ्यावं नासिकोन्मार्गगं तथा । विस्रं काञ्जिकसंकाशं सर्वकुष्ठकरं बहु ॥ १२ ॥

If vitiated by viṣa (poison) it becomes black, flows out of the nose; of unpleasant smell, assumes the consistence of kāñjikā and causes all kinds of kuṣṭha (leprosy and allied skin diseases) (12).

प्रकृतिस्थरक्तलक्षणमाह—

इन्द्रगोपप्रभं ज्ञेयं प्रकृतिस्थमसंहतम् ।

Normal blood should have the colour of indragopa insect (bright red) and not too thick in constistence (13).

येषु रक्तस्रावो विहितस्तानाह—

शोथे दाहेऽङ्गपाके च रक्तवर्णेऽसृजः स्रुतौ ॥ १३ ॥
वातरक्ते तथा कुष्ठे सपीडे दुर्जयेऽनिले । पाणिरोगे श्लीपदे च विषदुष्टे च शोणिते ॥ १४ ॥
ग्रन्थ्यर्बुदापचीक्षुद्ररोगरक्ताधिमन्थिषु । विदारीस्तनरोगेषु गात्राणां सादगौरवे ॥ १५ ॥
रक्ताभिष्यन्दतन्द्रायां पूतिघ्राणास्यदेहके । यकृत्प्लीहविसर्पेषु विद्रधौ पिटिकोद्गमे ॥ १६ ॥
कर्णौष्ठघ्राणवक्त्राणां पाके दाहे शिरोरुजि । उपदंशे रक्तपित्ते रक्तस्रावः प्रशस्यते ॥ १७ ॥
एषु रोगेषु शृङ्गैर्वा जलौकालाबुकैरपि । अथवापि सिरामोक्षैः कुर्याद्रक्तस्रुतिं नरः ॥ १८ ॥

Blood letting as a method of treatment is indicated in śotha (oedema), dāha (burning), pāka (pus formation), raktavarṇa (redness of the skin), asṛkasruti (bleeding conditions), vātarakta (gout), kuṣṭha (leprosy and other skin diseases), vāta diseases having severe pain, pāṇi roga (diseases of the hands), ślīpada (filariasis); blood vitiated with poisons, granthi (tumors), arbuda (malignant tumors) apacī (goitre), kṣudraroga (skin diseases), raktādhimantha (a kind of eye disease), vidārī (skin cracks), stanaroga (diseases of breasts); debility and heavyness of the body, raktābhiṣyanda (another disease of eye), tandrā (stupor), pūtighrāṇa (bad smell of the nose), pūtiasya (bad smell of the mouth), pūtideha

(foul smell of the body), yakṛt-plīhā (disease of liver and spleen), visarpa (erysepelas), vidradhi (abscess) piḍakas (eruptions), pāka of karṇa, oṣṭha, ghrāṇa, vaktra (ulceration of ears, lips, nose and mouth), śiroruja (headache), upadaṁśa (venereal diseases) and raktapitta (purpura).

In all these diseases blood letting can be done by either a śṛṅga (horn of animals), jalouka (leeches), alābu (gourd) or by cutting the śirā (vein) (13-18)

येषु सिरामोक्षो निषिद्धः तानाह—

न कुर्वीत सिरामोक्षं कृशस्यातिव्यवायिनः । क्लीबस्य भीरोर्गर्भिण्याः सूतिकापाण्डुरोगिणाम् ॥१९॥

पञ्चकर्मविशुद्धस्य पीतस्नेहस्य चार्शसाम् । सर्वाङ्गशोथयुक्तानामुदरश्वासकासिनाम् ॥ २० ॥

छर्द्यतीसारदुष्टानामितिस्विन्नतनोरपि । ऊनषोडवर्षस्य गतसप्ततिकस्य च ॥ २१ ॥

आघातस्रुतरक्तस्य सिरामोक्षो न शस्यते । एषां चात्ययिके रोगे जलौकाभिस्तु निर्हरेत् ॥ २२ ॥

तथा च विषदुष्टानां शिरामोक्षोऽपि शस्यते ।

Śirā mokṣaṇa (venesection) should not be done for persons who are emaciated, who indulge in too much of sex, who are impotant, frightful, pregnant women, women in parturition, persons who are anaemic, persons who have undergone the five purificatory therapies, who have taken snehapāna (oil drinking), persons suffering from arśas (haemorrhoids), sarvāṅga śotha (general anasarca), udara (abdominal enalargement), svāsa, kāsa (dyspnoea and cough), chardi (vomiting), atisāra (diarrhoeas), who are perspiring too much by sudation therapy, persons below the age of sixteen and above seventy years and persons who are bleeding heavily due to injury. Blood letting, if very necessary in the above diseases, leeches may be applied to suck blood while in cases of poisons, venesection is ideal (19-23).

वातादिदुष्टं केन स्रावयेदित्याह—

गोशृङ्गेण जलौकाभिरलाबुभिरपि त्रिधा ॥ २३ ॥

वातपित्तकफैर्दुष्टं शोणितं स्रावयेद्बुधः । द्विदोषाभ्यां तु संदुष्टं त्रिदोषैरपि दूषितम् ॥ २४ ॥

शोणितं स्रावयेद्युक्त्या शिरामोक्षैः पदैस्तथा ।

In cases of blood being vitiated by vāta, pitta and kapha doṣas, the blood should be let out by the use of cow's horn, leech and gourd respectively. In cases of vitiation by two or all the three doṣas together cutting the vein or making small incisions on the skin are to be adopted for letting out the blood (23-25).

गृह्णाति शोणितं शृङ्गं दशाङ्गुलमितं बलात् ॥ २५ ॥

जलौका हस्तमात्रं तु तुम्बी च द्वादशाङ्गुलम् । पदमङ्गुलमात्रस्य सिरा सर्वाङ्गशोधिनी ॥ २६ ॥

Application of cow's horn can bring out blood from an area of ten aṅgulīs around, leech can suck from an area of one hasta, the gourd from an area of twelve aṅgulis, cutting the skin from an area of one aṅguli, while venesection can purify the entire body (25–26).

शीते निरन्ने मूर्छायां तन्द्राभीतिमदश्रमैः । युतानां च स्रवेद्रक्तं तथा विण्मूत्रसङ्गिनाम् ॥ २७ ॥
अप्रवर्तितरक्ते च कुष्ठत्रिकटुसैन्धवैः । मर्दयेद्व्रणवक्त्रं च तेन सम्यक्प्रवर्तते ॥ २८ ॥

Blood does not flow out properly during cold season, on empty stomach, during fainting, during drowsiness, fright, intoxication, exhaustion and suppression of urine and faeces. In such cases a powder of kuṣṭha, trikaṭu and saindhava is to be rubbed into the wound by which blood flows out freely (27-28).

इदानीं सुखविस्रावणार्थं हितोपदेशमाह—

तस्मान्न शीते नात्युष्णे न स्विन्ने नातितापिते । पीत्वा यवागूं तृप्तस्य स्रावयेच्छोणितं बुधः ॥२९॥

Blood letting should not be attempted neither during cold season nor very hot season, neither before sudation therapy nor after too much of sudation. It should be adopted after the person has been satisfied with a drink of yavāgū (thin gruel) (29).

अथ केन हेतुना रक्तातिप्रवृत्तिस्तद्दर्शयन्नाह—

अतिस्विन्नस्योष्णकाले तथैवातिसिराव्यधात् । अतिप्रवर्तते रक्तं तत्र कुर्यात्प्रतिक्रियाम् ॥ ३० ॥
अतिप्रवृत्ते रक्ते च लोध्रसर्जरसाञ्जनैः । यवगोधूमचूर्णैर्वा धवधन्वनगैरिकैः ॥ ३१ ॥
सर्पनिर्मोकचूर्णैर्वा भस्मना क्षौमवस्त्रयोः । मुखं व्रणस्य बद्ध्वा च शीतैश्चोपचरेद्व्रणम् ॥ ३२ ॥
विध्येदूर्ध्वं सिरां तां च दहेत्क्षारेण वाग्निना । व्रणं कषायः संधत्ते रक्तं स्कन्दयते हिमम् ॥ ३३ ॥
व्रणास्यं पाचयेत्क्षारो दाहः संकोचयेत्सिराम् ।

Large quantity of blood flows out during and after excessive sudation therapy, during hot season or too prolonged venesection. In such cases it should be stopped by suitable methods such as application to the wound of powder of lodhra, sarjarasa, añjanas, yava, godhūma, dhava, dhanvana, gairika; or ash of peelings of snake skin, silk cloth and later bangaged tightly. The patient should be given cold foods and other cold comforts.

A fresh venesection should be done above the earlier wound or the wound is to be touched with a stick of kṣāra (alkalī) or red hot iron. Astringent substances close up the wound, cold things make the blood to clot, alkalies eat away the wound while fire constricts the veins (30-33)

वामाण्डशोथे दक्षस्य करस्याङ्गुष्ठमूलजाम् ॥ ३४ ॥

दहेत्सिरां व्यत्यये तु वामाङ्गुष्ठसिरां दहेत् । सिरादाहप्रभावेण मुष्कशोथः प्रणश्यति ॥ ३५ ॥

Dahana (branding with red hot iron) on the vein of the right hand below the thumb cures swelling of the left scrotum; in cases of swelling of right scrotum the left hand vein is to be burnt. By this muṣka śotha (scrotal swellings) will be cured (34-35).

Puṭapāka prepared out of breast milk, broth of flesh of jāṅgala animals, honey, ghee and drugs of bitter taste, constitute ropaṇa puṭapāka and it should be retained for a duration of three times as of lekhana puṭapāka.

Any complications during this therapy should be treated similar to those of tarpaṇa (60-61).

अञ्जनम्—

अथ संपक्वदोषस्य प्रातमञ्जनमाचरेत् । हेमन्ते शिशिरे चैव मध्याह्नेऽञ्जनमिष्यते ॥ ६२ ॥
पूर्वाह्ने चापराह्णे च ग्रीष्मे शरदि चेष्यते । वर्षासु नाभ्रे नात्युष्णे वसन्ते च सदैव हि ॥ ६३ ॥

Añjana (collyrium) is applied to the eyes when the doṣas have become pakva; in the afternoons during hemanta and śiśira ṛtus; during mornings in grīṣma and evening in śarat; when there is neither too cold nor too much of heat during varṣā; and any time during vasanta (62-63).

लेखनं रोपणं चैव तथा स्यात्स्नेहनाञ्जनम् । लेखनं क्षारतीक्ष्णाम्लरसैरञ्जनमिष्यते ॥ ६४ ॥
कषायतिक्तरसयुक्तस्नेहं रोपणं मतम् । मधुरं स्नेहसंपन्नमञ्जनं तु प्रसादनम् ॥ ६५ ॥

Añjana (collyriums) is of three types, lekhana (scarifying), ropaṇa (healing) and snehana (oleating) añjana prepared with kṣāras, tīkṣṇa and amla drugs constitute lekhana; that prepared with drugs of kaṣāya (astringent) and tikta (bitter) tastes and oil or ghee constitute ropaṇa, and añjana containing drugs of madhura (sweet) and oil or ghee constitute snehana añjana (64-65).

गुटिकारसचूर्णानि त्रिविधान्यञ्जनानि च । कुर्याच्छलाकयाऽङ्गुल्या हीनानि च यथोत्तरम् ॥ ६६ ॥

Añjanas can be prepared in the form of pill, liquid or powder and are applied to the eyes with a rod or fingers, each succeding one is poorer in efficacy than the previous (66).

श्रान्ते प्ररुदिते भीते पीतमद्ये नवज्वरे । अजीर्णे वेगघाते च नाञ्जनं संप्रशस्यते ॥ ६७ ॥

Añjana shonld not be applied to persons who are tired, weeping, frightful, intoxicated with alcoholic drinks, in early stages of fevers; indigestion and during suppression of urges (67).

हरेणुमात्रां कुर्वीत वर्तिं तीक्ष्णाञ्जने भिषक् । प्रमाणं मध्यमेऽध्यर्धं द्विगुणं तु मृदौ भवेत् ॥ ६८ ॥

Varti añjana (paste) if very powerful, should be applied in doses of one hareṇu, if of medium potency one and half hareṇus, and if of mild potency two hareṇus (68).

रसक्रिया तूत्तमा स्यात्त्रिविडङ्गमिता हिता । मध्यमा द्विविडङ्गा स्याद्धीना त्वेकविडङ्गिका ॥ ६९ ॥

Rasakriyā (liquid collyrium) in doses of three viḍaṅgas is considered as maximum, two viḍaṅgas as medium and one viḍaṅga as least (69).

वैरेचनिकचूर्णं तु द्विशलाकं विधीयते । मृदौ तु त्रिशलाकं स्याच्चतस्रः स्नैहिकेऽञ्जने ॥ ७० ॥

Cūrṇa añjana (powder) if possessing purgative action to the eyes should be applied twice in a metallic rod, if of mild potency thrice and if possessing snehana action four times (70).

मुखयोः कुण्ठिता श्लक्ष्णा शलाकाष्टाङ्गुलोन्मिता । अश्मजा धातुजा वा स्यात्कलायपरिमण्डला ॥७१॥
ताम्रलोहाश्मसंजाता शलाका लेखने मता । सुवर्णरजतोद्भूता शलाका स्नेहने मता ॥ ७२ ॥
अङ्गुलीव मृदुत्वेन कथिता रोपणे बुधैः ।

The śalākā (applying rod) should be eight aṅgulīs in length and it's applying end resembling a flower bud.

The rod prepared with copper, iron or stone is ideal for lekhana action, that of gold or silver for snehana action and finger itself best for ropaṇa action (71-73).

सायं प्रातर्वाञ्जनं स्यात्तत्सदा नैव कारयेत् ॥ ७३ ॥
नातिशीतोष्णवाताभ्रवेलायां संप्रशस्यते । कृष्णभागादधः कुर्यादपाङ्गं यावदञ्जनम् ॥ ७४ ॥

Anjana can be done either in the morning or evening but not always, neither during too much heat nor too much cold, heavy breeze or clouds is also not suitable. Añjana drug should be applied below the kṛṣṇabhāga (cornea) upto the outer corner of the eye (73-74).

चन्द्रोदया—

शङ्खनाभिर्विभीतस्य मज्जा पथ्या मनःशिला । पिप्पली मरिचं कुष्ठं वचा चेति समांशकम् ॥ ७५ ॥
छागीक्षीरेण संपिष्य वर्तिं कृत्वा यवोन्मिताम् । हरेणुमात्रां संघृष्य जलैः कुर्यादथाञ्जनम् ॥ ७६ ॥
तिमिरं मांसवृद्धिं च काचं पटलमर्बुदम् । रात्र्यान्ध्यं वार्षिकं पुष्पं वर्तिश्चन्द्रोदया जयेत् ॥ ७७ ॥

Śaṅkha nābhi, marrow of vibhītaka, pathya, manaśila, pippali, marica, kuṣṭha and vaca—all equal parts are nicely macerated with goat's milk, rolled into pills and dried. At the time of applying it is made into a paste with water and a quantity of one hareṇu is applied as añjana into the eyes. This recipe known as *Candrodaya varti* cures timira (blindness), māṃsavṛddhi (pterygium), kāca (opacity of lens), paṭala (coverings), arbuda (tumors), rātryāndhya (night blindness) and even long standing puṣpa (ulcers on sclera or cornea) (75-77).

करञ्जवर्तिः—

पलाशपुष्पस्वरसैर्बहुशः परिभाविता । करञ्जबीजवर्तिस्तु दृष्टेः पुष्पं विनाशयेत् ॥ ७८ ॥

Seeds of karañja macerated for many times with juice of flowers of palāśa and applied as añjana cures puṣpa (scars in the eye) (78).

समुद्रफेनादिवर्तिः—

समुद्रफेनसिन्धूत्थशङ्खदक्षाण्डवल्कलैः । शिग्रुबीजयुतैर्वर्तिःशुक्रादींश्छस्त्रवल्लिखेत् ॥ ७९ ॥

Samudraphena, saindhava, śaṅkha, shell of hen's egg and śigru bīja—made as an añjana removes śukra (scars) just like a knife (79).

दन्तवर्तिः—

दन्तैर्दन्तिवराहोष्ट्रगोहयाजखुरोद्भवैः । शङ्खमुक्ताम्भोधिफेनयुतैः सर्वैर्विचूर्णितैः ॥ ८० ॥
दन्तवर्तिः कृता श्लक्ष्णा शुक्राणां नाशिनी परा ।

Teeth of elephant, pig, camel, cow, horse, goat and ass, śaṅkha (couch), muktā (pearl), ambuphena (cuttle fish) all nicely powdered, made into a stick and applied with water cures śukra (scars in the eyes) (80–81).

नीलोत्पलवर्तिः—

नीलोत्पलं शिग्रुबीजं नागकेशरकं तथा ॥ ८१ ॥
एतत्कल्कैः कृता वर्तिरतिनिद्रां निवारयेत् ।

Nīlotpala, śigru bīja, nāgakeśara, made into a paste and used as añjana stops excess sleep (81).

पुष्पवर्तिः—

तिलपुष्पाण्यशीतिः स्युः षष्टिः पिप्पलितंडुला ॥ ८२ ॥
जातीकुसुमपञ्चाशान्मरिचानि च षोडश । सूक्ष्मं पिष्ट्वा जले वर्तिः कृता कुसुमिकाभिधा ॥ ८३ ॥
तिमिरार्जुनशुक्राणां नाशिनी मांसवृद्धिहृत् । (एतस्याश्चाञ्जने मात्रा प्रोक्ता सार्धहरेणुका ॥ ८४ ॥)

Flowers of tila, eighty in number, sixty in number of grains of pippalī, fifty in number of flower of jātī, sixteen in number of marica—all are made into a nice paste, rolled into pills and dried. This puṣpavarti made as añjana in doses of half hareṇus cures timira (blindness) arjuna (cyst), śukra (scars) and māṃsavṛddhi (pterygium) (82-84).

रसाञ्जनवर्तिः—

रसाञ्जनं हरिद्रे द्वे मालतीनिम्बपल्लवाः । गोशकृद्रससंयुक्ता वर्तिर्नक्तान्ध्यनाशिनी ॥ ८५ ॥

Rasāñjana, the two haridrās, mālati, tender leaves of nimba made as añjana with juice of fresh cowdung cures naktāndhya (night blindness) (85).

धात्र्यादिवर्तिः—

धात्र्यक्षपथ्याबीजानि एकद्वित्रिगुणानि च । पिष्ट्वा वर्तिं जलैः कुर्यादञ्जनं द्विहरेणुकम् ॥ ८६ ॥
नेत्रस्रावं हरत्याशु वातरक्तरुजं तथा ।

Seeds of dhātrī, akṣa, pathya, one, two and three parts respectively and made into a pill with water and applied in doses of two hareṇu stops excessive discharge from the eyes and diseases arising from rakta and pitta (86–87).

रसक्रिया—

तुत्थमाक्षिकसिन्धूत्थं सिताशङ्खमनःशिलाः ॥ ८७ ॥
गैरिकोदधिफेनं च मरिचं चेति चूर्णयेत् । संयोज्य मधुना कुर्यादञ्जनार्थं रसक्रियाम् ॥ ८८ ॥
वर्त्मरोगार्मतिमिरकाचशुक्रहरां पराम् ।

Tuttha, mākṣika, saindhava, sitā, śaṅkha, manaśila, gairika, udadhiphena and marica are nicely powdered and made into añjana with honey for the cure of diseases of eyelids, arma (pterygium), timira (blindness), kaca (opacity) and śukra (scars) (87–89).

तथाच लेखनी रसक्रिया—

वटक्षीरेण संयुक्तो मुख्यः कर्पूरजः कणः ॥ ८९ ॥
क्षिप्रमञ्जनतो हन्ति कुसुमं तु द्विमासिकम् ।

Good variety of comphor rubbed with sap of vaṭa (baniyan tree) destroys śukra (sears) within two months (89–90).

अतिनिद्रायां योगः—

क्षौद्राश्वलालासंघृष्टैर्मरिचैर्नेत्रमञ्जयेत् ॥ ९० ॥
अतिनिद्रा शमं याति तमः सूर्योदयादिव ।

Honey, saliva of horse and marica made into a nice paste and applied to the eyes relieves excess sleep just like the sun dispells the darkness in the morning (90-91).

प्रबोधनाञ्जनम्—

जातीपुष्पं प्रवालं च मरिचं कटुकी वचा ॥ ९१ ॥
सैन्धवं बस्तमूत्रेण पिष्टं तन्द्राघ्नमञ्जनम् ।

Flowers of jātī, pravāla (coral), marica, kaṭukī, vaca and sandhava made into a paste with goat's urine and applied cures tandrā, (stupor, sleepiness) (91-92).

शिरीषबीजगोमूत्रकृष्णामरिचसैन्धवैः ॥ ९२ ॥
अञ्जनं स्यात्प्रबोधाय सरसोनशिलावचैः ।

Seeds of śirīśa, cow's urine, kṛṣṇa, marica, saindhava, rasona, manaśila and vaca—made into añjana is best to arouse a person from sleep (92–93).

दार्व्यादिरसक्रिया—

दार्वी पटोलं मधुकं सनिम्बपद्मकोत्पलम् ॥ ९३ ॥
प्रपौण्डरीकं चैतानि पचेत्तोये चतुर्गुणे । विपाच्य पादशेषं तु श्रृतं नीत्वा पुनः पचेत् ॥ ९४ ॥
शीते तस्मिन्मधु सितां दद्यात्पादांशिकां नरः । रसक्रियैषा दाहाश्रुरक्तरागरुजो हरेत् ॥ ९५ ॥

Dārvi, paṭola, madhuka, nimba, padmaka, utpala and prapouṇdarīka—are cooked in four times of water and reduced to one quarter. Further it is made into a rasakriyā (thick consistence of añjana)' honey and sugar are added after it cools. Used as añjana, this recipe relieves burning, lacrimation, redness and pain of the eyes quickly (93–95).

रसाञ्जनादिरसक्रिया—

रसाञ्जनं सर्जरसो जातीपुष्पं मनःशिला । समुद्रफेनो लवणं गैरिकं मरिचानि च ॥ ९६ ॥

एतत्समांशं मधुना पिष्ट्वा प्रक्लिन्नवर्त्मनि । अञ्जनं क्लेदकण्डूघ्नं पक्ष्मणां च प्ररोहणम् ॥ ९७ ॥

Rasāñjana, sarjarasa, jātīpuṣpa, manaśila, samudraphena, lavaṇa, gairika and marica all equal parts rubbed with honey and used as añjana cures praklinna vartma, kleda and kaṇḍū. It helps growth of eye lashes (96–97).

गुडूचीरसक्रिया—

गुडूचीस्वरसः कर्षः क्षौद्रं स्यान्माषकोन्मितम् । सैन्धवं क्षौद्रतुल्यं स्यात्सर्वमेकत्र मर्दयेत् ॥ ९८ ॥
अञ्जयेन्नयनं तेन पिल्लार्मतिमिरं जयेत् । काचं कण्डूं लिङ्गनाशं शुक्लकृष्णगतान्गदान् ॥ ९९ ॥

One karṣa of fresh juice of guḍūci, one māṣā each of honey and saindhava are made into an añjana. It cures pilla (blurred eye), arma (pterygium), timira (defective vision), kāca (opacity of lens), kaṇḍū (itching), liṅganāśa (blindness) and diseases of śukra (scleera) and kṛṣṇa (cornea) (98–99).

पुनर्नवारसक्रिया—

दुग्धेन कण्डूं क्षौद्रेण नेत्रस्रावं च सर्पिषा । पुष्पं तैलेन तिमिरं काञ्जिकेन निशान्धताम् ॥ १०० ॥
पुनर्नवा जयेदाशु भास्करस्तिमिरं यथा ।

Just like the sun dispells darkness, punarnavā if used as añjana with milk dispells kaṇḍū (itching); with honey, discharges from the eyes; with ghee, puṣpa (corneal sears); with oil the defects of vision and with kañjika (rice-wash) night blindness (100–101).

बब्बूलरसक्रिया—

बब्बूलदलनिःक्काथो लेहीभूतस्तदञ्जनात् ॥ १०१ ॥
नेत्रस्रावं जयत्येष मधुयुक्तो न संशयः ।

Juice of leaves of babbūla made into a thick consistance by boiling and used as añjana with honey surely relieves discharges of the eye (101–102).

हिज्जलरसक्रिया—

हिज्जलस्य फलं घृष्ट्वा पानीये नित्यमञ्जनम् ॥ १०२ ॥
चक्षुः स्रावोपशान्त्यर्थं कार्यमेतन्महौषधम् ।

Fruit of hijjala is rubbed on stone with water and put into the eyes cures excessive discharges from the eye (102–103).

कतकरसक्रिया—

कतकस्य फलं घृष्ट्वा मधुना नेत्रमञ्जयेत् ॥ १०३ ॥
ईषत्कर्पूरसहितं स्मृतं नेत्रप्रसादनम् ।

Kataka bīja is made into a paste and mixed with honey and little quantity of karpūra. Application of this paste cleanses the eyes (103–104).

अथ शिरोत्पाते रसक्रिया—

सर्पिः क्षौद्रं चाञ्जनं स्याच्छिरोत्पातस्य शान्तये ॥ १०४ ॥

Añjana with ghee and honey relieves sirotpāta (net work of blood vessels) in the eye (104).

कृष्णसर्पवसारसक्रिया—

कृष्णसर्पवसा शङ्खः कतकात्फलमञ्जनम् । रसक्रियेयमचिरादन्धानां दर्शनप्रदा ॥ १०५ ॥

Fat of black cobra, śaṅkha (conch) and seeds of kataka made into a rasakriyā and applied as añjana gives sight to the blind quickly (105).

लेखनाञ्जनम्—

दक्षाण्डत्वक्शिलाकाचशङ्खचन्दनसैन्धवैः । द्रव्यैरञ्जनयोगोऽयं पुष्पार्मादिविलेखनः ॥ १०६ ॥

Shell of hen's egg, manaśila, kāca (rock crystal), śaṅkha (conch), candana and saindhava applied as añjana cures puṣpa (scars) and ārm a (pterygium) by scraping them out (106).

कणारसक्रिया—

कणा छागयकृन्मध्ये पक्त्वा नेत्रयुगेऽञ्जिता । अचिराद्धन्ति नक्तान्ध्यं तद्वत्सक्षौद्रमूषणम् ॥१०७॥

Kaṇā (pippalī) is kept inside the liver of a goat and cooked well. This pippalī taken out and used as añjana quickly relieves night blindness; marica done like-wise also acts similarly if applied with honey (107)

चूर्णाञ्जनम्—

शाणार्धं मरिचं द्वौ च पिप्पल्यर्णवफेनयोः । शाणार्धं सैन्धवं शाणा नव सौवीरकाञ्जनात् ॥१०८॥

पिष्टं सुसूक्ष्मं चित्रायां चूर्णाञ्जनमिदं शुभम् । कण्डूकाचकफार्तानां मलानां च विशोधनम् ॥१०९॥

Half śāṇa of marica, two śāṇas each of pippalī and samudraphena, half śāṇa of saindhava, nine śāṇas of souvīra añjana are powdered nicely during the period of citrā nakṣatra., This applied to the eye relieves kaṇḍū (itching) kāca (opacity) and disorders of kapha (108–109).

इदानीं रोपणचूर्णाञ्जनमाह—

(मृदुचूर्णाञ्जनम्)

शिलायां रसकं पिष्ट्वा सम्यगाप्लाव्य वारिणा । गृह्णीयात्तज्जलं सर्वं त्यजेच्चूर्णमधोगतम् ॥११०॥

शुष्कं च तज्जलं सर्वं पर्पटीसंनिभं भवेत् । विचूर्ण्य भावयेत्सम्यक्त्रिवेलं त्रिफलारसैः ॥ १११ ॥

कर्पूरस्य रजस्तत्र दशमांशेन निक्षिपेत् । अञ्जयेन्नयने तेन सर्वदोषहरं हि तत् ॥ ११२ ॥

सर्वरोगहरं चूर्णं चक्षुषोः सुखकारि च ।

Rasaka (kharpara) is placed in a stone pestle and macerated with plenty of water. After sometime the supernatant water is drained off and the thick precipitate is dried in sun and macerated three times with decoction of triphalā. Finally one tenth of it's weight of powdered karpūra (camphor) is added and stored. This powder used daily as añjana cures all diseases of the eyes and keeps it healthy (110–113).

प्रसादनाञ्जनम्—
(सौवीराञ्जनम्)

अग्नितप्तं हि सौवीरं निषेच्यं त्रिफलारसैः ॥ ११३ ॥
सप्तवेलं तथा स्तन्यैः स्त्रीणां सिक्तं विचूर्णितम् । अञ्जयेत्तेन नयने प्रत्यहं चक्षुषोर्हितम् ॥ ११४ ॥
सर्वानक्षिविकारांस्तु हन्यादेतन्न संशयः ।

Souvirāñjana (white antimony sulphate) is heated and immersed in the decoction of triphalā for seven times. Afterwards it is rubbed nicely with breast milk and stored. This powder used daily is good for the eye and cures all eye diseases without doubt (113–115).

अथ दृष्टिप्रसादनी नागशलाका विख्याता, तामपि दर्शयन्नाह—
त्रिफलाभृङ्गशुण्ठीनां रसैस्तद्वच्च सर्पिषा ॥ ११५ ॥
गोमूत्रमध्वजाक्षीरैः सिक्तो नागः प्रतापितः । तच्छलाका हरत्येव सर्वान्नेत्रमवान्गदान् ॥ ११६ ॥

Thin sheets of nāga (lead) are heated red and immersed in decoction of triphalā and juices of bhṛṅgarāja, śuṇṭhi, ghee, cow's urine, honey, goat's milk and used as añjana cures all diseases of eyes. Even a rod made out of it has the same effect (115–116).

प्रत्यञ्जनम्—
गतदोषमपेताश्रु संपश्यन्सम्यगम्भसि । प्रक्षाल्याक्षि यथादोषं कार्यं प्रत्यञ्जनं ततः ॥ ११७ ॥

By application of añjanas when the eyes have become free of doṣas, the tears are washed with water and the patient is asked to look into a jar of water for some time and later on pratyāñjana is done (117).

न वाऽनिर्गतदोषेऽक्षिण धावनं संप्रयोजयेत् । प्रत्यञ्जनं तीक्ष्णतप्ते नेत्रे चूर्णं प्रसादनम् ॥ ११८ ॥

Washing should not be done if the eye is not free from symptoms of doṣas. For the eyes which are tired by powerful añjanas, prasādana cūrṇa (cooling powders) is to be put in (118).

नयनामृताञ्जनम्—
शुद्धे नागे द्रुते शुद्धं तुल्यं सूतं विनिक्षिपेत् । कृष्णाञ्जनं तयोस्तुल्यं सर्वमेकत्र चूर्णयेत् ॥ ११९ ॥
दशमांशेन कर्पूरं तस्मिश्चूर्णे प्रदापयेत् । एतत्कृताञ्जनं नेत्रगदजिन्नयनामृतम् ॥ १२० ॥

Equal parts of purified nāga (lead) and sūta (mercury) are mixed by melting them together; equal amount of kṛṣṇāñjana (black antimony sulphate) is also added. Karpūra (camphor) is also added in one tenth the above quantity and stored. This is a good nayanāmṛta añjana for all eye diseases (119–120).

सर्पविषे संजीवनाञ्जनम्—

जयपालभवां मज्जां भावयेन्निम्बुकद्रवैः। एकविंशतिवेलं तु ततो वर्तिं प्रकल्पयेत् ॥ १२१ ॥
मनुष्यलालया घृष्ट्वा ततो नेत्रे तथाञ्जयेत्। सर्पदष्टविषं जित्वा संजीवयति मानवम् ॥ १२२ ॥

Jayapāla seeds macerated with lemon juice for twenty one times and made into a stick. This applied as a paste with human saliva relieves the effects of cobra poison and restores life to the bitten person (121–122).

अथ दृष्टिप्रसादनार्थं सार्वकालिकं योगद्वयमाह—

भुक्त्वा पाणितलं घृष्ट्वा चक्षुषोर्दीयते यदि। जाता रोगा विनश्यन्ति तिमिराणि तथैव च ॥१२३॥

After taking meals the hands are washed, the palms are rubbed briskly and applied warm to the eyes. This cultivated as a habit helps to cure diseases like timira blindness etc. (123).

शीताम्बुपूरितमुखः प्रतिवासरं यः कालत्रयेण नयनद्वितयं जलेन।
आसिञ्चति ध्रुवमसौ न कदाचिदक्षिरोगव्यथाविधुरतां भजते मनुष्यः ॥१२४॥

Person who washes his face with cold water three times a day and while doing so, throws cold water into the eyes, not only gets relieved of eye diseases but also becomes healthy with it (124).

'चक्षूरक्षायां सर्वकालं मनुष्यैर्यत्नः कर्तव्यो जीविते यावदिच्छा।
व्यर्थो लोकोऽयं तुल्यरात्रिर्दिवानां पुंसामन्धानां विद्यमानेऽपि वित्ते ॥'

Every person should try to protect his eyes always throughout his life, because the world is useles for, the day is as good as night for persons who are blind, though they might possess plenty of wealth.

आयुर्वेदसमुद्रस्य गूढार्थमणिसंचयम्। ज्ञात्वा कैश्चिद्बुधैस्तैस्तु कृता विविधसंहिताः ॥१२५॥
किंचिदर्थं ततो नीत्वा कृतेयं संहिता मया। कृपाकटाक्षनिक्षेपमस्यां कुर्वन्तु साधवः ॥ १२६ ॥

Wise men composed books collecting together many a precious gems fro... the ocean of Āyurveda. I have collected here a few efficient recipes from several such books and prepared this treatise. Let good men show their benevolence to it (125–126).

विविधगदार्तिदरिद्रनाशनं या हरिरमणीव करोति योगरत्नैः।
विलसतु शार्ङ्गधरस्य संहिता सा कविहृदयेषु सरोजनिर्मलेषु ॥ १२७ ॥

The many efficient recipes of this book dispel the diseases just as goddess Lakṣmī dispels diseases and poverty. Let this Saṃhitā (treatise) of Sāraṅgadhara shine in the pure hearts of good men (127).

अल्पायुषामल्पधियामिदानीं कृतं समस्तश्रुतिपाठशक्त्या ।
तदत्र युक्तं प्रतिबीजमात्रमभ्यस्यतामात्महितं प्रयत्नात् ॥ १२८ ॥

This treatise is written for the use of men who are of short span of life, and of poor intellegence who cannot read the whole literature of Āyurveda. Let such persons study this treatise which is an epitome and acquire benefit from it (128).

इति श्रीदामोदरसुनुना शार्ङ्गधराचार्येण विरचितायां शार्ङ्गधरसंहितायामुत्तरखण्डे नेत्रकर्मविधिर्नाम त्रयोदशोऽध्यायः ।

Thus ends the thirteenth chapter.

शार्ङ्गधरसंहिता समाप्ता

Thus ends the Saṁhitā of Śāraṅgadhara.

APPENDIX I

Weights and Measures

		Gm. equivalents
6 Trasarenus	1 Marichi	0.22 mg (Approx)
6 Marichis	1 Rajika	1.30 mg (Approx).
3 Rajikas	1 Sarshapa	3.12 mg (Approx).
8 Sharshapas	1 Yava	31.25 mg.
4 Yavas	1 Gunja	125 mg
6 Gunjas	1 Masha	750 mg
4 Mashas	1 Shana	3 gms
2 Shanas	1 Kola	6 gms
2 Kolas	1 Karsha	12 gms
2 Karshas	1 Shukthi	24 gms
2 Shukthies	1 Pala	48 gms
2 Palas	1 Prasrithi	96 gms
2 Prasrithies	1 Anjali or Kudava	192 gms
2 Kudavas	1 Manika or Sharava	384 gms
2 Sharavas	1 Prastha	768 gms
4 Prasthas	1 Adhaka (64 palas)	3072 gms
4 Adhakas	1 Drona	12, 288 gms

APPENDIX II

Diseases mentioned in Chapter 7 of Prathama Khanda with their nearest modern equivalents

1. Jwara—Fevers (25 in number)

   (a) Vatajwara—ordinary fever, fever due to aggravation of Vata
   (b) Pittajwara— ,, ,, Pitta
   (c) Kapha jwara— ,, ,, Kapha
   (d) Vata + Kapha jwara—Mild toxic fevers Vata + kapha
   (e) Pitta + Kapha ,, ,, Vata + Kapha
   (f) Vata + Pitta ,, ,, Vata + Kapha
   (g) Sannipata ,, —Highly toxic and septic fevers

(h) Vishama jwara —Intermittent fevers like Malaria, Filariasis, etc.

1. Santata „ — „ „ of seven day periods
2. Satata „ — „ „ rise of temp daily twice
3. Anyedyushka — „ „ rise of temp daily once
4. Triteeyaka — „ „ tertian alternate day
5. Chaturthaka — „ „ quartan every fourth day.

(i) Agantu jwaras (fevers due to injury, stress and other external causes)

1. Abhichara jwara (fever due to witchcraft)
2. Grahavesha („ possession by evil spirits)
3. Shapa jwara („ due to curses)
4. Shram jwara („ due to exertion)
5. Cheda jwara (fever due to injury by sharp weapons)
6. Kshata jwara (fever due to assault by blunt weapons)
7. Daha jwara (fever due to exposure to heat)
8. Kama jwara (fever due to excessive lust)
9. Bhaya jwara (fever due to freight)
10. Shucha (chinta) (fever due to mental worry)
11. Rosha (fever due to anger)
12. Visha (fever due to poisons)
13. Oushadhigandhaja (fever due to infestation with pollen, strong smell of plants products, drugs, chemicals etc.)

2. Atisaras (7) Diarrhoeas

Vataja—due to aggravation of vaṭa
Pittaja—due to aggrevation of pitta
Kaphaja—due to aggravation of Kapha
Sannipataja—due to combination of all three doshas
Amaja—due to indigestion
Shokaja—due to sorrow
Bhayaja—due to fright/nervous diarrhoea

3. Grahani (5) (Sprue)

Vataja
Pittaja
Kaphaja
Sannipataja
Amaja

4. Pravahika (4) Dysentery
   Vataja
   Pittaja
   Kaphaja
   Sannipataja
   Asrija (due to aggravation of Rakta)
5. Ajeerna (3) Indigestion
   Vishtabda
   Vidagdha
   Ama
   Vishajeerna
   Alasa
6. Vishoochi (3) Gastro-enteritis
   Vataja
   Pittaja
   Kaphaja
7. Dandakalasaka—severe form of Indigestion
8. Vilambika—severe form of Indigestion
9. Arshas (6) Haemorrhoids; piles
   Vataja
   Pittaja
   Kaphaja
   Raktaja
   Samsargaja
   Sannipataja
10. Charmakeela (3) warts on the skin
11. Krimis (20) Helmenthiasis. Intestinal parasites; external parasites like lice etc.
12. Panduroga (5) Anaemia
    Vataja
    Pittaja
    Kaphaja
    Sannipataja
    Mrittikaja (anaemia due to ingestion of mud etc.)

13. Kamala (1) Jaundice

14. Kumbhakamala (1) jaundice with enlargement of abdomen; Hepatomegaly, Cirrhosis of liver

15. Haleemaka (1) chlorosis

16. Raktapitta (3) purpura, Haemorrhagic diatheses
Urdhwaga—bleeding from orifices in the face (nose, throat, ears, eyes)
Adhoga—bleeding from urethra, anus or vagina
Dwimarga—both directions, even through skin

17. Kasa (5) cough—Bronchitis, pertusis
Vataja
Pittaja
Kaphaja
Urakshataja (cough due to trauma to the lungs)
Kshayaja (cough due to consumption)

18. Kshaya (5) consumption—emaciation, pulmonary tuberculosis
Vataja
Pittaja
Kaphaja
Sannipataja
Urakshataja (consumption due to injury to the lungs)

19. Shosha (6) Emaciation—phthisis
Vyavayaja—due to excess sexual activity
Shokaja—too much of grief
Vranaja—chronic ulcers
Adhwaja—too much of walking
Vyayamaja—strenuous excercises
Vardhakyaja—old age. senility

20. Swasa (5) dyspnoea
Kshudra—dyspnoea on exertion
Tamaka—bronchial Asthma
Oordhwa—dyspnoea with predominant expiration
Maha—dyspnoea of very severe degree
Chinna—discontinued, interrupted breathing

21. Hikka (5) Hiccough
Kshudra—very mild, occasional

Annaja—due to food (entering into trachea, spicy foods)
Gambheera—deep seated, arising from down below
Yamana—coming on in pairs
Mahati—powerful. very severe

22. Agnivikara (4) Disorders of digestion—Dyspepsia
Vishamagni—irregular activity
Teekshnagni—hyperactive digestion
Mandagni—hypo active digestion
Bhasmaka—unsatiable hunger, gluttony; hyperthyroidism ?

23. Arochaka (5) Anorexia
Vataja
Pittaja
Kaphaja
Sannipataja
Manasika—psychological/Neural

24. Chardi (7) Vomitting
Vataja
Pittaja
Kaphaja
Sannipataja
Krimija—due to intestinal parasites
Dweshta—due to aversion, hatred—psychological
Douhrida—due to pregnancy,—Hyperemisis gravidarum

25. Swarabheda (6) Hoarseness or loss of voice
Vataja
Pittaja
Kaphaja
Sannipataja
Medaja—accumulation of fat in the body (obesity)
Kshayaja—tubercular hoarseness.

26. Trishna (6) Thirst
Vataja
Pittaja
Kaphaja
Sannipataja

Upasargaja

Dhatukshayaja—due to tissue depletion—specially water depletion

27. Moorcha (4) Fainting

Vataja, Pittaja, Kaphaja, Sannipataja.

28. Bhrama (1) Dizziness

29. Nidra (1) Sleepishness

30. Tandra (1) Drowsiness

31. Sanyasa (1) Unconcsicusness

32. Mada (7) Intoxication

Vataja, Pittaja, Kaphaja, Sannipataja

Asrija (due to blood—i.e. hypertension

Vishaja—Poisonous.

Madyaja—Alcoholic

33. Madatyaya (4) Alcoholism

Vataja, Pittaja, Kaphaja, Sannipataja

Paramada
Panajeerna
Panavihbrama
Panatyaya } Different stages ol alcoholism

34. Daha (7) Burning sensation in the body.

Raktapittaja—due to purpura

Raktaja—due to diseases ol blood

Trishnaja—due to thirst

Pittaja—due to increase of pitta

Dhatukshaya—due to loss of tissues, dehydration etc.

Marmaghata—injury to vital parts

Rakta sanchaya in udara—due to internal bleeding

35. Unmada (6) Insanity

Vataja, Pittaja, Kaphaja, Vatakapha, Pittakapha, Vatapitta

Vishaja—poisonous

Manovikaraja—disorder of the mind

Bhootonmada—due to possession by evil spirits, etc.

Deva (gods), Danava (demons), Gandharva, Kinnara, Yaksha, Pitru (ancestors), gurushapa (curse of teachers), Preta (spirits of the dead), Guhyaka

(Bhoota, pishacha) Jaladevata, Naga, Brahmarakshasa, Kooshmanda, Vetala Eteo.
Kopa of Vriddhas—Wrath of elders
Kopa of suddhas—Wrath of ascetics
Krityonmada—Insanity due to witchcraft

36. Apasmara (4) Epilepsy
Vataja, Pittaja, Kaphaja, Sannipataja.

37. Amavata (4) Rheumatism
Vataja, Pittaja, Kaphaja, Sannipataja.

38. Shoola (8) Colic
Vataja, Pittaja, Kaphaja, Vatakapha, Pittakapha, Vatapitta, Sannipata.
Amaja—due to indigestion, accumulation of Ama
Annadrava shoola }
Parinama shoola } Colic due to peptic ulcers

39. Udavarta (13) Oppression in chest/abdomen.
One each from suppression of Kshut (hunger), Trisha (thirst), Nidra (sleep), Swasa (respiration), Chardi (vomiting), Kshavathu (sneezing) Jrimbha (yawning), Udgara (belching), Asru (tears), Shukra (semen) Mootra (urine), Mala (faeces), Vata (flatus).

40. Anaha (2) Distention of abdomen.
Pakwashayaja—intestinal
Amashayaja—gastric

41. Urograha (1) pain in the chest

42. Hridroga (5) diseases of heart
Vataja, Pittaja, Kaphaja, Sannipataja.
Krimija—due to worms, parasites, bacteria.

43. Udara (8) Enlargement of abdomen.
Vataja, Pittaja, Kaphaja, Sannipataja.
Jalaja—Ascites
Pleehaja—Splenomegaly
Kshataja—Perforations of viscera
Baddhaguda—intestinal obstruction, intusussuption.

44. Gulma (8) Abdominal tumors
Vataja, pittaja, kaphaja, vatapitta, vatakapha, kaphapitta, sannipata
Raktaja—uterine haematoma tumors.

45. Mootraghata (13) obstruction of micturition
Vatakundalika (due to) stricture
Vatashteela (due to) enlargement of prostate
Vatabasti (due to) retention
Mootrateela (due to) incontinence
Mootrajatara (due to) atony of bladder
Mootrakshaya (due to) suppression of urine, uremia.
Mootrotsarga (due to) uretheral stricture ?
Mootragranthi (due to) tumor of bladder
Mootrashukra (due to) spermatorrhoea
Mootrasada (due to) chronic cystitis
Vidwighata (due to) intestinal obstruction
Ushnavata (due to) haematuria
Bastikundala (due to) cystitis

46. Mootrakrichra (8) Dysurea
Vataja, pittaja, kaphaja, sannipataja
Shukraja—obstruction by semen
Vidha—trauma
Ghataja—by obstruction of passages
Ashmarija—calculus (vesical)

47. Ashmari (4) Urinary calculus
Vataja, pittaja, kaphaja, shukraja.

48. Meha (prameha) (20) Polyuria/Diabetes
Ikshu—alimentary glycosuria
Sura—phosphaturia
Pishta } colloidal urine
Sandra }
Shukra—spermatorrhoea
Udaka—diabetis inspidus
Lala—albuminuria
Sheeta— ?
Sikata—Crystaluria
Shanai ?
Manjishta urobilinuria
Haridra

Rakta—haematuria
Krishna—a symptom in black water fever, trypansomiosis ?
Kshara—alkalin uria
Hasti—diabets tuniflues
Vasa— ?
Majja— ?
Madhu—diabetes mellitus.

49. Prameha Pitaka (10) diabetic carbuncles
Sharavika—ulcer resembling a soucer
Kachapika—ulcer resembling tortoise shell
Putrinee—ulcer with smaller ulcers round about
Vinata—ulcer with depressed edges
Alajee ?
Masoorika—ulcer resembling chicken pox
Sarshapika—ulcer resembling mustard seed
Jalini—ulcer resembling a seive
Vidarika—lacerated ulcer
Vidradhi—Abscess.

50. Somaroga (1) Leucorrhoea.

51. Medodosha (1) Obesity

52. Shotha (9) Oedema. Anasarca.
Ekadoshaja, Dwandwaja, Sannipataja.
Abhighataja—traumatic
Vishaja—poisonous

53. Vriddhi (7) Scrotal enlargement.
Vataja, pittaja, kaphaja—
Raktaja—haematocele
Medaja—omentocele
Mootraja—hydrocele
Antraja—intestocele (inguino-scrotal hernia)

54. AndaVriddhi (1) Orchitis.

55. Gandamala (1) Cervical lymphadenitis, scrofula.

56. Gandalaji (1) Thyroiditis or tumours of thyroid. Tubercular lymphadenitis.

57. Granthi (9) Benign tumors.
Ekadoshaja
Raktaja—Haematoma.
Siraja—Haemangioma.
Medaja—Lipoma.
Vranaja—Tumour after an ulcer.
Asthija—Ostema, Osteo-sarcoma.
Mamsaja—Myoma, Sarcoma.

58. Arbuda (6) Malignant tumors, Cancer.
Vataja, Pittaja, Kaphaja.
Raktaja—Haematomatus cancer.
Mamsaja—Sarcomatus cancer.
Medoja—Lipomatus cancer.

59. Shleepada (3) Filariasis, Elephantiasis.
Vataja, pittaja, kaphaja.

60. Vidradhi (6) Abscess.
Vataja, pittaja, kaphaja, sannipataja.
Raktaja—
Kshataja—

61. Vrana (15) Ulceration.
Agantu—Traumatic.
Dehaja—Organic.
Vataja, pittaja, kaphaja, vatapitta, vatashleshma, pittakapha, sannipata.
Raktaja—
Vataraktaja
Raktapitta
Kapharakta
Vatapittarakta
Vatakapharakta
Pittakapharakta
Sannipatarakta

62. Sadyovrana (8) Traumatic wounds
Aviklipta
Vilambina
China—Excised wound

Bhinna—Incised wound
Prachalita—
Ghrishta—Lacerated wound
Viddha—Punctured wound
Nipatita—

63. Koshtabheda (2) Visceral trauma
Chinnantra—Intestinal perforation.
Nisritantra—Intestinal protrusion, Herniation.

64. Asthi Bhanga (8) Fracture of bones.
Kanda Bhagna—Fracture of shaft of long bones
Prishta
Vidarita
Vivartita
Vishslishta
Tiryakshipta—
Adhogata
Urdhwagata
Sandhi bhagna—Dislocation of joint.

65. Vanhidagdha (4) Burns and scalds
Degree 1. Plushta—
2. Atidagdha—
3. Durdagdha—
4. Samyakdagdha—

66. Nadivrana (5) Sinus ulceration.
Vataja, pittaja, kaphaja, tridoshaja.
Shalyaja—Osteomyclitis.

67. Bhagandara (8) Fistula in-Ano.
Shataponaka—Multiple fistula.
Ushtragreeva—curved fistula.
Parisravi—exudative fistula
Ruju—Straight sinus
Prakshepi—bleeding
Arshaja—Fistila in Ano due to haemorrhoids

68. Upadamsha (5) (syphilis).
Vataja, pittaja, kaphaja, sannipataja, raktaja.

69. Shooka roga (24) Diseases of penis due to application of poisonous drugs.
Lingarshas—polypus of the penis
Gratitha—Tumour of penis.
Nivritta—Protruded glans
Avamantha—In flamed glans
Mridita—Bruised glans
Shataponaka—perforated skin (prepuce).
Ashteelika—Hard prepuce
Sarshapika—multiple, red swellings of penis.
Twakpaka—ulceration of the prepuce
Avapatika—Polaceration of the prepuce.
Mansapaka—sloughing of prepuce
Sparshahani—Numbness.
Niruddhamani—Phimosis, concealed glans.
Uttama—maculae on the glans
Mamsarbuda—Myoma
Raktarbuda—Haematoma.
Pushkarika—multiple petechae
Sammodapidaka—Painless petechae
Alaji—A swelling of the size of seed of cardomem
Vidradhi—Abscess of the penis
Kumbhika—Abscess resembling a small pot.
Tilakalaka—Wart of penis.
Niruddhaprakasha—Phimosis.
Parivartika—Paraphimosis.

70. Kushta (18) Leprosy and allied skin diseases.
Kapalika—Erythematous leprosy
Oudumbara—Glandular leprosy
Mandala—Anglryred patched leprosy
Vicharchika—Eczema (weeping)
Rishyajiswa—Papilliparous growths.
Vipadika—Severe dermatosis of extremities.
Sidhma—Cloasma, ptyriasis
Eka—Localised patch
Kitibha—Psoriasis
Alasa—Lichen

Dadru —Ring worms
Pama—Scabies
Visphota—Impatigo
Maha—Leprosy
Charmadala—Xeroderma
Pundereeka—Psoriasis
Shataru—Rupia ulcers
Kakana—Lepromatous leprosy

71. Switra (3)—Leucoderma. Viteligo
Vataja, pittaja, Kaphaja.

72. Kshudra Rogas (6o)—Minor diseases.
Sharkararbuda—sebaceous horn, cyst.
Indraviddha—circular pustular ulcer.
Panasika—Fistula inside the ear.
Vivrita—Pustular ulcer.
Andhalaji—Hard, closed papule.
Varaha damshtra—Ulcerative parotitis.
Valmeeka—actinomycosis of foot, madur a foot.
Kacchapa—Hard growth, cysts.
Tilakalaka—Black mole.
Gardabhi—Erythematus rash.
Jala gardhabha—Lymphangitis—
Pashana gardabha—Mumps, parotitis
Rakasa—Dry eczema
Yavaprakhya—hard mole
Vidarika—Axillary or inguinal bubo.
Kadara—Corn in the sole.
Mashaka—Elevated mole.
Neelika—Bluish patch
Irivelli—Painful pustule in the head.
Jatumani—Congenital mole, birthmark.
Gudabhramsba—Prolapse of rectum.
Sanniruddhaguda—Stricture of rectum.
Agni Rohini—Plague.
Kota—Erythema, Rashes.
Anushayee—Deep abscess of the foot.

Padmini kantaka—Papilloma of the skin.
Chippa—Whitlow, Paronychia.
Kunakha—Onchogryphosis.
Alasa—Dhobies itch, Ulceration between toes.
Mukhadooshika—Pimple, Acne.
Kaksha—Axillary Lymphadenitis.
Vrishana kacchu—Scrotal eczema.
Ganda—Enlargement of lymph glands.
Rajika—Pustules.

73. Vyanga (4)—Black pigmentation of the face.
Vataja, Pittaja, Kaphaja, Raktaja.

74. Visphota (8)—Small pox, exanthima.
Ekadoshaja Dwandwaja, Sannipataja, Raktaja.

75. Masoorika (14)—Chicken pox
Ekadoshaja, Dwandwaja, Sannipataja.
Twakgata—residing in the skin
Raktaja—residing in the flood
Mamsaja—residing in the muscle
Medoja—residing in the fat
Asthija—residing in the bone
Majjaja—residing in the marrow
Shukraja—residing in the semen

76. Visarpa (9)—Eresypelas.
Ekadoshaja, Dwandwaja, Sannipataja.
Dahaja—due to burns
Abhighataja—due to injury

77. Udarda (1)—Erythema, Allergic rashes

78. Sheetapitta (1)—Neurotic oedema, Allergic rashes.

79. Amlapitta (3)—Hyperchlorhydria.

80. Vatarakta (8)—gout.
Ekadoshaja, Dwandwaja, Dwandwaja.

81. Vatarogas (80)—Diseases due to increase of vata. Nervous disorders.
Akshepaka—Convulsions.
Hanusthambha—Trismus. Lock jaw.

Oorusthambha—Stiffness of the leg.

Shirograha—Stiffness and pain in the neck and head (wry neck).

Bahyayama—Opisthotanos.

Antarayama—Emprosthotanos.

Parshwashoola—Pain in the flanks.

Katigraha—Lumbago. Back pain.

Khallee—Contractures of fingers and toes.

Jihwasthambha – Glossal palsy. Paralysis of the tongue.

Ardita—Facial paralysis.

Pakshaghata—Hemiplegia.

Kroshtukasheersha—Inflammation of knee joint.

Manyasthambha—Stiff neck, wry neck, torticollis.

Panguta—Lameness by both legs, paraplegia.

Toonee—Pain in the urinary bladder, renal colic.

Pratitoonee—urinary colic moving upwards.

Khanjata—Lameness by one leg.

Vatakantaka—Sprain.

Gridhrasi—Sciatica.

Viswachi—Monoplegia brachialis.

Apabahuka—Ankylosis of shoulder.

Apatana—Tetanus.

Dandapatanaka—Tetanus-orthrostotonos.

Vranayama—Tetanus as a sequel of ulcer.

Apatantraka—Convulsions.

Minminatwa—Nasal talk.

Gadgadatwa—Stammering.

Mookatwa—Mutism, inability to speak, aphasia.

Ashteela }
Pratyashteela } Prostatic pain.

Vamanatwa—Dwarfism.

Kubjata—Kyphosis, hunch back.

Angabheda—Cutting pain in the body parts.

Angashosha—Emaciation, wasting, dryness of the body parrs.

Angapeeda—Squeezing pain in the body parts.

Angashoola—Pain in the body parts.

Sankocha—Contractures, shortening of parts.

Sthambha—Stiffness, loss of movement.
Rookshata—Dryness.
Angabhanga—Cutting pain.
Anga vibhramsha—Drooping of body parts, looseness.
Vidgraha—Constipation.
Baddha vitkata—Constipation-scabelous stools.
Ati jrimbha—Excessive yawning.
Ati udgara—Excessive belching.
Antra koojana—Intestinal gurglings.
Vata apravritti—Retention of flatus.
Sphurana—Excessive fullness of blood vessels, pulsation.
Kampa—Tremors.
Karshya—Emaciation.
Shyavata—Bluish discolouration.
Pralapa—Excessive irrelevant talk.
Kshipra mootrata—Frequency of micturition.
Nidranasha—Loss of sleep, Insomnia.
Swedanasha—Loss of perspiration-Androsis.
Durbalatwa—Debility.
Bala kshaya—Loss of strength.
Shukra Atipravritti—Excessive seminal discharge-Spermatorrhoea.
Retonasha—Loss of semen (non-production).
Anavasthita chitta—Unsteady mind.
Kathinya—Hardness of body parts.
Virasasyata—Bad taste in the mouth.
Kashayavakrata—Astringent taste
Adhmana—Tympanitis of lower abdomen.
Pratyadhmana—Tympanitis of upper abdomen.
Sheetata—Coldness of body parts.
Romaharsha—Horripulations.
Bheetatwam—Phobia, fright.
Toda—Pricking pain.
Kandoo—Itching.
Rasa ajnata—Loss of taste, Agensia.
Bhabola ajnata—Loss of hearing, Deafness.
Prasupti—Loss of feeling, loss of sensation of touch-Anesthesia.

Gandha Agnata—Loss of smell-Anosmia.
Drishti kshaya—Loss of sight-Blindness.

82. Pitta Rogas (40)—Diseases due to increase of pitta.
Dhoomodgara—Hot erectations.
Vidaha—Burning sensation in the stomach.
Ushnangatwa—Increased warmth of the body.
Mati bhrama—Loss of mental balance.
Kanti hani—Loss of lustre.
Kanthashosha—Dryness of the throat.
Mukhashosha—Dryness of the face.
Alpashukrata—Scanty seminal discharge.
Tiktasyata—Bitter taste in the mouth.
Amla vaktrata—Sour taste in the mouth.
Loha gandhasyata—Iron smell in the mouth.
Sweda srava—Excessive perspiration.
Anga paka—Ulceration of body parts.
Klama—Debility even without exertion.
Haritvarna—Greenish colouration.
Atripti—Restlessness non-contentment.
Peetagatrata—Yellowish discolouration.
Peetamootrata—Yellow urine.
Peetavitkata—Yellow faeces.
Peetanetrata—Yellow eyes.
Peetavalokana—Yellow vision.
Peetadanta—Yellow teeth, gums.
Peetanakhata—Yellow nails
Haritvarna—Greenish discolouration.
Raktrasrava—Bleeding tendency.
Angadarana—Cracking pain.
Dourgandhya—Foul odour of the body.
Arati—Restlessness.
Sheetaicha—Desire for cold things.
Tejodwesha—Hatred for hot things.
Alpa nidrata—Scanty sleep.
Kopa—Anger.
Gatrasada—Debility.

Bhinnvitkata—Loose motions.
Andhata —Blindness.
Ushnamootrata—Hot urine.
Ushnochhwasa—Hot respiration.
Ushnamalata—Hot faeces.
Tamodarshana—Seeing darkness, loss of sight.
Peetamandala—Yellow patches on the skin.
Peeta darshana—Seeing yellow rings.
Nissahatwam—Incapacity to withstand.

83. Kapharogas (20)—Diseases due to increase of kapha
Tandra—Drowsiness.
Atinidra—Excessive sleep.
Gouravam—Heavyness of the body.
Mukhamadhurya—Sweet taste of the mouth.
Mukhalepa—Coating on the tongue.
Praseka—Excessive salivation.
Shweta avalokana—Seeing things white.
Sweta vitkata—Whitish faeces.
Sweta mootrata—Whitish urine.
Sweta angata—Whitish skin.
Shiatya—Coldness.
Ushnaicha—Desire for hot things.
Tikta kamita—Desire for bitters.
Maladhikya—Excessive waste products from the body.
Shukrabahulya—Excessive seminal production.
Bahumootrata—Excessive urination—Polyuria.
Alasya—Lazyness.
Manda bhuddhi—Dullness of mental activity.
Tripti—Feeling of satisfaction (abnormal).
Ghurghura vakyata—Husky voice.
Achaitanya—Inactivity, Docility.

84. Rakta rogas (10)—Diseases due to aggravation of blood.
Gourava—Heavyness of the body.
Raktamandala—Appearance of red rashes on the skin.
Raktanetra—Reddish eyes.
Rakta motra—Reddish urine. (Haematuria).

Rakta stheevana—Reddish sputum (Haemptysis).
Rakta pitaka—Reddish eruptions.
Oushnya (vriddha)—Increased body temperature.
Pootigandhata—Bad smell of body.
Peeda—Pain in the body.
Paka—Ulcerations.

85. Oshtha rogas (11)–Disease of lips.
Vataja, Pittaja, Kaphaja, Tridoshaja, Raktaja.
Kshataja—Traumatic.
Khandoshtha—Harelip.
Mamsarbuda—Sarcoma of the lip.
Medorbuda—Lipma of the lip.
Jalarbuda—Tumour of the lip.
Arbuda—Cancer of the lip.

86. Danta roga (10)—Diseases of teeth.
Dalana—Cracks on the teeth.
Krimidanta—Caries.
Dantaharsha—Tingling.
Danta sharkara—Tartar.
Karala danta—Irregular teeth.
Danta chala—Shaking of teeth.
Adhi danta—Extra teeth, over-riding teeth.
Shyava danta—Black discolouration of teeth.
Dantabheda—Breaking, cracking.
Kapalika—Wearing out, Atrophy of enamel.

87. Dantamoola rogas (13)—Diseases of gums.
Sheetada—Spongy gums, scurvy.
Upakusha—Ulceration of gums.
Dantavidradhi—Gum abscess, Alveolar abscess.
Dantapupputa—Gingivitis.
Adhimamsa—Impacted wisdom tooth.
Vidarbha—Gingivitis.
Mahasoushira—Gangrenous stomatitis.
Saushira—Gingivitis.
Dantanadi—Dental sinus.

88. Jihwa rogas—Diseases of the tongue.
Vataja, Pittaja, Kaphaja—Itcheosis.
Alasa—Sublingual abscess.
Adhi jihwa—Epiglottitis.
Upajihwa—Ranula or salivary cyst.

89. Talu rogas (8)—Diseases of the palate.
Arbuda—Cancer of the palate.
Talupitaka—Pustule in the palate.
Kachchapi—Tumor of the palate.
Talu samhati—Tumor of the palate.
Gala`shundhi—Enlargement of uvula
Talu shosha—Dryness of the palate.
Talu paka—Ulceratun of the palate.
Talu pupputa—Cupils of the palate.

90. Gala rogas. (13)—Diseases of the throat.
Rohini—Diphtheria.
Vataja, Pittaja, Kaphaja, Tridoshaja.
Medorohini—Diptheria.
Vrinda—Mild sore throat.
Galougha—Sore throat blocking the food passage.
Gala vidradhi—Pharyngeal abscess.
Swaraha—Laryngitis.
Tundikeri—Enlargement of tonsils.
Shataghni—Throat cancer.
Shalooka—Adenoids.
Arbuda—Cancer.
Gilayu—Tonsillitis.
Valaya—Dysphagia due to tumor.
Ganda—Enlarged lymph gland, thyroid enlargement.
Vataja, Pittaja, Kaphaja.

91. Mukha roga (8)—Diseases of the oral cavity.
Mukhapaka—Stomatitis
Vataja, Pitttaja, Kaphaja, Raktaja, Sannipataja.
Pootyasya—Hallitosis.
Oordhwagada—Inflammation of buccal cavity
Arbuda—Oral cancer.

92. Karna rogas (18)—Diseases of the ear.
Vataja, Pittaja, Kaphaja, Raktaja, Sannipataja.
Vidradhi—Abscess in the ear.
Shotha—Inflamed ear, Otitis.
Arbuda—Tumor.
Pooti karna—Otorrhoea; foetid discharge from the ear.
Kares—Polypus of the ear.
Karna hallika—polypus of the ear.
Badhirya—Deafness.
Tantrika—Tinetus.
Kandoo—Itching.
Shashkulee—Obstuction by wax.
Krimikarna—Maggots in the ear.
Karna nada—Tinnitus.
Karna pratinaha—Melting of cerumen.

93. Karnapali rogas (7)—Diseases of pinna of the ear.
Utpata—Inflammation.
Palishosha—Emaciation.
Vidari—Tumor.
Dukhavardhana—Hard pinna.
Paripota—Swelling of the pinna.
Lehi—Pustules of the pinna.
Pippali—Warts on the pinna.

94. Karnamoola roga (5)—Diseases of root of the ear.
Vataja, Pittaja, Kaphaja, Sannipataja, Raktaja.

95. Nasa Rogas (18)—Diseases of the nose.
Pratishyaya—Common cold, coryza.
Vataja, Pittaja, Kaphaja, Raktaja, Sannipataja.
Apeenasa—Atrophic rhinitis.
Dushtapeenasa—Ch. Rhinitis.
Pootinasa—Ozeana.
Nasarshas—Nasal polyp.
Bhramshathu—Vasomotor rhenorrhoea.
Kshavathu—Sneezing.
Nasanaha—Deviation of the septum.

Pootirakta—Traumatic epistaxis.
Nasarbuda—Tumor in the nose.
Nasa shosha—Rhinitis sicca.
Pooti srava—Exudation of pus.
Deepti—Acute coryza.
Ghranapaka—Nasal ulceration.

96. Shirorogas (10)—Headaches.
Vataja, Pittaja, Kaphaja, Sannipataja, Raktaja, Krimija.
Ardhavabheda—Hemicrania.
Sooryavarta—Migraine.
Shira kampa—Shaky head.
Shankhaka—Temporal headache.

97. Kapala rogas (9) —Diseases of the scalp.
Upasheershaka—Caput cephalus.
Aroomishika—Scabies of the scalp, seborrhoea.
Vidradhi—Abscess on the scalp.
Daruna—Dandruff.
Pitaka—Pustules on the scalp.
Arbuda—Tumor of the scalp.
Indralupta—Alopacea aereata.
Khalittya—baldness.
Palita—Premature greying of hairs.

98. Netra rogas—diseases of the eye.
Vartma roga—Diseases of eye lids.
Krichronmeela—Difficult opening.
Kaphot Klishta—mucoid lids.
Raktotklishta—Bleeding lids.
Lohita—Blepharitis.
Arugnimesha—ulcerative Blepharitis.
Kukoonaka—Ophthalmis neonatarum.
Pakshma pata—Falling off of eye lashes.
Pakshmarshas—Polyp of the eye lid.
Pakshmarodha—Prestricted movement of lids due to oedema.
Pittotklishta—Yellow exudation.
Klishtavartma—Exudative lids.
Pothakee—Trachoma.

Bahala vartma—Blepharitis-non-Inflammatory.
Pakshotsanga—Eversion of lids.
Arbuda—Tumor of the lid, cancer.
Kumbhika—Follicular cojunctivitis.
Sikatavartma—Tracoma.
Lagana—Chalazion
Anjananamika—Hardeolum, stye.
Kardama—Eczema of the lids.
Shyava vartma—Acute eczema of the lids.
Bisa vartma—Eczematus conjunctivitis.
Alaji—Pecetinules of lids.
Utklishtavartma—Ch. Blepharo-conjunctivitis

99. Netra sandhi rogas (9)—Diseases of fornices of the eye.

Jala srava —Excessive lacrymation.
Kapha srava
Rakta srava
Poopa srava —Ch. Lacrocystitis.
Parvani—Phlyctenule at the limbus.
Krimigranthi—Blepharitis Acarica.
Upanaha—Lacrymal cyst, mucocele.
Alaji—Episcleritis.
Pooyalasa—Dacrocystitis, sac. abscess.

100. Shukla rogas (13)—Diseases of the sclera.

Sirotpata—Pannus, Hyperemia.
Siraharsha—Indolent ulcer, chemosis.
Sirajala—Pannus.
Shuktika—Xerosis.
Shuklarma—Pseudo-pterygium, cicatrical.
Adhimamsarma—A wide pterygium.
Pishtika—Conjunctival cyst.
Sirajachippita (pitaka)—Multiple follicular conjunctivitis.
Kapha granthi—
Arjuna—Subconjunctival haemorrhage.
Snayuarma—Symblepheron.
Shonitarma—Pannus.

101. Krishna rogas (5)—Diseases of the cornea-Keratitis.

Shudhashukra—Keratitis without ulceration.
Sirashukra—Engorged arteries aud veins.
Kshatashukra—Injury to cornea.
Ajaka—Prolapse of iris, staphyloma.
Sirasanga—Venous thrombosis in the cornea.

102. Kacha rogas (6)—Diseases of the Lens.

Vataja, Pittaja, Kaphaja, Samsargaja, Sannipataja, Raktaja.

103 Timira rogas (6)—Disorders of vision.

Vataja, Pittaja, Kaphaja, Samsargaja, Sannipataja, Raktaja, Upasargaja.

104. Drishti Mandala rogas (8)—Diseases of pupil/vision.

Pitta vidagdha drishti—Retinitis pigmentosa, Hemenalopia.
Amla vidagdha drishti—Retinitis ophthalmia.
Ushna vidagdha drishti—Erythropia.
Nakulandhya —Glioma of the retina.
Dhoosarandhya—Asthenopia.
Ratryandhya—Night blindness, Nyctalopia.
Hraswadrishti—Dissiminated choroditis.
Gambheera drishti—Paralysis of sixth cranial nerve.

105. Adhimantha (4)—Glaucoma.

Vataja, Pittaja, Kaphaja, Raktaja.

106. Abhishyanda (4)—Conjunctivitis.

Vataja, Pittaja, Kaphaja, Raktaja.

107. Sarvakshi rogas (8)—Diseases affecting the entire eye-Opthalmia.

Vata viparyaya—Supra orbital neuralgia.
Alpa shopha—Ophthalmia.
Anyatovata—Neuralgia of V cranial nerve.
Pakatyaya —Hypopion ulcer.
Shushkakshipaka—Ophthalmoplegia.
Shopha—Oedema of the eye.
Adhyushita—Ophthalmia.
Hatadhimantha—Panophthalmitis.

108. Pumsthwa rogas (5) Impotence.

Irshyaka
Asekya
Kumbheeka — different kinds of impotence.
Sugandhi
Shandata

109. Shukra doshas (8)—Disorders of semen.

Vataja, Pittaja, Kaphaja.
Kunapagandhi—Having cadaveric smell.
Pooyabha—Resembling pus.
Ksheena—Scanty.
Grenthila—Mucoid.
Malabha—Dirty, Floculant.

110. Artava doshas (8)—Diseases of menstruation.

Vataja, Pittaja, Kaphaja.
Kunapa—Having cadaveric smell.
Pooyabha—Resembling pus.
Granthila—Mucoid.
Ksheena—Scanty flow.
Malabha—Dirty, floculant.

111. Raktapradara (4)—Metrorrhagia.

Vataja, Pittaja, Kaphaja, Sannipataja.

112. Yoni rogas (20)—Diseases of female urogenital tract.

Vataja, Pittaja Kaphaja, Sannipataja, Raktaja.
Raktakshayaja—Due to loss of blood.
Shushka yoni—Dryness of vaginal passage.
Vaminee—Abortive tendency.
Khandita—Lacerated Vagina.
Antarmukhee—Retroverted passage.
Soochimukhee—Pin hole vagina.
Vipluta—Dysperunia.
Putraghnee—Habitual abortion.
Paripluta—Dysperunia.
Upapluta—Dysmenorrhoea.
Prakcharana—Perineal laceration.

Mahayoni—Wide vaginal tract.
Karninee—Mass in the vagina.
Ananda—Excessive libido.
Aticharana—Inability to conceive.

113. Yoni Kandas (4)—Cervicitis.
Vataja, Pittaja, Kaphaja, Sannipataja.

114. Garbhashaya rogas (8)—Diseases of uterus.
Upavishtaka—Arrest of foetal growth.
Nagodara—Poor foetal growth.
Makkalla—Post partum colic.
Vishkambha—Obstruction of foetal passage.
Moodagarbha—Abnormal foetal presentation.
Gooda garbha—Protracted foetal movement.
Jarayu dosha—Disorders of placenta.
Garbha pata—Abortion, Miscarriage.

115. Stana rogas (5)—Diseases of breasts.
Vataja, Pittaja, Kaphaja, Sannipataja.
Kshataja—Due to injury.

116. Sootika rogas—Diseases of purperium.

117. Stree doshas (3) Mental disorders of women.
Adaksha purushotpanna—Due to company of inefficient male partner.
Sapatni vihita—Due to other co-wives.
Devaja—Due to providential causes.

118. Bala rogas (22)—Diseases of children.
Dushtaksheera (3)—Due to bad milk.
Vataja, Pittaja, Kaphaja.
Dantodbheda—Primary teething.
Dantaghata—Biting tendency.
Dantasabda—Grinding of teeth.
Akala danta—Premature dentition.
Ahipootana—Sore buttock, Napkin rash.
Muksh sarva—Excessive salivation.
Guda paka—Ulceration of rectum.
Upasheershaka—Cephalic haematoma.
Parshwaruna (ja)—Pain in the flanks.

Talukantaka—Adenoids.
Vichinna—Early stage of adenoids.
Parigarbhika—Disease due to milk of pregnant women.
Dourbalya—Debility.
Gatrashosha—Marasmus.
Shyyamootra—Bed wetting.
Kukoonaka—Opthalmia Neonatorum.
Rodana—Excessive crying.
Ajagallika—Painless papules on the skin.

119 Bala grahas (12)—Paediatric diseases due to possession by evil spirits.

Skanda
Vishakha
Shwagraha
Pitrugraha
Naigameya
Shakuni
Sheetapootana
Mukha mandatika
Pootana
Andhapootana
Revathi
Shushka Revathi

120. Panchakarmaja rogas (15)—Diseases resulting from improper therapies such as purgation, emesis, etc.

Heena yoga—Inadequate dosage, course, etc.
Mithya yoga—Improper dosage, course, etc.
Ati yoga—Excessive dosage, course, etc.

121. Upadravas (4)—Effects of

Sheetaja—Cold.
Ushnaja—Heat.
Shalyaja—Foreign body.
Ksharaja—Alkalies.

122. Visha rogas (3)—Diseases due to poisons.

Sthavara—Vegetables, mineral and metallic origin.
Jangama—Animal origin.

Kritrima—Synthetic, homicidal.

Upavishas—Intoxication from minor poisonous materials (drinking polluted water, poisoned weapons, etc.).

123. *Kandoo*—Itching/pruritus.

From Kapikachu—Mucuna prurens.

From Bhallataka—Semicarpus anacardium.

From Soorana—Amarphophallus campanulatus.

124. Mada—(Intoxication) due to.

Pooga—Arcunut/Areca catechu.

Bhanga—Cannabis indica.

Aksha—Terminalia belerica.

Kodrava—Parpalum Scorbiculatum.

Dhatura—Datura alba.

APPENDIX III

INDEX OF DRUGS

A

Abda (musta)—Cyperus rotundus

Abhaya—Terminalia chebula

Abhraka—Mica, Biotite

Agaru—Aquilaria agalocha

Agastya—Sesbania grandifolia

Agni (chitraka)—Plumbago zeylanica

Agni(ka) (bhallataka)—Semicarpus anacardium

Agnimantha—Premna integrifolia, clerodendron phlomidis

Ahi (naga)—Lead

Ahiphena—Opium

Ahinirmoka—Snake peel

Aja dugdha (ksheera)—Goat's milk

Aja mootra—Goat's urine

Ajaji—Cuminum cyminum

Ajagandha—Gynandropis gynandra, peucedenum grande

Ajamoda—Carium Roxburghinum, Tachyspermum ammi

Ajashringi—Pistacia integrima

Ajya—Cow's ghee

Akarakarabha
Akkalaka } —Anacyclus pyrethrum

Aksha (vibhitaki)—Terminalia belerica

Ala (haritala)—Orpiment, Arsenous sulphide

Alabu—Lagenaria siceraria, L Vulgaris

Alambusha—Cucurbita lagenaria

Amalaki—Phyllanthus emblica

Ambu (hreebera)—Coleus Vettiveroides

Ambuda (musta)—Cyperus rotundus

Amalavetasa—Garcinia pedanculata

Amra—Mangifera indica

Amra asthi—Kernel of mango fruit

Ananta—Hemidesmus indicus

Ankota (Ankola)—Alangium lamarki

Anjana (souveeranjana)—Black sulphide of antimony

Anjeera—Ficus carica

Apamarga—Achyranthus aspera

Aparajita—Clitoria ternata

Ara—Brass

Aralu (ka)—Ailanthus excelsa, A. malabarica

Ardraka—Green ginger. Zingiber officinale

Aragwadha—Cassia fistula

Arishta (nimba)—Azadirechta indica

Arjuna—Terminalia arjuna

Arka—Calatropis procera, C. gigantica

Arka moola—Roots of calotropis procera

Artagala—Barleria serigosa

Asana—Terminalia tomentosa

Ashmabheda—Bergania ligulata, Aerva lanata

Ashoka—Saraca indica

Ashwagandha—Withania somnifera

Ashwakhura—Horse's hoof

Aswatha—Ficus religiosa

Atasi—Linum usitatissimum
Atibala—Sida rhombifolia
Ativisha—Aconitum heterophyllum
Atmagupta—Mucuna pruriens
Avalguja (bakuchi)—Psorelia corylifolia
Avimootra—Sheep's urine
Ayoraja—Iron filings

B

Babbula—Acacia arabica
Badara, Badaramla—Zizyphus Jujube, Z. sativa
Bakuchi—Psorelia corylifolia
Bala—Sida cordifolia, S. acuta
Balaka—Coleus vettiveroides
Basta mutra—Goat's urine
Beejaka, Beejasara (asana)—Pterocarpus marsupium
Beejapoora—Citrus medica
Bhadraila—Amomum subulatum
Bhadramusta—Cyperus tuberosis
Bharngi—Clerodendron indicum, C. serratum
Bhallataka—Semecarpus anacardium
Bhoomyamalaki—Phyllanthus neruri
Bhoonimba—Andrograyhis paniculata
Bhringaraja—Eclipta alba
Bida (lavana)—Black salt, salt from mines
Bidala vishta—Excreta of cat
Bilwa—Aegle marmelos
Bimbi—Coccinia indica, Cephandra indica
Bisa—Nelumbo nucifera
Brahmi—Centella asiatica, Bacopa monnira
Brihati (brihat simhi)—Solanum indicum
Brihati dwaya (two brihatis—Brihati and Kantakari)—Solanum indicum and Solanum Xanthocarpum

C

Chaga Ksheera—Goat's milk
Chaga roma—Goat's hairs
Chakramarda—Cassia tora
Chanaka—Cicer arietinum
Chandana—Santalum album
Chandra
Chandraprabha } Karpoora—Camphor
Changeri—Oxalis corniculata
Chaturjataka (combination of Twak, Ela, Patra and Nagakesara)—Combination of Cinnamomum zeylanicum, Elettaria cordomomum, Cinnamomum tamala and Mesua-ferra
Chavika-chavya—Piper chaba
Chincha—Tamarindus indicus
Chinna—Tinospora cardifolia
Chirabilwa—Pongamia glabra; Haloptelia integrifolia
Chitraka—Plumbago zeylanica

D

Dadhi—Curds
Dadima—Punica granatum
Dadrughna—Cassia tora, C.alata
Danta—Elephant's tooth
Danti—Baliospermum monatum, Croton seeds
Darada—Cinnabar, ore of mercury
Daru (devadaru)—Cedrus deodar
Daru nisha
Darvi }—Berberis aristata
Dashamoola—Group of the following ten drugs
(1) Bilwa—Aegle marmelos
(2) Agnimantha—Clerodendron phlomoides
(3) Syonaka—Uroxylum indicum
(4) Kashmari—Gmelina arborea
(5) Patala—Stereospermum souvelens
(6) Saliparni—Desmodium gangeticum

(7) Prishniparni—Uraria picta
(8) Brihati—Solanum indicum
(9) Kantakari—Solanum xanthocarpum
(10) Gokshura—Tribulus terrestris
Devadali—Luffa eccinata
Devadaru / Devakashta }—Cedrus deodar
Dhanvayasa (ka)—Fagonia cretica
Dhanyaka—Coriandrum sativum
Dhanwana—Grewia tillifolia
Dhataki—Woodfordia floribunda, W.fruticosa
Dhatura—Datoora metel, D.alba, D.stramonium
Dhatri—Phyllanthus emblica, Emblica officinalis
Dhurta—Dhatoora stramonium, D.meta, D.alba
Dindighosha (Rakta eranda)—Ricinus communis (red variety)
Dipyaka—Carium copticum, Tachyspermum ammi
Draksha—Vitis vinifera
Drona pushpi—Leucos cephalotes
Druma (kutaja)—Holerrhina antidysenterica
Dugdhika—Euphorbia microphylla; oxystelma esculentum
Duralabha / Dusparsha }—Fragonia cretica
Durva—Cynodon dactylon

E

Edagaja (chakra marda)—Cassia tora
Ela—Elettaria cardamomum
Elavaluka—Prunus avium; P. cerasus
Eranda—Ricinus communis

G

Gada lavana (romaka lavana)—Salt of sambhar lake
Gairika—Red ochre
Gambhari (kashmari)—Gmelina arburea
Gandhaka—Sulpher
Gandhatrina—Saccarum cilliare
Gandharva hasta—Ricinus communis

Gangeruki—Grewia populifolia
Ghana (musta)—Cyperus rotundus
Ghrita—Cow's ghee
Girikarnika—Clitoria ternata
Godhooma—Wheat
Gokanta / Gokshura }—Tribulus terrestris
Goksheera / Go dugdha }—Cow's milk
Go mutra—Cow's urine
Go rochana—Ox gall; ox bile
Go shakrit—Cow dung
Gostana (draksha)—Vitis Vinifera, dried grapes.
Goura sarshapa—Brassica alba
Granthika (tagara)—Vallerina Wallachi
Guda—Jaggery, treacle, mollases
Guduchi—Tinospora cardifolia
Guggulu—Commiphora mukul
Gundra—Saccharum ciliare
Gunja—Abrus precatorius

H

Hamsapadi—Coldenia procumbens; Adiantum lumulatum
Hapusha—Juniperus communis
Haritaki—Terminalia chebula
Harenuka—Vitex-agnus castus
Haridra—Curcuma longa
Haridra—Dwaya—Curcuma longa and Berberis aristata
Harinashringa—Stag's horn
Haritala—Orpiment, yellow sulphide of arsenic
Hasti danta—Elephant's tooth
Hasti pippali—Scindaspus officinalis
Hataka—Gold
Hayamara-hayari—Narium indicum
Hemahwa-hemaksheeri—Argimona mexicana
Hijjala—Barringtonia acutangula

Himsra—Capparis sepiaria
Hingu—Asofoetida-Ferula foetida
Hingupatri—Gardenia lucida
Hribera—Pavonia odorata

I

Ikshu— Sugar cane-Saccharum officinasum
Ikshuraka (kokilaksha)—Asterecantha longifolia
Ileya (kumari)—Aloe barbadensis
Indivara—Nelumba nucifera
Indradaru—Cedrus deodar
Indravaruni—Citrullus colocynthis
Indrayava—Seeds of Hollerhina antidysentrica
Ingudi—Balanites roxburghi
Iravati (nagabala)—Sida veronicafolia
Irimeda (Vitkhadira)—Acacia leucophloea

J

Jala (vaḷaka)—Coleus vettiveroides
Jaladhara (musta)—Cyperus rotundus
Jalini (Koshataki)—Luffa acutangula
Jambira—Lemon, Citrus acida
Jambu—Eugenia jambolona
Jatamamsi—Nardostachys jatamamsi
Jati—Jasmine flower, Jasminum officinale
Jati patra—leaves of Myristica fragrans
Jatiphala—Nutmeg. Fruit of Myristica fragrans
Jayapala—Croton taglium
Jayanthi (Jwalamukhi)—Sesbania sesbamum, S. aegyptica
Jiraka—Cuminum Cyminum
Jiraka Dwaya (Two Jeerakas) }—Cuminum Cyminum and Nigella Sativa
Jivanti—Dendrobium macrei, Leptadania reticulata
Jivaka—Microstylus musifera
Jyotishmati—Calastrus paniculatus, Cardiospermum halicalum

K

Kacha—Extract of Acacia catechu
Kadali—Musa sapientum
Kadamba—Anthocephalus cadamba
Kakamachi—Solanum nigrum
Kakanasa—Pentatropis microphylla, Hygrophilia-augustifolia
Kokodumbarika—Ficus hispida
Kakoli—Lilium polyphylum
Kakubha (arjuna)—Terminalia arjuna
Kalanusariva (tagara)—Valeriana wallachi
Kalaya—Pea, Lathyrus sativus
Kaleyaka—Coscinium fenestratum
Kalinga yava—Seeds of Hallerrhina antidysenterica
Kamala—Lotus, Nelumbium speciosum
Kambhari (Kashmari)—Gmelina arborea
Kampillaka—Mallotus phillipensis
Kamsya—Bell metal, bronze
Kana (Pippali)—Piper longum
Kanamoola—Roots of piper longum
Kanaka—Gold
Kanaka—Datura metal, D. abla
Kanchanara—Bauhinia variegata
Kankola—Piper cubeba
Kankushta—Latex of Garcinia morella or
Latex of Argemona mexicana
Kantakari—Solanum xanthocarpum
Kanya—Aloe barbadensis; Aloe indica
Kapikachu—Mucuna pruriens
Kapitha—Feronia elephantum; F.limonia
Karanja—Pongamia glabra
Karavella—Memordica chirantia
Karavira—Nerium indicum; N. odorum
Karkata—Pistacia integrrima
Karpasa—Cotton, Gossypium herbaceum
Karpura—Camphor, Cinnamomum camphora
Kaseesa—Ferrous sulphate

Kaseruka—Seirpus kysoor; S.grossus
Kasha—Saccharum spontaneum
Kashmari—Gmelina arborea
Kasturi—Musk
Katakaphala—Strychnos potatorum
Katphala—Myrica nagi
Katuki } —Piccrorrhiza kurroa
Katurohini }
Katu taila—Mustard oil
Kesara (kumkum kesara)—Saffron, Crocos sativus
Kesara (Naga kesara)—Mesua ferrea
Kesharaja (bhringaraja)—Eclipta alba
Ketaki—Pandanus tectorius
Khadira—Acacia catechu
Khadira Sara—Extract of A. catechu
Khakhasa beeja—Seeds of Papaver somniferum
Kharjoora—Dates, Phoenix sylvestris
Kharpara—Calamite, Zinc ore
Khanda sita—Sugar candy
Kinwa—Yeast, brewing agent
Kirata tikta—Swertia chirata
Kodrava—Paspalum scorbiculatum
Kola—Ziziphus jujube
Kosha Amra—Schleichera oleosa
Koshataki—Luffa acutangularis
Kounti (Renuka)—Vitex agnus castus
Kramuka—Betel nut, Areca catechu
Krimighna—Embelia ribes
Krishna—Piper longum
Krishna Agaru—Aqularia agallocha
Krishna Anjana—Black Sulphide of antimony
Krishna Jiraka—Nigella sativa
Krishnamrit—Black mud
Krishna lavana—Black salt
Krishna tila—Sessamum indicum
Krishna vrinda—Stereospermum swavelens

Kshara dwaya (two ksharas)—Two Alkalies
(1) Yavakshara—Potassium carbonate
(2) Sarjikshara—Sodium carbonate
Ksheera kakoli—Frittilaria royle
Kshoudra—Honey
Kshudra—Solanum xanthocarpum
Kuchala (vishamushti)—Strychnos nuxvomica
Kukkuta pureesha—Excreta of cock
Kukkuta Anda twak—Shell of hen's agg
Kulattha--Dolichos biflorus, horse gram
Kumari—Aloe indica; Aloe vera
Kumkuma—Crocus sativus
Kupilu—Strychnos nuxvomica
Kurabaka (rakta sairepaka)—Barleria cristata
Kurantaka (peeta saireyaka)—Barleria prionitis
Kusha—Demostachyia bipinnata; Eragrotis cynosuroides
Kusha Dwaya (two kushas)— „ „
Kushmanda—Benincasa cerifera; B.hispida
Kushta—Soussurea lappa
Kushtumburu—Coriandrum sativum
Kutaja—Holerrhina antidysenterica
Kuteraka—Ocimum basilieum; O.gratissimum

L

Laghupanchamoola—Combination of—
(1) Shaliparni—Desmodium gangeticum
(2) Prishniparni—Uraria picta
(3) Brihati—Solanum indicum
(4) Kantakari —Solanum Xanthocorpum
(5) Gokshura—Tribulus terrestris
Laja—Fried paddy
Lajjalu—Mimosa pudica
Laksha—Lac
Langali—Gloriosa superba
Lashuna—Allium sativum, garlic

Lavana-saindhava—Rock salt, potassium + sodium chloride
Lavana panchaka (five salts)—Five salts-viz.,
(1) Saindhava—Rock salt
(2) Souvarchala—Salt from soil
(3) Samudra—Sea salt, common salt
(4) Bida—Black salt
(5) Oudbhida—Salt from mines, marshy places.
Lavanga—Syzygium aromaticum; Eugenia caryophyllata
Lodhra (Sabara)—Symplocos racemosa
Lodhra Dwaya (Sabara and pattika)—Symplocos recemosa and S. crataegoides
Loha—Iron
Loha kitta—Iron flax, waste of molten iron

M

Madanaphala—Randia dumetorum
Madhu—Honey
Madhuka
Madhuyashti } —Glycerhiza glabra
Madhooka—Bassia latifolia
Madhuparni—Teramnus labialis
Madhurasa (moorva)—Marsenia tenassisima
Magadhi (ka)—piper longum
Maha daru—Cedrus deodar
Maha meda—Polygonatum cirrhifollium
Maha nimba—Ailanthus excelsa; Melia azadirechta
Mahat panchamoola—Group name of five viz.,
(1) Bilwa—Aegle marmelos
(2) Agnimantha—Premna integrifolia
(3) Syonaka—Oroxylum indicum
(4) Kashmari—Gmelina arborea
(5) Patala—Sterospermum swaveolens
Maherana (Sallaki)—Boswellia Serrata
Mahoushada—Ginger, Zingiber officinale
Makanda phala (machiphala)—Atalantia monophylla
Makshika—Honey

Makshika dhatu—Chalcopyrites
Malakangani—Celastrus paniculata
Malati—Jasminum officinale
Malayu (Kashtoudumbarika)—Ficus hispida
Mamsi—Nardostochys jatamamsi
Manashila—Realgar, Red sulphide of arsenic
Mandura—Iron flax, waste of molten iron
Manjishta—Rubia cardifolia
Maricha—Piper nigrum
Markati (Kapikachu)—Mucuna pruriens
Masha—Black gram, phaseolus mungo
Mashaparni—Teremanus labialis
Mastu—Whey, water of buttermilk
Masura—Lens esculanta; L. Culiuaris
Matulunga—Citrus medica; C.decumena
Mayurapucha—Peacock's feather
Meda—Litsea sebiteria
Mesha sringi—Gymnema sylvestre; Helecteres isora
Mishi—Foeniculum vulgare
Minakshi—Alternanthera sessalis.
Mocha (kadali)—Musa sapientum
Mocharasa—Extract of Bombax malabarieum
Mridweeka (draksha)—Vitis vinifera, grapes.
Mrigamada—Musk
Mrigashringa—Stag's horn
Mrinala—Nelumbo nucifera
Muchukunda pushpa—Pterospermum acerifolium
Mudga—Green gram; phaseolus rediatus
Mudga parni—Phaseolus trilobus
Mukta—Pearls
Mulaka—Raddish, Raphinus sativus
Mundi (Munditaka)—Spharanthus indicus; S. hirtes
Mura (gandha dravya)—Erythrina stricta
Murva—Marsenia tenassisma
Musali—Chlorophyllum tuberosum; Asparagus ascendens
Mushaka karni—Merremia emerginata
Musta—Cyperus rotundus

N

Naga—Lead

Nagabala—Sida spinosa; S. veronicaefolia

Nagakesara—Mesua ferea; ochrocarpus longifolius

Nagara—Ginger, Zingiber officinale

Naktamala—Cassia fistula

Nala—Arundo donax; phragmites karaka

Nalada—Nardostychis jatamamsi

Nata—Valeriana wallachii

Navaneeta—Butter

Navasara (navasadara)—Sal ammoniac, Ammonium Chloride

Navasara—Potassium Nitrate

Neelanjana—Lead Sulphide

Neeli (ka)—Indigofera tinctoria

Neelotpala—Nymphaea stellata; N.nouchali

Nichula (Jalavetasa)—Barringtonia acutangula

Nidigdhika—Solanum xanthocarpum

Nimba—Azadirachta indica; Melia azadirachta

Nirgundi—Vitex nigundo

Nisha—Termuric, Curcuma longa

Nisha dwaya (two nishas)—Curcuma longa and Berberis aristata

Nyagrodha—Ficus bengalensis

P

Padmaka—Prunus Cerasoides; P. puddum

Palasha—Butea frondosa; B.monosperma

Pancha kola—five drugs viz.,

(1) Pippali—Piper longum

(2) Pippali moola—Roots of piper longum

(3) Chavya—Piper chaba

(4) Chitraka—Plumbago zeylanica

(5) Nagara—Zingiber officinale

Pancha Valkala—Five barks of

(1) Nyagrodha—Ficus bengalensis

(2) Udumbara—Ficus glomerata

(3) Aswatha—Ficus religiosa

(4) Plaksha—Ficus infectoria
(5) Vetasa—Calamus viminalis; Salix capera
Parada—Mercury
Parisha pippali—Thesparia populenea
Parasika yavani—Hyosyamus niger
Parushaka—Grewia asiatica
Parni dwaya—Two parnis
(1) Shali parni—Desmodium gangeticum
(2) Prishni parni—Uraria picta
Parni Chatasra—Four parnis
(1) Sali parni,—Desmodium gnngeticum
(2) Prishni parni—Uraria pita
(3) Masha parni—Teramnus labialis
(4) Mudga parni—Phaseolus trilobus
Parpata—Fumaria parviflora; Rangia repens
Pashana bheda—Bergania ligulta; Saxifraga ligulata
Patala garudi—Ophiorrhiza mungoos; Cooculs hirsutus
Pata—Cissampelus pereirá; Stephania hernado folia
Patola—Trichosanthes diocea
Pathya—Terminalia chebula
Patra—Cinnamomum tamala
Pattanga—Caesalpinia sappan
Paya—Cow's milk
Payasya (ksheera kakoli)—Frittilaria royle
Phala traya, p. trika—Three fruits of
(1) Haritaki—Terminalia chebula
(2) Vibhitaki—Terminalia belerica
(3) Amalaki—Phyllanthus emblica
Pinyaka—Oil cake of sesamum seeds
Pippala (Aswatha)—Ficus religiosa
Pippali—Piper longum
Pippali mula—Roots of p. longum
Pitaka (haridra)—Curcuma longa
Plaksha—Ficus infectoria, F. lacor
Prapoundarika—Nelumbo nucifera
Prapunnata—Cassia tora

Prasarini—Uraria logopoides; Sida verenecofolia
Prativisha—Aconitum palmatum
Pravala—Coral
Prishni parni/prishti parni —Uraria picta, U. logopides
Priyala beeja (chirounji)—Buchanania lauzan; B. latifolia
Priyangu—Aglalia roxburghiana
Puga—Areca catechu
Punarnava—Boerhavia diffusa
Pundarika—Nelumbo nuciferae
Puram (guggulu)—Comnifera mukul
Pushkara moola—Inula racemosa
Putika (putikaranja)—Cesalpinia banducella; C. Crista

R

Raja masha—Dolichos catiang
Rajani (haridra)—Curcuma longa
Rajani dwaya—two rajanis Haridra & Daru haridra }—Curcuma longa and Berberis arstata
Raja Vriksha—Cassia fistula
Raji (ka)—Mustard seeds, Brassica juncea
Rakta chandana—Pteroearpus santalinus
Rakta Karaveera—Narium indicum
Rambha (kadali)—Musa sapientum
Rasa—Mercury
Rasaka—Calamite, Zinc ore
Rasanjana—Extract of Berberis aristata
Rasna—(1) Alpinia galanga
(2) Vanda roxburghi
(3) Pluchea lanciolata
Rasona—Garlic, Allium sativum
Rata phala (madana phala)—Randia dumetorum
Ratna—Gems
Ravi priya—Leaves of Calotropis procera
Renuka—Vitex agnus castus
Reeti—Brass metal
Rodhra—Symplocas racemosus

Rohisha (gandha trina)—Andropogon schonanthus, Cymbopogan martini
Rohita (ka)—Amoora rohitaka
Romaka—A kind of salt
Roupya—Silver
Rubu (ka)-(eranda)—Ricinus communis
Rudanti—Capparis mooni
Ruddhi—Habenaria intermedia
Rushabhaka—Microstylis wallachii

S

Sahachara—Barleria cristata/B. Calurees
Sahadevi—Centratherum anthelmaricum, Vernonia Cinerea
Sahakara—Mangifera indica
Saindhava—Rock salt
Saireyaka—Barleria prionitis
Samanga (Manjishta)—Rubia cardifolia
Samudra lavana—Common salt
Samudra phena—Sea foam, cuttle fish
Saptachada (S. Parna)—Alstonia scholaris
Saptala—Acacia concinna
Sapta ranga—Salacia chinensis
Sarala—Pinus longifolia
Sarinee—Sida veronicaefolia
Sariva—Hemedesmus indicus
Sarjarasa—Vateria indica (resin of)
Sarjika Kshara—Sodium Carbonate
Sarshapa—Mustard, Brassica nigra
Saptala—Acacia concinna
Sehunda (Snuhi)—Euphorbia nerifolia
Sevya (Usheera)—Vettivera zizanoides
Shabara (lodhra)—Symplocos racemosa
Shadgrantha (vacha)—Acorus calamus
Shaileya—Permalia abyssinica
Shakotaka—Strebulus asper
Shalutu (Bilwa)—Aegale marmelos
Shali parni—Desmodium gangaticum

Shalmali—Bombax malabaricum
Shallaki—Boswelia serrata
Shami—Prosopsis spicigera
Shamyaka—Cassia fistula
Shana—Crotalaria juncea
Shankha —Conch shell
Shankha nabhi—Central spiral of conch shell
Shankha pushpi—Convolvulus microphylus/Canscora decussata
Shankhini—Tenolepis cerasiformis
Shara—Sacharum munja
Sharkara—Sugar
Shashtika—A kind of paddy maturing in 90 days
Shatahwa—Anethum sowa
Shata parni—Euphorbia dracunculoses
Shata patra (Sevantika)—Crysanthemum indicum
Shata pushpa—Anethum sowa
Shatavari—Asparagus racemosus
Shati—Hedychium spicatum; Curcuma zedoaria
Shelu—Cordia dichotoma, C. obliqua; C. mixa
Shephalika—Vitex nigundo
Shigru—Moringa pterygosperma
Shikhari (apamarga)—Acyranthus aspera
Shila (manshila)—Realgar, Red sulphide of arsenic
Shilajatu—Black bitumen
Shipha (pippali moola)—Roots of piper longum
Shirisha—Albizza lebbeck
Shiva (haritaki)—Terminalia chebula
Shleshmataka—Cordia mixa
Shobhanjana—Moringa pterygosperma
Shreyasi (haritaki)—Terminalia chebula
Shrichandana—Santalum album
Shringa (mriga sringa)—Stag's horn
Shringavera—Zingiber officinale
Shringi (Karkataka)—Rhus succedenea
Shringi (Ajasringi)—Odina wodier
Shringi (Sitasringi)—Aconitum heterophyllum

Shringi (meshasringi)—Gymnema Sylvestre, Helecteres isora
Shriphala (Bilwa)—Aegale marmelos
Shrivasa—Pinus longifolia
Shukanasa—Oroxyllum indicum
Shunti—Ginger, Zingiber officinale
Shyama (trivrit)—Ipomea terpethum
Shyamaka—Panicum italicum
Shyonaka—Oroxylum indicum
Siddharta (ka)—Brassica compestris
Siktaka—Bees wax
Simhi (brihati)—Solanum indicum
Sindhu—Rock salt
Sindhuvara—Vitex nigundo
Sindhura—Red oxide of lead
Sita—Sugar
Sitopala—Sugar candy
Shuhi—Euphorbia nerifolia
Sourashtraka—Alum
Souvarchala—A kind of salt, Sodium Sulphate + S. Chloride
Souveeranjana—Black sulphide of antimony
Souveeraka—Fermented gruel
Srotonjana—Antimony sulphide
Sthira (Shaliparni)—Desmodium gangeticum
Sthula babboola—Acacia arabica
Sthula Jiraka—Nigella sativa
Suradaru—Cederus deodar
Suranakanda—Amorphophallus campanulatus
Suta—Mercury
Suvarna—Gold
Suvarna pushpi (Gokshura)—Tribulus terrestris
Swadamshtra—Tribulus terrestris
Swarna makshika—Chalcopyrites
Sweta lodhra—Symplocos racemosa
Sweta maricha—White variety of pepper
Sweta sarshapa—White variety of mustard
Syonaka—Droxyllum indicum

T

Tagara—Valeriana wallichi
Taila—Sesamum oil, any oil
Takra—Butter milk
Taḷaka—Orpiment, yellow arsenous sulphide
Talisa patra—Abies webbiana
Tamboola patra—Leaves of piper betel
Tamra—Copper
Tandula—Rice, oryza sativa
Tanduleeyaka—Amaranthus viridis; A. polygamus
Tandulodaka—Rice washed water
Tankana—Borax
Tapya—Chalcopyrites
Tara—Silver
Tarkshya—Emerald
Tejohwa (tejani)—Cinnamomum tamala, Xanthoxylum armatum
Tikta—Picrorrhiza kurroa
Tikta Koshataki—Luffa acutangula
Tikta Patola—Trichosanthes diocia
Tikshna loha—Magnetic iron
Tila—Sessamum indicum
Tila parni—Gynandropis gynandra
Tinduka—Diospyros perigrina, D. embroptyris
Tintidika—Rhus parviflora
Trayanti-Trayamana—Gentiana kurroa
Trikantaka—Tribulus terrestris
Trikatu-Katu traya, Tryooshana —Three pungents viz.,
Shunti—Ginger
Maricha—Pepper
Pippali—Piper longum
Trilavana—Three salts viz.,
Saindhava—Rock salt
Souvarcha—Salt from lakes
Bida—Black salt

Triphala—phalartraya } —Three fruits viz.
Phaltrika }

Haritaki—Terminalia chebula

Vibhitaki—Terminalia belerica

Amalaki—Phyllanthus emblica

Trisugandha—Three fragrants viz.

Twak—Cinnamomum zeylanieum

Patra—Cinnamomum tamala

Ela—Elettaria cordomomum

Trivrit—Ipomea terpethum, Opereculina terpethum

Tugaksheeri (vamsarochana)—Bamboo manna; White crystals inside big bamboo

Tulasi—Occimum sanctum

Tumburu } (tejovati)—Xanthoxylon alatum
Tuni }

Tuntuka—Oroxylon indicum

Tutha—Copper sulphate

Tuvaraka—Hydnocarpus Wightiana/Hydnocarpus lavrifolia

Tuvari—Alum

Twak—Cinnamomum zeylanicum

U

Udadhiphena—Seafoam, cuttle fish

Udichya—Coleus Vettiviroides

Udumbara—Ficus glomerata

Upakunchika—Nigella sativa

Urna—Sheep's wool

Urubuka—Ricinus communis

Urumana—Pronus asmeniaca

Ushana (Maricha)—Piper nigrum

Ushana (Pippali)—Piper longum

Ushira—Andropogon squarrosus, Veteveria zizanoides

Utingana (Sunishannaka)—Marselia cardifolia, Blepharis edulis

Utpala—Nymphea stellata

V

Vacha—Acrous calamus

Vahni (Chitraka)—Plumbaga Zeylanica

Vaikranta—Tourmuline, Manganese Oxide
Vajra—Diamond
Vajri (Snuhi)—Fuphorbia Nerifolia
Vakuchi—Psorelea corylifolia
Valaka—Coleus vettiveroides, pavonia odorata
Valuka—Sand
Vamsarochana—Bamboo manna
Vanari beeja—Seeds of mucuna pruriens
Vandhya Karkotaki—Memordica disica
Vanga—Tin
Vanita (priyangu)—Collicarpa microphilla
Vara (triphala)—See triphala
Varatika—Cowri shells
Vari—Asparagus racemosus
Varshabhoo (punarnava)—Boerhavia diffusa
Varuna—Crataeva nuruvula; C. religiosa
Vasa (ka)—Adathoda vasaca
Vata—Ficus bengalensis
Vata Ankura-Rohaka—Shoots or areal roots of F. bengalensis
Vatsaka (kutaja)—Holerrhina antidysenterica
Vayasee (kakamachi)—Solanum nigrum
Vayasya (amalaki)—Emblica officinale
Venu—Bambusa arundanacea
Vetasa—Calamus Viminalis
Vibhitaka—Terminalia belerica
Virataru—Dichostachys Cinera
Vidanga—Embelia ribes
Vidari—Pueraria tuberosa
Vijaya (bhanga)—Cannabis indica
Vimala—Iron pyrites
Visha (Vatsanabha)—Aconitum ferox
Vishala—Cytrullous colocynthis
Vishamushti—Strychnos nuxvomica
Vishnukranti—Clitoria ternata
Viswa
Viswa bheshaja } —Ginger, Zingiber officinalis

Vriddhadaru—Ipomea pataloidea
Vriddhi—Habenaria intermedia
Vriksha Vrinda—Dioscoria bulbifera
Vrisha—Adathoda Vasaca
Vrischikali—Tragia involulata
Vyaghri—Solanum indicum
Vyaghranakha—Capparis Zeylanica, C. horrida
Vyosha—See Trikatu
Vayastha (Haritaki)—Terminalia Chebula
Vayastha (Amalaki)—Emblica officinalis
Vayastha (Brahmi)—Herpestes monneira

Y

Yamya (rakta chandana)—Pterocarpus santalinus
Yasti/Yastimadhu—Glycerrhiza glabra
Yava—Berley. Hardeum Vulgare
Yavasa—Alhagi maurorum
Yavakshara—(1) Alkali from barley straw
(2) Potassium Carbonate
Yavani—Carium Copticum
Tachyspermum ammi

INDEX

A

B

T

U

V

SOME IMPARTANT WORKS ON AYURVEDA

1. **Introduction to Dravyaguna** Prof. P.V. Sharma
2. **Fruits and Vegetables in Ancient India** Prof. P.V. Sharma
3. **Current Trends in the Study of Sārira** (Illustrated) Dr. D. G. Thatte and G. P. Tewari
4. **Some Controversial Drugs in Indian Medicine** Dr. Bapalala Vaidya
5. **Caraka-Saṁhitā Text With English translation**
   Editor-translator Prof. P.V. Sharma. 1– 4 Vols. complete
   Vol. I–**Sūtrasthāna to Indriyasthāna**.
   Vol. II–**Cikitsāsthāna to Siddhisthāna**
   with Important seventeen classified appendices
   Vol. III–**Sūtrasthāna to Indriyasthāna.**
   Vol. IV–**Cikitsāsthāna to Siddhisthāna**
   Critical notes (Incorporating the commentaries of jejjata.
   Cakrapāni, Gaṅgādhara and Yogindranātha).
6. **Clinical Methods in Āyurveda** Prof. K. R. Srikantha Murthy
7. **Śarṅgadhara Samhitā** of Pt. Śarṅgadharacārya Son of Pt. Dāmodara.
   Sanskrit Text with English Translation. Critical Introduction and Appendix
   By Dr. K. R. Srikantha Murthy
8. **Mādhava-Nidānam.** (Roga-Viniścaya) of Madhavakar. Text with English Translation,
   Critical Introduction and Appendices. by- Dr. K. R. Srikantha Murthy.
9. **Acupuncture Marma other Asian Therapeutic Techniques** by D. G. Thatte.
10. **Aṣṭāṅga Samgraha of Vāgbhaṭa** (Text, English Translation, Notes,
    Index etc.) By Prof. K. R. Srikantha Murthy Vol. I – III complete
    Vol. I **Sūtrasthāna**
    Vol II **Sārīra, nidāna, cikitsita and Kalpasthāna**
    Vol III **Uttarasthana**

11. **A Critical Study of Yogāratnākara** by Dr. Nirmal Saxena
12. **Diabetes Mellitus in Indian Medicine (Illustrated)** by Dr. Virendra Keshav Shah
13. **Luminaries of Indian Medicine (From the earliest times of the Present day)** By Dr. K. R. Srikantha Murthy Foreword By Dr. P. M. Mehta
14. **Introduction to Kāyacikitsā** By C.Dwārakānātha
15. **New Horizones of yoga and Tantra (Illustrated)** By Dr. Raman Das Mahatyagi
16. **Indian Medicinal Plants in Children diseases (Illustrated)** by Dr. C. S. Yadav
17. **Suśruta-Saṃhita. Illustrated.** Text with English Translation.
    By K. R. Srikantha Murthy Vol. I to IV Complete
    Vol I. Sūtrasthāna and Nidansthana
    Vol II. Sārira Sthāna
    Vol III. Cikitsa and Kalpsthan
    Vol IV. Uttar Sthana
18. **Āyurvedokta Ouṣhadha Niruktamala** Etymological Derivations of Single Drugs in Āyurveda. English and HindiTranslation By Dr. J.L.N. Sastry
19. **Introduction to oncology (Cancer) in Ayurveda** By Dr. J.L.N. Sastry
20. **Research Methodology for Ayurvedic** Post-Graduate Scholars/Researchers and Doctors (According to CCIM Syllabus prescribed for M.D/M.S. courses By Dr. S. Suresh Babu M.D (Ayur.)
21. **Geriatrics in Āyurveda** By Dr. S. Suresh Babu (M.D) Ayur.
22. **Myopathy Ayurvedic Perspective** By Dr. S. Suresh Babu
23. **Dravyaguna Vijñāna** By Dr. J.L.N. Sastry
    FundamentalPrinciples of Pharmacotherpeutics in Ayurveda Vol. I
    Comprehensive Study of the Essential Medicinal Plants in Ayurved Vol. II
24. **Guide For Competitive Exams in Ayurveda** By Dr. J.L.N. Sastry
25. **Kayacikitsa:** The Principles and Practice (Ayurveda's Internal Medicine) According t CCIM Syllabus By Dr. S. Suresh Babu M.D. (Ayu.)
26. **Ayurvedic Management for Heart Diseases** by Dr. J.L.N Sastry and Dr. K. Nistesw
27. **Synopsis of Suśruta Saṁhita.** Dr. Rajneesh V. Giri
28. **Animal Drugs.** (Illustrated) (Dravya Guna-vijñana part B) Introduction, Properties, actions and used (As per syllabus approved by C.C.I.M.) Dr. C.S.Yadav
29. **A Concise text book of Aṣṭānga samgraha (Sūtrasthana).** Dr. P. Ramesh Bhat
30. **Caraka Saṁhitā.** Text with English Translation and Critical notes based on **Cakrapānidatta's Ayurvedadipikā** By Dr. K. R. Srikanth Murthy
    Vol. I. **Sutrasthanam**
    Vol. II **Nidana, Vimana and Indriyasthana**
    Vol. III **Cikitsasthana**
    Vol. IV **Siddhi, kalpasthana**
    Vol. V **Sarirasthana**
31. **Aṣṭāñga Samgraha of Vāgbhaṭa. (Sūtrasthāna)** student English edition by Dr. S. Suresh Babu
32. **Rasa Shāstra (M.C.Q.)** By Dr. Ajit Kadam

GA

(1)5